Managing
Back Pain

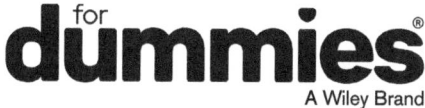

for
dummies®
A Wiley Brand

Managing
Back Pain

by Patrick Roth, MD & Phil Ross, MS

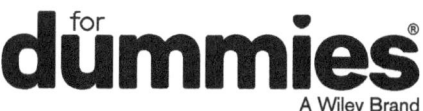

Managing Back Pain For Dummies®

Contents at a Glance

Table of Contents

Introduction

Your back hurts, and you have two questions: "What's causing it?" and "What can I do about it?" Chances are good that you've already tried to get answers to those questions. Maybe you asked your doctor about it, searched the Internet, had your back cracked by a local chiropractor, tried hanging upside down on an inversion table, bought an expensive new mattress, or even had spinal surgery. Despite your best efforts, your back still hurts, and you have no idea what to do about it. Chances are good that your doctor doesn't know either.

So, now, here you are, book in hand, hoping it can answer those two questions. We hate to break it to you, but you may never get a clear, definitive answer to that first question. You may never know what's causing your back pain. Its cause can be elusive. It doesn't always show up clearly on medical imaging or a lab test, and it can be the result of several factors, some of which modern medicine has no way of determining for sure. The good news is that knowing what's causing your back pain often doesn't matter. You can do a lot on your own to manage it effectively, maybe even make it go away, without having any idea what's causing it.

The fact is that almost regardless of what's making your back hurt, being healthier and stronger and having the right mindset make your back feel better. And it feels better because it *is* better — it's stronger, more mobile, more flexible, and more resilient.

About This Book

In this book, we offer a unique patient-centered approach to managing back pain that puts you at the head of your treatment team. Here, you discover how to build a powerful mind-body synergy that makes your back healthier, more mobile, and more resilient. You do most of the heavy lifting by educating yourself and building a healthier, stronger mind and body, and you consult providers when you need professional assistance — physical therapy, pain meds, surgery, chiropractic adjustment, fitness training, and so on.

The way we structured the information and guidance presented in this book reinforces our patient-centered philosophy. Had we followed a traditional approach, we would have covered diagnosis and medical treatments first and then discussed what you, as a patient, could do to enhance your recovery. Instead, we focus first on education and self-help and then discuss diagnoses, treatments, and therapies that healthcare professionals can provide to augment *your* efforts.

Admittedly, such an approach may seem counterintuitive. Logically, diagnosis comes first, followed by treatment. Sometimes, that is the best course of action. If your back pain is so severe that you can't move, or it's accompanied by weakness in a limb (arm or leg), diagnosis and medical treatment may be the first steps. However, diagnosis can, and often does, lead patients down a path of unnecessary surgeries and other treatments that can do more harm than good and burden them with a hefty and avoidable expense. In addition, diagnosis often makes people mistakenly believe that fixing back pain is simply a matter of identifying and treating physical injury or damage (a pain generator), and that's often not the case. The fact is that most people with back pain would be better off *not* seeking a diagnosis first. More often than not, the pain will subside in a few days to a couple of weeks. If the exercise, stretching, and other do-it-yourself remedies do not provide relief or if the condition worsens, seek medical attention.

REMEMBER

We are not suggesting that you "self-diagnose," but realize that many strains and pains may go away on their own or by employing tactics other than an immediate visit to the doctor. In Chapter 5, we provide guidance to help you decide the right approach for you — seeing a doctor first or starting with a do-it-yourself approach.

This book has two authors with vastly different backgrounds — one a neurosurgeon and the other a personal trainer — a Master Trainer. You get the benefits of both perspectives, along with comprehensive coverage of all aspects of managing back pain. Together, we bring you up to speed on the anatomy and physiology of back pain and equip you with the knowledge, insight, and tools you need to manage it effectively. We don't expect you to do everything we recommend all at once, all the time, or in the order we present it. Feel free to skip around and try different things. Everybody's different, and *everybody* is different. Additionally, you may need to focus on different aspects of back pain at different points in time as your needs change. Incorporating a broad range of exercises and activities is also great for keeping things interesting and stimulating adaptation (your mind and body's natural ability to adapt to stress).

Foolish Assumptions

As you'll soon discover when you start reading this book, we discourage people from making assumptions about anything related to their health, such as assuming that the doctor is always right or that your back pain is due to an injury. However, to better serve your needs, we make the following foolish assumptions about you:

>> Your back hurts, and you want to know how to make the pain go away.

>> You're tired of having your back pain prevent you from living a full and active life. You have things to do, places to go, and people to love!

>> You're not looking for a quick fix that merely masks the pain or makes it go away for a few days or weeks. You want a more permanent solution — and a better back.

>> You're willing to take responsibility for your own health and invest time and effort into becoming healthier, stronger, and more resilient.

Icons Used in This Book

Throughout this book, icons in the margins highlight certain types of valuable information that call out for some special attention. Here are the icons we use and a brief description of each.

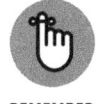

REMEMBER

Of course, we'd love for you to remember everything you read in this book, but if you can't quite do that, then remember the important points we flag with this icon.

TIP

Tips are tidbits of information and insight that we've gathered from our many years of education, training, and experience that are distilled to save you time and effort.

WARNING

"Pump the brakes!" Before you take another step, read these warnings. We provide this cautionary content to help you avoid the common pitfalls that are otherwise likely to slow your progress or set you back on your road to recovery.

Beyond the Book

As if we didn't already pack this book with a ton of great information on managing back pain, you can access the book's Cheat Sheet at Dummies.com. This Cheat Sheet provides quick and handy info and tips you can use on the go. It includes guidance on when to see a doctor, reasons to avoid a diagnosis, a common-sense approach to back pain diagnosis, six essential exercises for mobilizing the back, and a list of professionals who can help manage back pain. To access this Cheat Sheet, simply go to https://www.dummies.com/ and search for "back pain cheat sheet."

You can also find videos for several of the exercises we cover in Chapters 8 and 9 by visiting Phil's YouTube channel @TheMasterPhil.

Where to Go from Here

As with all *For Dummies* guides, you can read this book from cover to cover or skip around to the topics you find most interesting or applicable to your situation. If you choose to skip around, use the table of contents at the front of the book or the extensive index at the back of the book as your guide.

To make our book easier to navigate, we divided the content into the following four parts:

>> **Part 1: Getting Started with Back Pain Management** brings you up to speed on the basics, introduces you to common anatomical injuries and anomalies that can trigger back pain, explains the powerful role the mind can play in both creating and relieving back pain, and provides guidance on where to start — whether you should see a doctor first or try to resolve your back problem on your own.

>> **Part 2: Taking a Do-It-Yourself Approach to Back Pain** presents a host of self-care therapies for building a stronger, healthier back. Here, we cover everything from improving diet and making lifestyle changes to doing exercises focused specifically on strengthening the back to home remedies and healthy breathing. If you do half of what we encourage you to do in Part 2, you may not need to see a doctor.

>> **Part 3: Exploring Professional Back Pain Treatment Options** explains how different healthcare professionals who specialize in treating various aspects of back pain can help you get back on your feet and enable you to engage in the

self-care therapies we recommend in Part 2. Here, we cover topics including medical imaging, pain management, physical therapy, chiropractic care, spinal surgery, and psychological therapies. These pockets of professional care can do wonders to jump-start and accelerate your self-healing. You may not need them but they're great to have if you do.

» **Part 4: The Part of Tens** presents ten tips to help you stick with your personalized pain management program and ten hard-to-believe facts about back pain.

Browse through the part titles and chapter titles, or simply flip through the book to find something that catches your eye. Feel free to explore the pages and dip into what seems most relevant to you at the moment. You don't need to read the book cover to cover, although you may find yourself compelled to do so as the many aspects of back pain management combine to form a comprehensive guide.

1
Getting Started with Back Pain Management

Understanding where pain comes from.

Comparing the conventional, illness-centered approach to managing back pain with our personalized, patient-centered approach.

Taking a crash course on back anatomy and anatomical triggers of back pain.

Using the power of your mind to combat pain and build a healthier, stronger back.

Figuring out when you should probably see a doctor and when it's probably best not to.

Chapter **1**

Brushing Up on Back Pain Basics

B ack pain is ubiquitous, and treatment for it is inadequate and expensive, despite the healthcare community's extensive experience dealing with it and the remarkable technology available to diagnose and treat it. Modern medicine's failure with back pain is frustrating for patients and providers. It can significantly diminish the quality of life, and it's rarely improved with a "quick-fix" — a simple correction of a misalignment in the spine, a surgical procedure, a better mattress, or a muscle relaxer. Doctors can order X-rays and magnetic resonance images (MRIs) that remarkably reveal the patient's inner anatomy, yet they often can't decipher from those images what's causing the pain. The pain can magically go away without treatment and then, just as magically, return three months later worse than ever before without a precipitating event.

Doctors sometimes conclude that they can "find nothing wrong," the implication being that the pain is all in the patient's head. Even worse, it suggests that the only choice is to live with the pain or try a prescription medication or an injection to dial it down. These treatments are not without a downside. They have side effects, they're temporary, and they do nothing to address the underlying pain generator or make the back healthier.

The good news is that regardless of whether your doctor can find a cause, you can do a great deal on your own and with the help of various healthcare professionals to successfully manage your back pain and get your life back. In this chapter, we bring you up to speed on the basics.

Exploring Possible Causes of Back Pain

When most people set out to answer the question of what's making their back hurt, they assume something is broken, perhaps a musculoskeletal issue that's putting pressure on a nerve — a slipped disc, a compression fracture, arthritis, osteoporosis, something structural or mechanical like that. However, sources of back pain can be far more wide-ranging and elusive to decipher. Here's a short list of less obvious factors that can cause or contribute to back pain and the perception of pain:

>> **Diet:** Diets high in processed foods, sugars, refined carbohydrates, and unhealthy fats (such as trans fats) can contribute to arthritis and other inflammatory conditions, which may affect the spine. (*Arthritis* means joint inflammation.)

>> **Dehydration:** For reasons not fully understood, dehydration can cause back pain. We've seen it happen with athletes who intentionally lose water weight to qualify for competition in a certain weight class.

>> **Posture:** Poor posture when sitting, standing, lifting, or doing anything can strain muscles and ligaments. In Chapter 7, you discover how to keep your spine in a neutral position, which is the most stable contour of the spine when you're standing, sitting, and even when you're "bending over."

>> **Sleep:** How you sleep (on your back, side, or belly), the mattress you sleep on, how long you sleep, and the quality of your sleep can all contribute to back health. Keep in mind that when you're sleeping, your body is busy detoxing, repairing damaged cells and tissues, and engaging in numerous other activities that impact every system in your body.

>> **Body weight:** Carrying extra weight isn't necessarily bad for the back in and of itself. In fact, in some ways, it can help strengthen the spine. However, being overweight can be a sign of other underlying health issues that can contribute to back pain. In addition, excess weight can amplify the negative effects of poor posture.

>> **Lifestyle factors:** Use of nicotine products (smoking, vaping, chewing tobacco), a sedentary lifestyle, excessive alcohol consumption, and other unhealthy lifestyle factors can cause back pain or make it worse.

UNDERSTANDING CENTRAL SENSITIZATION

Back pain is generally divided into two categories — acute and chronic. *Acute pain* usually occurs suddenly. It can have a specific cause but often presents without an obvious cause. *Chronic pain* is ongoing, typically lasting longer than three months, and often persists even after the injury or underlying cause has healed or had adequate time to heal. (Note that acute back pain rarely resolves completely and often recurs.)

A concept that may explain why pain persists even after the cause has been resolved is *central sensitization* — a tendency for the nervous system to become more sensitive to pain signals due to chronic pain. When back pain becomes chronic, the brain may persist in signaling pain or become hyper-responsive, amplifying pain signals even when the underlying issue has improved.

>> **Other medical conditions:** Certain medical conditions can cause back pain, including urinary tract infection (UTI), kidney stones, hernia, gastrointestinal issues, tumors, and fibromyalgia. Obviously, these conditions need to be ruled out before jumping to the conclusion that the origin of the pain is musculoskeletal.

>> **Psychological and emotional factors:** Depression, anxiety, and emotional distress can all cause or contribute to back pain. On the positive side, your mind can play a powerful role in successfully managing back pain.

See Chapter 3 for more about the possible anatomical and biological causes of back pain, and turn to Chapter 4 to discover more about the mind–body relationship and how to leverage it to enhance your recovery.

Looking Into the Conventional Approach to Back Pain Management

The conventional approach to back pain management involves using several therapies, alone or in combination, depending on the nature, severity, and duration of the back pain and underlying conditions. Conventional back pain therapies and treatments include the following:

>> **Rest:** Traditionally, doctors have recommended periods of rest and avoiding strenuous physical activities. More enlightened healthcare providers now recommend short periods of rest only for severe, acute back pain, a gradual

return to normal activities as the pain subsides or even before the pain subsides, and exercise to strengthen the back for long-term recovery.

>> **Cold/heat:** Cold diverts blood supply away from the back and stifles both inflammation and healing, and heat recruits blood supply to the back, increasing both inflammation and healing.

>> **Chiropractic care:** Chiropractic adjustments and other manual interventions can provide short-term relief for acute back pain, but adjustments may not be sufficient for protecting against future back pain, and they do nothing to strengthen the back and structures that support the spine.

>> **Physical therapy:** Physical therapy can help with flexibility, break up scar tissue and knots, improve poor posture, and strengthen the core, which can reduce back pain. It should always include exercise and a home-based plan for long-term recovery, but this is something therapists and patients often fail to follow up on.

>> **Medication:** Medication is useful for short-term relief. Think of it as a means for enabling you to exercise your back for more long-term and sustainable back pain management. Medication carries a risk of side effects and developing a dependence on it.

>> **Spinal injections:** Spinal injections involve the targeted delivery of medication, such as a corticosteroid (to reduce inflammation) or an anesthetic (to block the pain). Spinal injections may be used therapeutically (to provide relief) or diagnostically (to confirm a suspected pain generator prior to performing a more invasive procedure such as surgery).

>> **Surgery:** Surgery can be very effective for relieving back pain in cases in which the doctor can clearly identify a structural or mechanical abnormality that's clearly associated with the pain, such as a herniated disc or bone and ligament pressing on the spinal cord or a nerve. However, surgery is overprescribed for back pain, as explained in the nearby sidebar, "Tread Carefully."

TREAD CAREFULLY

People often think of modern medicine as purely scientific, but it's a business that's susceptible to human nature and corruption like any other business. When seeking treatment, be well-informed, skeptical, and assertive. Keep in mind that treatment decisions are ultimately your call, and don't be swayed by the belief that the doctor is always right. Here are some points to make you consider a provider's treatment recommendation more carefully:

- Most providers follow a fee-for-service model, so they're incentivized to recommend the services they provide. As a result, your diagnosis and treatment may be decided more by where you start looking for answers than by what's actually wrong. We're not suggesting that doctors are greedy and driven solely by a profit motive — only that the way they're incentivized can subtly influence their treatment recommendations.

- Doctors are human and are driven to help their patients in the best way they know how. They provide the treatment they've been trained to provide, which may not always be what's best.

- Patients generally don't like to hear, and doctors hate to say, "I don't know," when the question of what's causing the pain and what will make it go away comes up, so doctors often give the best possible answer they can think of, which isn't always the best answer.

- Conventional medicine is focused more on treating illnesses or suppressing symptoms, and less on improving health, so doctors tend toward prescribing medication, surgery, and other medical interventions instead of offering advice on diet, lifestyle, and other self-care interventions.

- Doctors often assume, sometimes correctly, that patients won't put the time or effort into improving their own health or will continue to make unhealthy choices, so they provide what they think their patients want — a quick fix.

- Health insurance companies provide little time for doctors to spend with their patients getting to know them and educate them. Doctors often have just enough time to review the patient's symptoms, come up with a diagnosis, and prescribe something or make a referral. The fee-for-service system incentivizes doctors to pack in as many patients as possible.

- Medical imaging, such as X-rays and magnetic resonance imaging (MRI) can show anomalies that are incidental to the back pain a patient is experiencing, and the doctor may jump to the conclusion that the anomaly is the cause of the back pain without any ability to confirm it. This is a common practice that results in a great deal of unnecessary procedures.

The take-home message here is to be skeptical about any diagnosis or treatment recommendation you receive. Get a second opinion before proceeding with any major surgery or costly or invasive medical procedure.

Taking a Novel Approach to Back Pain Management

Conventional treatments for back pain are provider-centered and focused on illness (pain and what's causing it), with the patient being a passive recipient of treatment. Our novel approach to back pain management is personalized and patient-centered, with the patient playing an active and supervisory role and providing substantial self-care (for example, diet and exercise). Providers (chiropractors, surgeons, pain management professionals, physical therapists, and so on) are at the periphery, being called in to provide services on an as-needed basis. In this model, you take on more of the responsibility for managing your back pain.

In the following sections, we explain this model in more detail.

Embracing self-efficacy: You can do it!

Self-efficacy is the belief that you can accomplish what you set out to do. It is an independent determinant of health; in other words, all other things being equal, those who are confident in their ability to overcome health challenges have better outcomes than those who don't. Make a commitment to yourself that you're not going to let back pain get you down and that you'll do whatever it takes, and then stick to it.

WARNING

Don't confuse self-efficacy with self-reliance. You may need some help along the way — a chiropractor, surgeon, physical therapist, or pain specialist can play a key role in empowering you to achieve your back pain management goals. For more about self-efficacy, see Chapter 4.

Shifting your focus from combating illness to restoring health

One of the biggest mistakes both patients and doctors make in the context of back pain management is that when they fail to identify a clear anatomical or biological cause of the back pain, they assume that nothing can be done to reduce the pain. The truth is that almost regardless of what's making your back hurt, you can build back strength and mobility and reduce the pain, mostly with self-care, including the following:

>> Eating healthy foods

>> Staying hydrated

>> Improving sleep quantity and quality

>> Improving your posture

>> Building core strength, especially your hidden core (the back muscles that support your spine)

>> Making healthy lifestyle choices, such as not smoking or vaping, drinking alcohol in moderation (if at all), and maintaining a healthy weight

>> Managing stress, which may involve addressing relationship and work-place issues

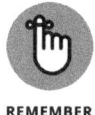

REMEMBER

Restoring health may also involve combatting illness, but as you become healthier, you're going to find that your body resolves some illnesses on its own and requires less medication and medical treatment overall.

Taking a do-it-yourself approach

Our approach to managing back pain is mostly do-it-yourself (DIY) with the addition of pockets of assistance from various healthcare providers as needed. In Chapter 5, we provide guidance for determining when starting with a healthcare provider is best — for example, when you can't move without experiencing excruciating back pain or when your back pain is accompanied by weakness in your arms or legs. In most cases, however, you can safely start with a DIY approach.

For easy reference, we packed most of our DIY advice in Part 2 (Chapters 6–11). Here's our overall advice in a nutshell:

>> **If you smoke, vape, chew tobacco, consume excessive amounts of alcohol, or bring other nasty stuff into your body, stop that.**

>> **Eat healthy, mostly plants (vegetables, nuts, fruits, and grains), along with healthy proteins and fats.** Steer clear of sugar, baked goods, highly processed foods, and any foods that make you feel lousy (for example, many people have trouble with dairy products).

>> **Drink mostly water and enough of it, but not too much.** (When you're getting enough water, your pee is pale yellow — not clear and not dark yellow or orange.)

>> **Get off your butt.** Your body is designed to move and is a lot healthier when it does, even when you're in pain.

>> **Be mindful of your posture.** Stand straight, sit up, shoulders back and down. If you need to pick something up, squat, keeping your back straight (see Chapter 7 for details).

>> **Build core strength, especially your hidden core (the back muscles that support the spine).** See Chapters 7, 8, and 9 for details and specific exercises that strengthen and mobilize the hidden core.

REMEMBER

Most people think of the spine as the framework of support for the back, but muscles, tendons, and ligaments provide a network of support for the spine, as well — they have a relationship based on mutual support. Even if nothing can be done to "fix" the spine, plenty can be done to strengthen the muscles that support it.

>> **Incorporate homespun remedies to decompress the spine, massage your back muscles, increase circulation, and relieve pain.** By "homespun remedies," we mean DIY techniques involving inexpensive items such as foam rollers, a yoga/physio ball, over-the-counter pain-relief ointments, and other equipment and supplies that are readily available. (See Chapter 10 for details.) You can do this while watching TV instead of melting into your recliner.

>> **Improve your breathing.** Every cell in your body needs a constant supply of oxygen and a continuous release of carbon dioxide (a waste product). In Chapter 11, we provide several techniques to optimize breathing. Maintaining good posture also helps by giving your lungs more room to inflate.

Embracing the five components of fitness

Many doctors' offices, especially those of orthopedic and spinal surgeons, have a model of a skeleton or spine hanging in every examination room (or at least a poster hanging on a wall). This gives the false impression that the spine is somehow separate from the body. The truth is that the body is an organic whole. To have a healthy spine, you need a healthy body. One approach is to focus on the five components of fitness, as explained in the following sections.

TIP

Start with the movements and exercises we recommend in Chapters 8 and 9. As you build strength and endurance, consider looking into high-intensity interval training (HIIT). HIIT workouts address several of the five components of fitness at once. Other workout types generally address only one or two. For example, weightlifting improves both muscular fitness and body composition.

Muscular fitness

Muscular fitness has three components of its own:

>> **Explosive power:** Single or multiple high-exertion motions that move weight quickly; for example, jumping, punching or kicking a heavy bag or pads, performing Olympic weightlifts, and putting shot (shotput).

>> **Absolute strength:** The movement of a maximum amount of weight a certain distance; for example, bench pressing the most weight you can or

lifting the heaviest stone you can to the top of a wall — the tests of strength common in strongman competitions.

>> **Muscular endurance:** The ability to move the body or a weight many times over a sustained period of time; for example, doing 10 pullups, 20 push-ups, or 15 curls with a 10-pound dumbbell.

REMEMBER

Most of the exercises we recommend in Chapters 8 and 9 build muscular endurance, which has the biggest positive impact, specifically on everyday back health and fitness.

Cardiovascular fitness

Cardiovascular fitness is the ability of the heart, lungs, and blood vessels to deliver oxygen to the muscles during sustained physical activity. To build cardiovascular fitness, you typically need to engage in strenuous physical activity for at least 20 minutes at a time. Activities and exercises that build cardiovascular fitness include running (or walking at a fast pace), dancing, bicycling, rowing, climbing stairs, jumping rope — anything that makes you breathe heavily for 20 minutes or more.

Mobility and flexibility

Mobility is the ability of the joint to move and is commonly referred to as "range of motion." *Flexibility* is the ability of a muscle to stretch. Both are essential for muscle strength and performance and for mitigating the risk and severity of injury.

REMEMBER

During the initial stages of improving your back, focus first on building mobility and strength and then on increasing your flexibility. Even during workout sessions, mobilizing and strengthening muscles first warms them up and makes them more pliable, optimizing the benefits of any stretching you do while mitigating the risk of injury from stretching. Don't stretch cold muscles.

Body composition

Body composition is the ratio of body fat to the rest of the body (muscle, bone, organs) by weight. Excessive body fat is an indicator of poor health. We're not going to get into an in-depth discussion of what's considered excess body fat, what constitutes "ideal" body composition, body mass index (BMI), or other such topics. Too much focus on body weight can take the focus off of building strength, and we're not sure how relevant it is to back pain. Besides, most people who need to be conscious of the health implications of being overweight know when their weight issue is significant enough to be negatively impacting their health.

Neuromuscular fitness

Neuromuscular fitness is the ability of the nervous and muscular systems to work together to produce physical movement. You can think of it in terms of reflexes, balance, and coordination. In addition to ensuring well-coordinated physical movement, neuromuscular fitness helps to lower blood pressure, enhance mobility, and increase flexibility. Disciplines such as yoga, Pilates, tai chi, qi gong, and other martial arts are all effective in building neuromuscular fitness. Dancing, surfing, skiing, and other fun athletic activities are also helpful.

REMEMBER

We like to think of neuromuscular fitness as part of the mind-body connection that we discuss in Chapter 4. Everything in your life that impacts how you think and feel, including your job, relationships, and overall outlook impacts your health in some way, positively or negatively.

Augmenting self-help with professional care

We view self-care as the core treatment for back pain and look at other treatments, not as ends in themselves but as the means to enabling self-care. The purpose of whatever treatment you receive — surgery, chiropractic adjustment, pain management, physical therapy, acupuncture — is to get you back on your feet, re-engaged in physical activities, and back to the gym.

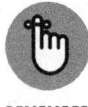

REMEMBER

The big question is where to start. If you have a serious spinal injury that's clearly causing your back pain, you probably want to start with a surgeon. You don't want to do anything that could possibly make a spinal injury or deterioration worse. However, in most cases, people with back pain are better off not being too hasty about seeing a medical professional, because a diagnosis can lead to unnecessary surgery or other medical interventions and plant seeds of illness in the mind of the patient, which can be counterproductive. We can't tell you where to start on your journey to more effectively managing your back pain, but in Chapter 5 we provide guidance that can help you make a more judicious decision.

In Part 3, we take you on a deeper dive into your provider options and other related topics, including the following:

>> Getting an accurate diagnosis and exploring the different types of providers who can enhance your recovery, including physical therapists, surgeons, chiropractors, personal trainers, and psychologists

- ❯❯ Understanding the unique benefits of different types of medical imaging technologies, including X-ray, magnetic resonance imaging (MRI), computed tomography (CT), and single-photon emission computerized tomography (SPECT)

- ❯❯ Deciding whether to treat the pain generator, the pain, or the patient and in what sequence

- ❯❯ Using medication to manage the pain

- ❯❯ Engaging in physical therapy to improve mobility and reduce pain

- ❯❯ Understanding the benefits and limitations of chiropractic care

- ❯❯ Exploring common surgical procedures that can help, estimating their predictability of success, and understanding their potential drawbacks

- ❯❯ Knowing what a psychologist or psychiatrist can do to help manage back pain

Opting for value-based care

Value-based care (VBC) is a healthcare delivery model that rewards healthcare providers based on the *quality* of the care they deliver rather than on the *quantity* of that care. The current healthcare system in the United States is a pay-for-service model that rewards providers for the quantity of care they deliver. You may not be able to do much to change the system, but you have the power to create your own VBC model by playing an active role in coordinating your treatment. Here are a few suggestions for ensuring that you're getting the most effective treatment options for you:

- ❯❯ **Get educated:** Reading this book is a great way to build your knowledge and understanding of back pain and make well-informed treatment decisions. Do additional research on your own if a provider recommends a treatment you're not familiar with.

- ❯❯ **Choose your providers carefully:** If you feel as though you're being rushed through appointments, your provider's not listening to you or doesn't "get you," or you're getting a diagnosis and prescription that seems too quick to be accurate, don't hesitate to change providers.

- ❯❯ **Communicate and collaborate closely with your providers:** Build strong relationships between you and your providers and encourage and facilitate communication among providers when appropriate. Be assertive. Let your providers know that you're more interested in long-term solutions than quick fixes, and you're willing to do the hard work it takes to achieve and maintain optimal health.

» **Make sure proposed treatments align with your bigger goals.** Providers are often focused on treating illness, which is appropriate at times, but be sure you're not getting quick fixes that set you up for bigger problems later (such as providing medication that relieves the pain but does nothing to improve your back). Understand the benefits and potential drawbacks of every treatment option and have a big-picture plan in place that supports your long-term personal, professional, health, and fitness goals.

Managing back pain isn't just about your back or your pain; it's about your life. This book is committed to empowering you to reclaim your life and live it more fully. Our hope is that your back pain gradually diminishes to the point at which it no longer crosses your mind.

IN THIS CHAPTER

» Tracing the pain to its root cause

» Comparing and contrasting acute and chronic back pain

» Looking at back pain as a symptom of modern living

» Getting up to speed on the three-tier theory of pain

» Taking a casual approach to back pain

Chapter **2**

Is Something Broken Inside Me?

When most people experience back pain, they suspect that something is broken inside — that they pulled a muscle, tore a ligament, fractured a vertebra, herniated a disc, "threw out their back," or experienced some other physical damage or misalignment. They head to the doctor to have it checked out, believing that the doctor can identify and then fix whatever's broken, and then they can return to their lives as though nothing had ever gone wrong. They think it's like taking their car to the local mechanic to have the wheels aligned.

Unfortunately, "identifying" the cause or "fixing" the back is rarely that simple. Numerous factors, alone and in combination, can cause back pain, contribute to it, and make a person more susceptible to it. Although back pain is often blamed on work conditions or activities, an uncomfortable mattress, injury from a fall, a sports injury, or having to drive for extended periods, other factors can cause or contribute to it, such as poor diet or posture, emotional or psychological stress, and sedentary living.

In this chapter, we focus on some of the most common causes of back pain so you can begin to consider factors in your life that could be causing or contributing specifically to *your* back pain, and you can start to decide on the approach you want to take to address it.

Finding the Pain Generator

Pain is an unpleasant sensory and emotional feeling resulting from injury or illness. It's a person's perception of *nociception* — the nervous system's response to actual or potentially harmful sensory stimuli. For example, suppose you fall and scrape your knee. Your peripheral nervous system senses the injury and sends a signal to your brain — that's nociception.

A person's back has numerous potential pain generators — structures or tissue types that can produce sensations that the brain interprets as pain, and not all of them are located in the spine itself. Common back pain generators include the following:

>> **Muscles:** Tight muscles or sprain or strain from overuse, improper lifting techniques, poor posture, or trauma can cause muscles to be damaged or inflamed and cause pain. Underuse and atrophy of muscles can also cause pain.

>> **Vertebrae and bones:** Fractures (cracks or compressions) in the vertebrae (the bones that form the spinal column, see Figure 2-1) caused by trauma and/or weak bones can be a significant source of pain.

>> **Discs:** Between the vertebrae are round fluid-filled cushions called "discs" that act like shock absorbers. When they rupture or bulge out of their normal position, they can press on nearby nerves, causing pain. Disc degeneration over time can also cause a loss of cushioning, resulting in neighboring vertebrae rubbing together or pressing against nerves. Disc inflammation can also be a source of pain.

>> **Facet joints:** *Facet joints* are the hinges between vertebrae that allow the spinal column to bend and twist. Inflammation or degeneration of these joints can result in vertebrae rubbing together or pressing on nerves. Pain from facet joint injury or degeneration is often worse when standing or twisting.

>> **Ligaments:** The ligaments that stabilize the spine can become overstretched, strained, or injured due to poor posture, improper lifting, or sudden movements. Ligament strain or injury is often accompanied by muscle spasms.

>> **Nerves:** Pinched or irritated nerve roots (due to spinal compression, for example) can cause pain that radiates down the arms or the legs, as in the case of *Radiculopathy* (irritation of the sciatic nerve roots, which can result in pain that travels from the butt down each leg to the foot). The pain is typically a sharp, shooting, or burning sensation.

>> **Sacroiliac (SI) joint:** The SI joint is located where the pelvis joins to the sacrum at the base of the spine. It's often implicated as a cause of back pain, but proving it to be so is difficult.

>> **Spinal canal stenosis:** This condition is a narrowing of the spinal canal, which puts pressure on the spinal nerve roots, resulting in pain, numbness, or occasionally weakness, especially of the arms and legs.

>> **Myofascial tissue:** "Myofascial" refers to the muscle (*myo*) and connective tissue (*fascia*) surrounding the muscle. *Myofascial pain syndrome* is a condition caused by tight, inflamed muscle fibers or fascia.

>> **Bone spurs (osteophytes):** These bone growths can result from osteoarthritis or other degenerative conditions, which can irritate spinal joints or nerves, causing pain.

>> **Referred pain:** Back pain can come from conditions outside the back, such as premenstrual syndrome (PMS), kidney stones, appendicitis, endometriosis, and inflammation of the gallbladder. Referred pain is perceived as occurring somewhere other than the location of the painful stimulus.

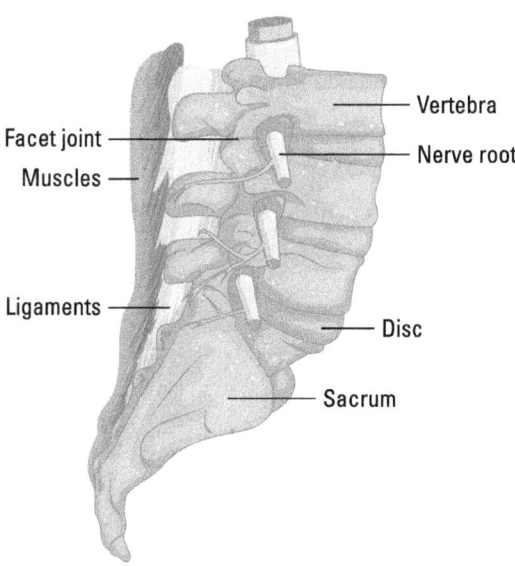

Facet joint

Muscles

Vertebra

Nerve root

Ligaments

Disc

Sacrum

FIGURE 2-1:
Some areas of the back commonly associated with back pain.

Visit your doctor for a full workup and medical imaging. Your doctor will perform a differential diagnosis to rule out unlikely causes, identify the most likely potential causes, and may make some treatment recommendations. Identifying and treating (or ruling out) conditions such as kidney stones, tumors, and fractures is an important early step in the process of reclaiming your life from back pain. However, don't be surprised if you end up back at square one with no definitive diagnosis and only a prescription for symptomatic relief. The root cause(s) of back pain can be difficult to pin down. However, even if you can't identify the root cause, you have a good chance of eliminating the pain by following the advice we give in this book.

GAUGING YOUR SUSCEPTIBILITY TO BACK PAIN

Almost everyone will experience back pain sometime in their life, but some people are more susceptible than others. The following are factors that may determine a person's susceptibility to back pain:

- **Fitness level:** Being physically fit reduces your susceptibility to back pain, which is no surprise; a strong core supports the spine. However, excessive activity after having been inactive for some time may strain your back.

- **Weight:** Back pain is more common among people who are overweight.

- **Job:** Jobs that require heavy lifting, pulling, pushing, or twisting increase a person's susceptibility to back injury, so too can jobs that require sitting or standing for long periods of time, such as desk jobs and occupations that involve a lot of driving.

- **Stress:** Stress and anxiety tend to tighten muscles and restrict blood flow, both of which can result in back pain and increase one's susceptibility to injury.

- **Age:** Back pain becomes more common with age, especially after the age of 45.

- **Heredity:** Genetics have been linked to a number of disorders associated with back pain, including *scoliosis* (curvature of the spine), *Spondylolisthesis* (vertebral shifting), degenerative disc disease, *kyphosis* (hunched back), and *ankylosing spondylitis* (a form of inflammatory arthritis).

Regardless of the nature and the number of factors you have working against you, you have the power to strengthen your back, increase mobility, and build resilience. In this book, we show you how.

Differentiating Acute from Chronic Back Pain — and Why It Matters

Pain comes in two types: acute (short-term) and chronic (long-term). In this section, we dig a little deeper into the differences and explain why it matters.

Acute back pain

Acute back pain has the following characteristics:

>> It lasts less than six weeks and resolves on its own or with proper care.

>> It's often caused by a specific event such as a strain, sprain, or trauma.

>> It's typically localized.

>> It often responds well to standard non-invasive therapies, such as rest, massage, cold/heat, and gradually increasing movement.

>> The pain subsides after the injured tissue heals.

>> It impairs one's ability to work or engage in enjoyable physical activities only temporarily.

REMEMBER

Although acute back pain is, by definition, only temporary, it tends not to resolve fully and to recur, so don't ignore it, even if it seems to be getting better. Be proactive. Follow up with the therapies we recommend in this book for strengthening your mind and body and improving your resilience.

TIP

Generally, you should treat acute back pain with rest and ice, getting back on your feet as soon as possible — which is usually sooner than most patients think. In some cases, 24 hours of rest is sufficient. In other cases, you may need more time. However, motion and exercise are usually better for long-term recovery than rest and ice. See Chapter 6 for details.

Chronic back pain

Chronic back pain is characterized by the following:

>> It lasts longer than three months. The pain may be constant or intermittent, but it's a lingering issue.

>> It is often associated with a long-term condition, such as a degenerative disease (osteoarthritis, for example), herniated disc, sciatica, or musculoskeletal imbalances. However, it can also result from an old injury, overuse, an inflammatory condition, emotional stress, or a combination of factors. Often, the underlying cause(s) remain a mystery.

>> The pain often persists even after the underlying cause(s) have healed.

>> It's often dull or aching with possible episodes of sharp pain and may be cyclical. It may also be accompanied by numbness, tingling, or weakness if nerves are damaged.

>> Successful treatment always requires a multifaceted approach involving cognitive behavioral therapy, physical therapy, pain management, dietary and lifestyle changes, stress management, and rarely, in cases involving structural damage or deformities, surgery. Conventional treatment typically aims to manage symptoms and improve function but often fails to identify and address the underlying cause(s).

>> Chronic pain is life-changing, and not in a good way! It can lead to depression, anxiety, poor physical and mental performance, decreased sex drive, and a host of other debilitating issues. People living with chronic back pain often avoid certain activities, situations, and occupational opportunities. Many people even dread waking the next day because they're aware of the looming pain awaiting them at daybreak.

Chronic back pain is much more than pain lasting more than three months. It represents changes in the brain, which make it much harder to treat. Modern medicine has done a poor job of helping patients with chronic back pain. We believe the most effective treatment is a multifaceted approach that targets both mind and body.

Why the difference matters

The difference between acute and chronic back pain matters because the approach to treating each type of pain is so different. Acute pain typically responds well to a conventional short-term treatment protocol focused on gradually restoring movement and strength while alleviating pain to prevent it from hindering the healing process. Look at acute back pain as a signal to start exercising your back; you can find exercises in Chapters 8 and 9. Don't expect it to resolve on its own; relief is typically incomplete, and recurrence is common. The right exercise can result in a more robust recovery.

Chronic pain typically requires a multifaceted approach over a much longer period. It may involve stress management, exercise to increase strength and mobility, testing and treatment for inflammatory conditions, and rarely, surgery to address any structural damage or impairments, and other treatment protocols.

REMEMBER

Don't settle for treatments that merely address symptoms and provide temporary relief, such as medications and injections. These treatments may be helpful for alleviating pain and inflammation that's preventing you from engaging in physical therapy and exercise, but a long-term solution requires treatments that target root causes that may have developed over years or even decades. The best way to treat chronic pain is to change your mind and your body.

Understanding the role that stability and mobility play in chronic back pain

An often unrecognized cause of back pain is the musculoskeletal imbalances that result from overusing some muscles while underusing others. For example, if you sit eight hours a day at work, your back muscles get stretched while the muscles in the front of your body are shortened. The antidote is to stretch the hip flexors (the muscles that bring the knee up closer to the chest) and strengthen the paraspinal and multifidus muscles (the muscles that run along the spinal column and align and support the spine).

Certain joints are designed for stability, while others are designed for mobility. Compare the shoulders and hips, for example. The shoulders are designed for mobility relative to the stability of the hips. The lumbar (lower) and cervical (upper, neck) spines are designed to allow for mobility, while the thoracic (middle) spine is designed for stability. The idea here is that any structure that is designed for mobility is stabilized by muscles more than by ligaments and tendons and, as such, is more responsive to rehab. Muscle building around a joint designed for mobility is a predictable and common-sense path to reducing pain through rehab.

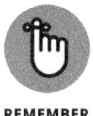

REMEMBER

Fortunately, we have a solution for restoring balance. See Chapters 8 and 9 for more about stability and mobility and exercises that address common musculoskeletal imbalances.

Counteracting the Curses of Modern Living

A great deal of back pain is self-inflicted, not willingly but simply through the course of modern living. Two of the biggest contributors to back pain these days are the modern sedentary lifestyle and the growing dependence on mobile electronic devices. These factors literally put us in a position (posture) that is bad for our backs and necks and our overall physical and mental health and well-being.

In this section, we delve a little deeper into each of these modern curses and provide guidance on how to counteract their deleterious effects.

Sitting is the new smoking

Humans are not designed to be sedentary creatures. By design, we are the world's best long-distance, hot-weather runners, but if you spend a little time people-watching at the local mall, grocery store, theme park, or state fair in the U.S., you're likely to be appalled at the physique of the average citizen. Over 72 percent of adults in the United States are overweight, and more than 43 percent are considered obese.

If you're out of shape, it's not entirely your fault. It's often the result of today's sedentary lifestyle combined with unhealthy foods laced with additives that make consumers crave more of it. Fortunately, although being out of shape isn't entirely your fault, you have the power to counteract the negative effects of modern living. Here are a few general recommendations:

>> **Eat whole foods, mostly plants — vegetables, nuts, and fruits — along with healthy proteins (such as chicken, fish, and grass-fed beef).**

>> **Avoid sugar and sweets.** The body stores excess sugar as fat, which is the most common cause of weight gain.

>> **If you're carrying too much weight, eat less. Intermittent fasting works wonders.** An easy approach is to stop eating at about 6 p.m. and eat a light breakfast around 8 a.m.

>> **Drink mostly water and avoid sweet beverages and alcohol.**

>> **Adopt a more physically active lifestyle.** Camp, hike, work in the garden, tinker in the garage — anything that gets your body moving instead of sitting or standing around.

>> **Do some physically strenuous activity or exercise for at least 30 minutes at a time most days of the week.** Do something that makes you breathe hard.

REMEMBER

We have become so sedentary in our lifestyles that sedentary living has surpassed smoking as the number one preventable cause of death in the United States. This lack of activity significantly increases the risk of coronary artery disease (CAD) and a host of other serious health conditions, including arthritis, depression, anxiety, gout, diabetes, and, of course, back pain.

Tech neck: A neckademic

Tech neck is a condition caused by continuously straining the neck muscles to support the head when looking down at a digital device such as a smartphone, tablet, or laptop computer. It's a musculoskeletal imbalance similar to the imbalance caused by excessive sitting. The neck extensor muscles are stretched and weakened, while the neck flexor muscles are shortened. The antidote is to stretch the front of the neck and strengthen the back of the neck.

Nearly everyone is guilty of spending too much time looking down. The only differences between people who get tech neck and those who don't are how frequently they do it, how far down they bend their heads, and whether they do anything to counteract the negative effects.

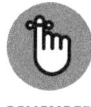

REMEMBER

Every inch your head is off its neutral position doubles the weight your neck muscles must support.

To prevent tech neck, take the following precautions:

>> Limit your screen time overall, especially time spent looking down at the device.

>> Position the screen/device at eye level.

>> Keep your ears aligned with your shoulders at all times. See Chapter 8 for guidance on how to maintain a *neutral spine* (the ideal contour of the spine when standing erect).

>> Take frequent breaks to look up and look around.

>> Spend some time developing your neck muscles. See Chapters 8 and 9 for specific exercises. Many doctors, physical therapists, and trainers neglect the neck muscles.

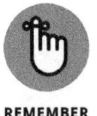

REMEMBER

You don't need the neck of a professional bodybuilder or boxer, but a strong neck makes you far less susceptible to developing tech neck, and it serves as a shock absorber in the event of a motor vehicle accident or fall.

Understanding the Three-Tier Theory of Pain

People have been trying to understand the nature and mechanism of pain for thousands of years. Physicians and philosophers have proposed numerous frameworks to explain how the body and mind process and respond to pain signals. One such framework is the three-tier theory of pain, which traces pain from its biological source to its cognitive and emotional interpretations, which affect how people perceive and manage the pain. The three tiers are as follows:

1. **Stimulus:** The physical experience of the event or condition that is ultimately perceived as painful. When tissue suffers trauma or damage, *nociceptors* (pain receptors) in the skin, muscles, joints, or internal organs or tissues are activated. The nociceptors transmit signals through the body's nervous system to the brain, where the sensation is perceived and processed. The stimulus may be a cut, burn, inflammation, pinched nerve, or other trauma or physical irregularity.

2. **Epiphenomenon:** The secondary physical adaptations that the body initiates as a result of the stimulus. This includes muscle spasms, swelling and inflammation, and *disuse atrophy* (a reduction in muscle mass usually from avoiding activity that hurts). These bodily adaptations can be a cause of pain independent of the stimulus.

3. **Judicial function:** The cognitive and evaluative role the brain plays in interpreting pain and determining the appropriate response. At this tier, the brain determines whether the pain is serious (for example, requiring medical attention) or whether it's a mild discomfort that can be self-managed without medical intervention.

The three-tier theory of pain explains why two people who have the same painful injury can experience and respond to the pain so differently. Generally, surgeons and pain management doctors address the stimulus; therapists and chiropractors address the epiphenomenon; and psychologists address the judicial function. Of course, all three tiers would ideally be addressed by a team of providers at the same time, as pain always involves all three tiers to some extent.

Approaching Routine Back Pain as You Would a Common Cold

The severity of a health condition and the degree to which it disrupts one's life is often determined by the person's perception and attitude. For example, most people who catch a cold work right through it. They get extra rest, drink plenty of fluids, eat chicken soup, supplement their diet with vitamin C and zinc, and maybe take an antihistamine, decongestant, or pain reliever to alleviate their symptoms. They know that the cold simply needs to run its course, and they'll be feeling back to normal in seven to ten days.

However, for some people, the common cold totally disrupts their life. They take a few sick days, lie in bed all day, and head to the doctor's office demanding a prescription for antibiotics (which are useless in treating viral infections like those that produce cold symptoms).

The same is true for most people who experience back pain, especially chronic pain that has no clear cause. If you're experiencing back pain, you need to decide how you're going to approach it — are you going to accept it as a disability or confront it as just another inconvenience on the road of life? Are you going to succumb to the pain and lie there like a slug, or will you take action to reduce the pain and reclaim your life?

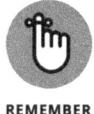

REMEMBER

Your body is an incredible creation that can repair and heal itself when given sufficient time and appropriate nutrition and therapeutics. Depending on the root cause of your back pain, medical intervention may be required. However, in most cases, the root cause of back pain is a musculoskeletal weakness or imbalance that you can correct by strengthening and mobilizing the back and addressing other contributing factors, such as diet and lifestyle.

Back pain is a part of life and in most cases, barring severe injury or trauma, it's best addressed by viewing it as a simple inconvenience of life and taking proactive, holistic measures to rectify the situation. You can help your body heal itself without the use of prescription drugs that merely mask the pain and provide no healing benefits whatsoever.

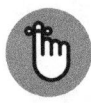

REMEMBER

In many ways, alleviating back pain is a case of mind over matter — if you don't mind, the pain doesn't matter. We're not implying that the pain is all in your head. We're just saying that the best approach is to live a healthy and active life, giving your body everything it needs to heal and strengthen itself — fresh air, clean water, healthy foods, and a range of strenuous physical activity. Thinking of your body as adaptable rather than vulnerable is essential.

TIP

Movement is the key! It increases blood flow, which stimulates the healing process.

Chapter **3**

Looking at Back Pain from an Anatomical Perspective

When most people experience back pain, they assume an anatomical cause — a pulled or strained muscle, a pinched nerve, a herniated disc, a compression fracture, arthritis, or maybe a tumor. As your understanding of back pain evolves, you will begin to recognize that the cause(s) of back pain can be far more complex than that. In addition, despite our advances in modern technology, the cause is often not identifiable. Causes may be related to diet, exercise (a lack thereof), weight, stress, poor posture, smoking, alcohol consumption, poor sleep, or other factors or a combination of factors. And back pain isn't just a physical sensation — how you experience pain is influenced by mental processes as well. And these mental processes can create additional stressors, such as muscle tension, that can exacerbate the pain and become an ongoing (and, in some cases, the primary) source of your chronic pain.

We cover the mind-body relationship in more detail in Chapter 4. In this chapter, we focus on the potential anatomical causes of back pain — structural defects, physical damage or deterioration, and illnesses that are commonly at the root of back pain.

REMEMBER

Diagnosing and treating back pain isn't a simple matter of spotting a spinal misalignment on an X-ray and then getting a chiropractic adjustment or having surgery to correct it. Nor does treatment boil down to popping a pill to dull the pain. Treatment is not so much about addressing the pain or its cause as it is about restoring health, strength, mobility, and resilience. However, we are not recommending that you or your doctor ignore or discount the possibility of injuries, anatomical anomalies, or illnesses that may be causing your back pain. These issues need to be considered and addressed when necessary as part of a personalized, holistic treatment plan focused on restoring back health and fitness.

Getting to Know Your Spine

Understanding the *etiology* of back pain (what causes it) often begins with understanding the structure and function of the spine and the pain generators (the components of the spine where pain often originates). In this section, we take you on a tour of the spine, identify the common pain generators, and share a couple of important insights that can help narrow a diagnosis to a specific pain generator.

Mapping the spine

No discussion of spinal anatomy is complete without a mention of its overall structure. By convention, the spine is divided into the following four parts (from top to bottom), as shown in Figure 3-1:

>> **Cervical spine (neck):** The cervical spine consists of the first seven vertebrae, labeled C1–C7. It supports the head and is the most flexible part of the spine, facilitating head movement, such as rotation, flexion, extension, and tilting.

>> **Thoracic spine (upper back):** The thoracic spine consists of the 12 vertebrae in the middle, labeled T1–T12. It provides support for the upper body, including the rib cage, which protects the heart and lungs. It's less mobile than both the cervical and the lumbar spines.

>> **Lumbar spine (lower back):** The lumbar spine consists of the five vertebrae, labeled L1–L5 near the bottom of the spine. It's the thickest and strongest part of the spine, bearing most of the weight of the upper body and providing mobility to the lower back.

>> **Sacrum:** The sacrum is the triangular-shaped structure at the base of the spine, consisting of five vertebrae fused together. It forms the back of the pelvis and connects the spine to the hip bones (ilium). It plays a crucial role in transferring weight from the upper body to the hips and the lower limbs.

At the very bottom of the spine is the *coccyx* (tailbone), which consists of four vertebrae fused together. The coccyx and the muscles and ligaments attached to it form the pelvic floor and serve as a support structure when sitting.

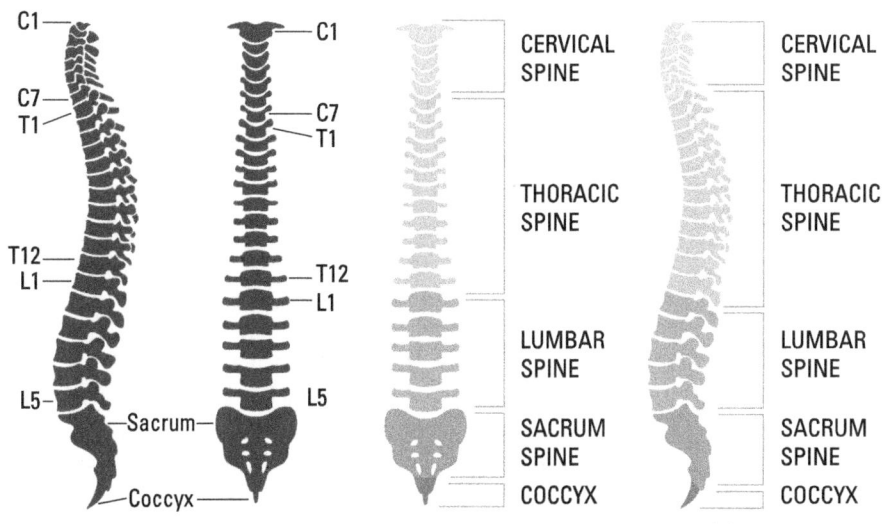

FIGURE 3-1: The spinal column is divided into four parts.

4zevar/Adobe Systems Incoprated

Zeroing in on the pain generators

Nearly everything in your back — bones, muscles, tendons, ligaments, and nerves — is capable of causing pain. Anything with a pain fiber is a potential source of pain. We refer to those many structures as the "pain players" and divide them into two groups:

>> **Structures that are part of the spine:** The *vertebral bodies* (the bones that make up the spinal column) and the *intervertebral discs* (the cushions between the vertebral bodies), as shown in Figure 3-2. The two major spinal pain players to focus on are the intervertebral discs and the facet joints.

>> **Supporting structures:** The structures outside the spine, including the nerves, muscles, and ligaments. These structures are the secondary pain players.

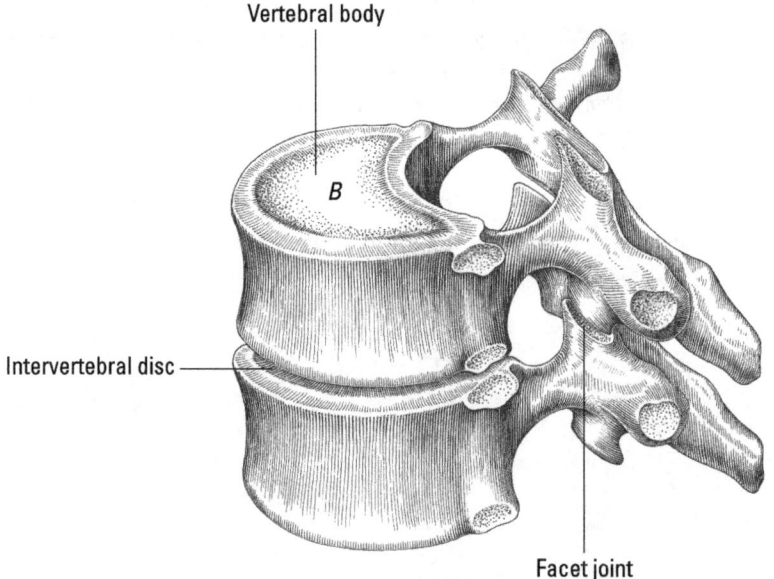

Vertebral body

B

Intervertebral disc —

Facet joint

channarongsds/Adobe Systems Incoprated

FIGURE 3-2:
The spinal column consists of vertebral bodies separated by intervertebral discs.

Bones: Vertebral bodies

The vertebral bodies are the large cylindrical bones that make up the main part of the vertebrae in the spine. They play a significant role in the structure and function of the spine, and they bear most of the load (especially in the lower back). One or more vertebral bodies can become a source of back pain when the following issues arise:

» **Degeneration:** Vertebral bodies can degenerate due to age, wear and tear, and conditions such as osteoporosis. Degeneration can cause the vertebrae to lose height or develop cracks or fractures that irritate the nerves.

» **Compression fractures:** Excessive pressure on the spine or weaknesses in the vertebral bodies (or a combination of the two) can cause fractures, resulting in pain and negatively impacting nerve function.

» **Alignment issues:** Vertebral bodies can shift out of alignment, which can cause pain directly, or cause it indirectly by triggering muscular imbalances to compensate for the shifting.

Intravertebral discs

Between the vertebral bodies are intravertebral discs that act as shock absorbers. Without them, walking would feel as though you were riding a scooter down a gravel road. Each disc is made up of two components, as shown in Figure 3-3:

>> **Nucleus pulposus** is the gel inside the disc. The gel is often described as being the consistency of gelatin or toothpaste, but it's more like crab meat.

>> **Annulus fibrosus** is a ligament containing pain fibers that holds the nucleus pulposus in place. When a disc is causing pain, the pain fibers in the annulus fibrosus are likely involved.

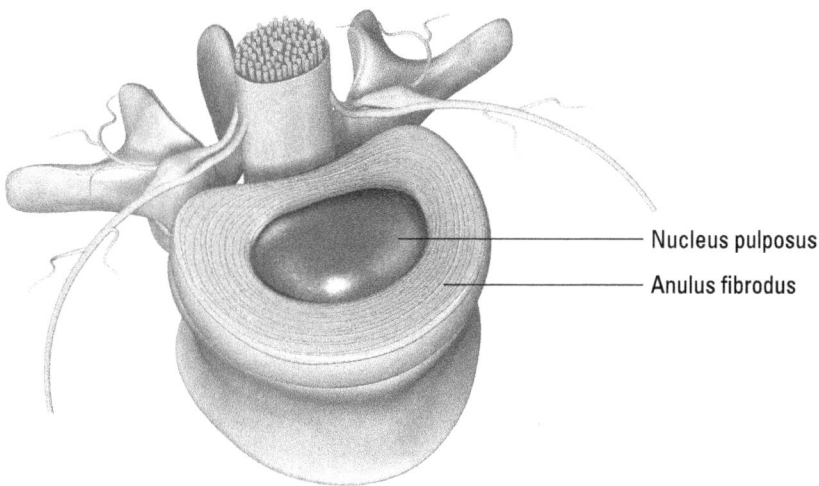

Nucleus pulposus

Anulus fibrodus

FIGURE 3-3: Intravertebral discs are a common source of back pain.

Axel Kock/Adobe Systems Incoprated

A disc-related nerve called the *basivertebral nerve* (see Figure 3-4) *innervates* (supplies nerve function to) the *endplate* of the vertebral body (the portion of the vertebral body that is attached and adjacent to the disc). The innervated endplate is another common contributor to back pain.

Several issues can negatively impact the health and function of one or more intravertebral discs, including the following:

>> **Disc degeneration:** The nucleus pulposus is 80 percent water when you're young but slowly starts to desiccate (lose water content) as you age. As discs desiccate, they become less flexible. They also lose height, which can cause the spine to compress, leading to other problems such as nerve impingement.

>> **Bulging or herniated disc:** When a nucleus pulposus bulges or herniates (ruptures) through the annulus fibrosus, it can press on nearby nerves, leading to sharp localized or radiating pain, numbness, or tingling sensations down the legs (if the bulging or herniation is in the lower back) or down the arms and into the hands (if the herniation is in the neck).

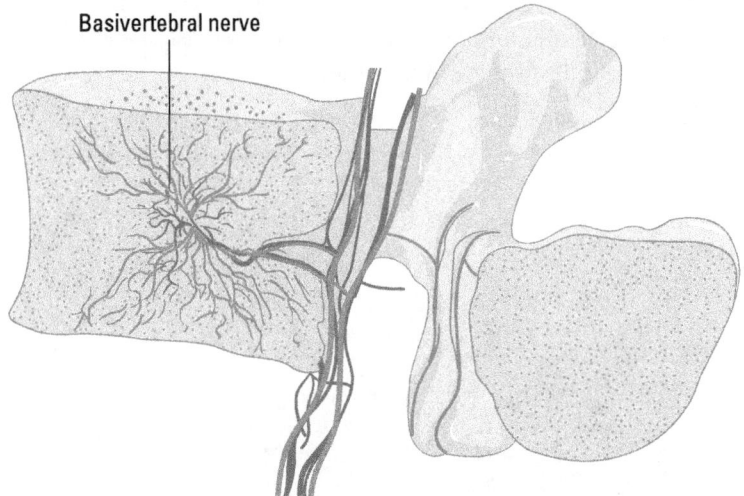

Basivertebral nerve

FIGURE 3-4:
The basivertebral nerve can also contribute to back pain.

>> **Infection/inflammation:** If a disc becomes infected or inflamed *(discitis)*, it can cause significant back pain, which tends to be intense, persistent, and often accompanied by fever as the body's immune system fights the infection.

>> **Mechanical stress:** Poor posture, improper lifting techniques, and other abnormal movement patterns can increase pressure and wear and tear on discs, resulting in degeneration, bulging, or herniation. (Discs often show signs of wear and tear related to a genetic tendency to age.)

TIP

Improving posture, practicing proper lifting techniques, and strengthening your back muscles all help to alleviate pressure on the discs and reduce daily wear and tear.

Facet joints

Vertebral bodies are joined by one disc (in front of the canal where the nerves traverse) and two facet joints (behind the canal where the nerves traverse). The facet joints stabilize the spine, but they also allow the spine to flex and rotate. Several issues related to facet joints can result in back pain, including the following:

>> **Inflammation/arthritis:** Inflammation of the facet joints (from overuse, injury, degeneration, or inflammation) can cause sharp or dull pain, typically in the neck or lower back. (*Arthritis* means "joint inflammation.")

>> **Degeneration:** Facet joints can wear down over time, which can result in pain and inflammation. When facets degenerate, they *hypertrophy* (enlarge), leading to nerve compression.

>> **Dysfunction:** When a facet joint becomes misaligned or doesn't move properly, it can cause pain. Dysfunction may result from injury, poor posture, or overuse.

>> **Nerve compression:** Enlarged facet joints can narrow the spinal canal (spinal stenosis), applying pressure to nearby nerves, which can result in pain, numbness, or weakness. These sensations can radiate pain to the legs or other parts of the body. For more about spinal stenosis, see the later section by that name.

Sacroiliac (SI) joint

The sacroiliac (SI) joints connect the sacrum to the pelvis (see Figure 3-5). They tend to have much less motion than the facet joints, but they're susceptible to two of the same issues — inflammation/arthritis and degeneration. People who've had spinal fusion are more likely to have SI joint issues.

WARNING

Be skeptical of a diagnosis that identifies the SI joint as the source of your back pain. We believe that SI joint issues are very over-diagnosed and that too many procedures are done to the SI joint based on limited information. It's a tempting diagnosis because the pain is often experienced directly over an SI joint, but it can lead to unnecessary procedures that may do more harm than good.

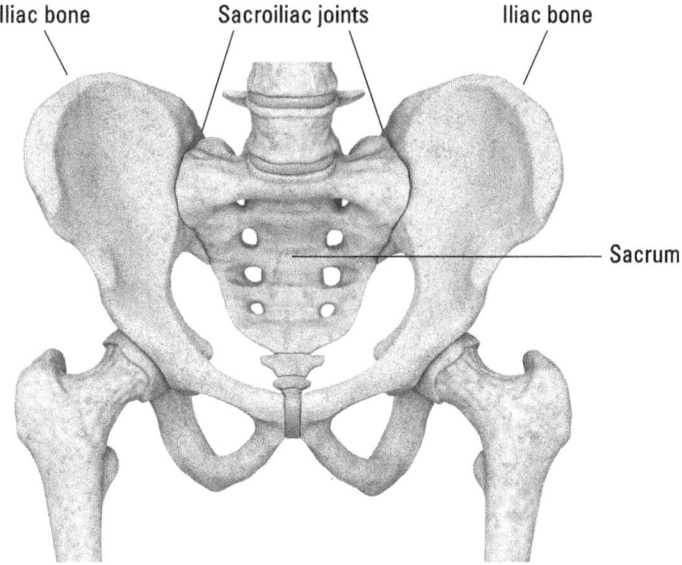

Iliac bone   Sacroiliac joints   Iliac bone

Sacrum

FIGURE 3-5:
Sacroiliac joints are often implicated as a source of back pain.

Matthieu/Adobe Systems Incoprated

Muscles

Although muscles can be a significant source of back pain, we prefer to think of them more positively — as a key ally in managing back pain. Your back muscles help to stabilize your spine and enable it to flex and rotate properly and safely. Despite the fact that muscles are awesome, various factors can make them a source of pain, including the following:

>> **Muscle strain or spasms:** Overstretching or overloading the muscles (for example, by lifting something heavy improperly); a sudden awkward movement; or poor posture can lead to muscle tightness, soreness, or spasms.

>> **Musculoskeletal imbalances:** If muscles in the back, core, butt, legs, or shoulders become too strong or too weak in relation to other muscles, misalignments can occur. Poor posture — such as slouching in a chair or looking down at a screen for long periods of time — is a leading cause of musculoskeletal imbalances. A common imbalance also develops when people exercise the muscles of their *anterior chain* (stomach and chest muscles) and neglect their *posterior chain* (back, butt, and shoulder blade muscles). In Chapters 8 and 9, we present movements and exercises that promote musculoskeletal balance.

>> **Chronic tension:** Emotional and psychological stress can lead to chronic muscle tension, a condition often referred to as "stress-related back pain." Stress can also reduce blood flow to tissues (muscles, bones, tendons, and ligaments), negatively impacting their overall health and function and your body's ability to heal any damage they've suffered.

REMEMBER

Your muscles are your not-so-secret weapon for battling back pain, and they're something *you* can control. Here are some of the ways muscles help to alleviate back pain and restore back health and mobility:

>> **Support your spine:** Strong muscles around the spine, including the deep stabilizing core muscles, carry some of the load so that your spine doesn't have to carry all the weight. In addition, muscles help to distribute the forces placed on your back more evenly. With your muscles doing more of the heavy lifting, your bones and joints suffer less wear and tear.

>> **Improve your posture:** Strengthening the muscles of the back, butt, shoulder blades, and core helps you maintain proper posture, reducing strain on your spine.

>> **Improve body mechanics:** Strong, flexible muscles enable you to move more efficiently and perform everyday tasks with less risk of injury.

>> **Increase blood flow:** Building muscle and engaging in regular physical activity improves blood circulation. Enhanced blood flow helps to deliver oxygen and nutrients to muscles and tissues and remove toxins, aiding recovery and reducing stiffness or inflammation in the back muscles.

>> **Reduce stress:** Well, muscles don't actually reduce emotional or psychological stress, but exercising to tone your muscles certainly does, and, as a result, it reduces muscle tension. Regular exercise, including strength training, is also known to release *endorphins* — natural painkillers.

>> **Enhance weight management:** Building muscle boosts your metabolism and helps you burn fat. You may not lose weight, and you may even gain some weight as you build muscle, but you'll be healthier overall, and your back will thank you for it!

>> **Engages mind-body synergies:** As you build muscle, you feel stronger and more resilient because you *are* stronger and more resilient. This mindset has a positive physical impact on your body that scientists and researchers are only beginning to understand. See Chapter 4 for more about the mind-body relationship.

Fascia

Fascia is the thin, dense connective tissue that surrounds and supports muscles, bones, and organs. *Myofascia* refers specifically to the fascia around muscles. It provides structure and stability while allowing for flexibility and movement. When fascia becomes tight, inflamed, or injured, it can lead to pain and discomfort. Here are two common fascia-related conditions that can be a source of back pain:

>> **Fascial (or myofascial) tightness:** Poor posture, repetitive movements, and stress can cause the fascia to become tight, restricting movement and resulting in stiffness, pain, and discomfort. Tightness can also create muscle "knots," which can be painful when pressed. Deep tissue massage, which we discuss in Chapter 16, can help eliminate this tension.

>> **Fascial adhesions:** Injuries, such as muscle strains and sprains, can result in *adhesions* — areas in which the fascia sticks to itself or surrounding tissues. This scar tissue often causes pain and limits mobility. Deep tissue massage can break up this scar tissue and promote healing.

Spinal nerves and nerve roots

From the brain down through the vertebral bodies runs the spinal cord, and between vertebral bodies, nerves branch off from the cord to other parts of the body (see Figure 3-6). Nerve roots can become irritated, inflamed, or compressed near the spine, causing back pain, which can also radiate to other areas of the body, such as the arms and legs.

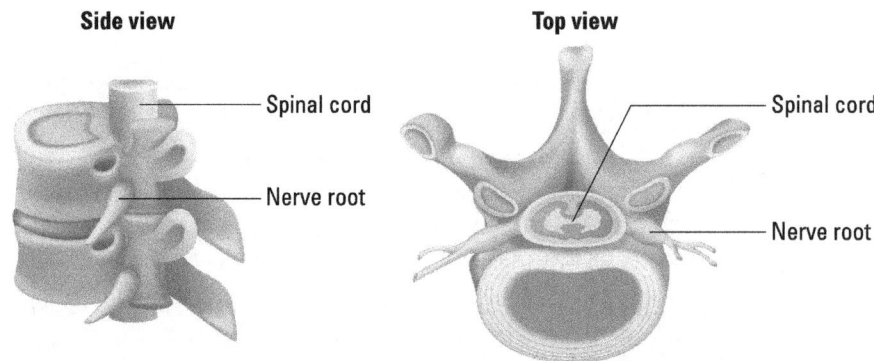

Side view

Spinal cord

Nerve root

Top view

Spinal cord

Nerve root

FIGURE 3-6:
Nerve roots can become irritated, inflamed, or compressed.

Macrovector/Adobe Systems Incoprated

TIP

Each nerve has a predictable radiation pattern, so where you feel the pain can help identify the nerve that's under stress. If pain is radiating to your arm, for example, the pain is coming from a nerve in the cervical spine. If your pain is radiating down your leg, it's probably coming from a nerve in the lumbar spine. The probability that the pain you feel in your arm or leg is related to your spine is greater if you also feel the pain in your back or neck. For example, you can reasonably assume that a nerve root near the spine is the origin of pain when you experience back and leg pain together or neck and arm pain together.

To trace pain to a specific nerve, look at where the pain terminates *distally* (at its farthest point from the origin of the nerve); for example, the pain terminates in specific fingers or toes. You can use a similar approach to trace muscle weakness to a specific nerve. These distal locations are called dermatomes and myotomes:

» **Dermatome:** An area of the skin that carries nerve signals to a specific spinal root. The dermatome where the pain terminates can help identify the nerve root where the pain originates.

» **Myotome:** A group of muscles that relies on a specific spinal root for innervation. The myotome experiencing muscle weakness can help identify the nerve root experiencing dysfunction.

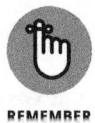

REMEMBER

Medical professionals often use a dermatome map, shown in Figure 3-7, to trace where pain terminates distally to the nerve root where the pain originates. They use a similar map to trace muscle weakness to a specific nerve root.

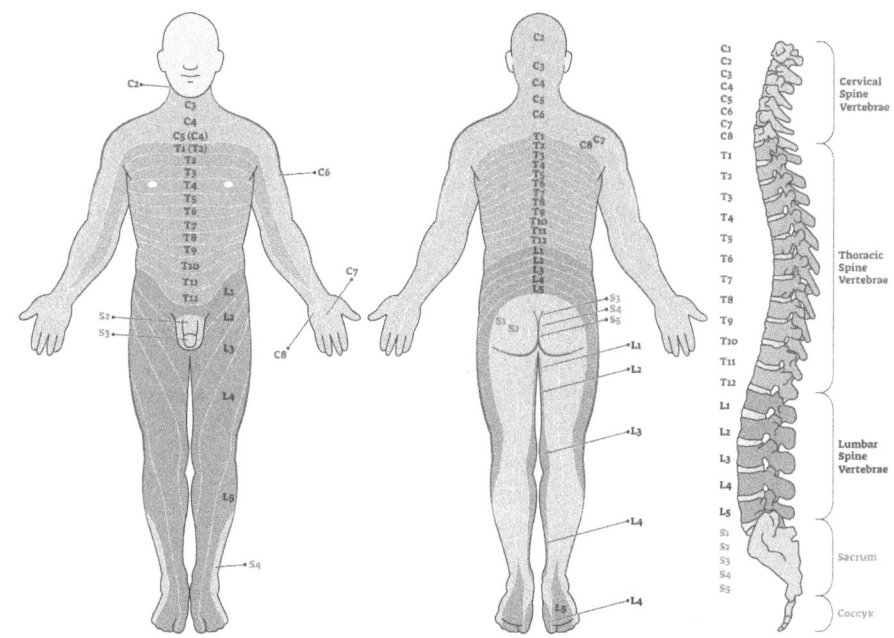

FIGURE 3-7:
A dermatome
map.

VectorMine/Adobe Systems Incoprated

Other spinal support structures

Although the discs and facet joints are the primary supporting structures of the spinal column, other structures provide additional support, including facet joint capsules, ligaments, tendons, and muscles. All of these have nerve supply and are capable of generating pain. Unfortunately, many anomalies related to these structures are beneath the threshold of magnetic resonance imaging (MRI), so they're not easily detectable. (See Chapter 13 for more about MRIs and other medical imaging technologies.)

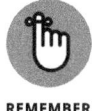

REMEMBER

Years ago, the healthcare industry typically recommended rest for an inflamed joint. Now, strengthening the muscles that subserve (protect and stabilize) the joint is the preferred treatment. Muscle atrophy is commonly associated with pain, which may be why bed rest, in and of itself, causes back pain. Make the muscles bigger and stronger, and the pain improves, regardless of the individual pain generator.

Distinguishing between disc pain and facet pain

As we mention at the beginning of this section, the major pain players in the realm of back pain are the discs and facet joints. A key first step in the diagnostic process is to determine which of those major pain players is the more likely cause of your back pain. Although every rule has exceptions, the following rules are very reliable:

>> Discs tend to be the source of pain when sitting is the most painful position for the patient. *Discogenic* (disc-related) pain generally improves when standing and lying down.

>> *Facetogenic* (facet-joint related) pain is characterized by pain that's worse when you stand or lie down and improves when you sit. Classic facet pain is felt when transitioning from sitting to standing, taking first steps out of bed in the morning, turning in bed, and standing or walking for a prolonged period. Patients with facet-driven pain will often note that they can walk in the food store for an extended period of time as long as they are using a cart allowing them to stoop forward a bit.

Disc pain and facet pain often overlap, especially with age. Over time, discs tend to degenerate — they lose height and water and ultimately form bony spurs called *osteophytes*. These changes to the discs alter the facet anatomy, causing facet pain. Conversely, facet joints can fatigue and stress the discs, causing disc degeneration. With age, these two main players tend to work against each other.

Understanding the role of motion

When you look at a picture of a spine, you see a static representation — an arrangement of discs, facet joints, and other support structures frozen in a frame of time. However, the spine serves both as a support structure and a means of movement. It bends, twists, and turns. For optimal function, it requires just the right balance of stability and mobility. If movement is overly restricted, you're not as flexible as you should be, but too much movement (instability) can cause pain.

One key to understanding pain *etiology* (what's causing the pain) is discerning normal motion from too much motion (instability). Some practitioners have gone so far as to believe that the presence of pain is proof of instability, but we don't subscribe to such a reductionist theory. Doing dynamic X-rays (having the patient flex and extend in a standing position while taking X-rays) can help to identify any abnormal motion. In addition, an MRI can provide clues to instability (for example, increased water content in support structures such as a disc). In most cases, containing the excess motion, primarily by strengthening muscles, helps resolve the pain.

WHY DOES MY BACK HURT?

Understandably, patients want to know why their back is hurting. What's causing their pain? Unfortunately, even with the incredible advances in medical imaging, the answer to the question often remains elusive. Identifying the cause is rarely a simple process of tracing the pain back to a nerve that's being stressed or spotting an anomaly on an X-ray or MRI, and treatment is rarely a quick fix — a pill, an injection, or a surgical procedure. In fact, in the pursuit of a quick fix, modern medicine has, from some perspectives, done more harm than good. To some extent, the recent opioid epidemic is rooted in the narrow goal of diminishing pain, and today's enthusiasm for cannabinoid relief of pain may lead patients down a similar path to short-term pain relief, psychological dependency on a substance, and no long-term improvement to their backs. Certain surgical procedures may be helpful, but these, too, can be overprescribed and cause additional problems.

We believe that the most effective approach to evaluating back pain and proposing treatment is to try to understand what the pain generator is while at the same time trying to understand the patient and the context in order to propose solutions that address both the pain and the patient's experience of the pain. The best solutions are holistic and rarely limited to a quick fix. The focus should be on improving back strength and mobility over eliminating pain.

Patients are often disappointed and discouraged when their doctors cannot tell them why their back is hurting or identify a specific problem that's causing the pain. Even more frustrating is receiving several different diagnoses from several doctors and enduring multiple courses of treatments, none of which have worked. In many (perhaps most) cases, your doctor has no way of knowing what's causing the pain, and it often really doesn't matter. By focusing instead on improving back strength and mobility, you enable your body to heal itself and build muscle that can compensate for any weaknesses or defects in other supporting structures.

Identifying Spinal Conditions Commonly Associated with Back Pain

The spine is an incredible support structure that's very strong and highly resilient, but it's not immune from illness, injury, age, or wear and tear. Several medical conditions can negatively impact its health and function, resulting in acute or chronic pain. In this section, we highlight some of the more common medical conditions that can trigger or contribute to back pain.

"Arthritis"

As we mention earlier in the "Facet joints" section, arthritis literally means "joint inflammation," and it makes sense in reference to facet joints. However, many people misuse the word to refer to any sort of degenerative condition of the spine.

What's often called "arthritis" is better described as "degenerative aging." Spines age naturally. Over time, discs lose water and height, facet joints expand, supporting ligaments thicken, and bone spurs form. These changes, alone or collectively, can press on or irritate nerves, resulting in back pain.

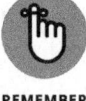

REMEMBER

Don't let the notion of "wear and tear" discourage you from exercising your back. Lifting weights isn't going to accelerate the degenerative processes. In fact, it's more likely to slow them down by building muscle to carry more of the weight and improve your posture. Most patients assume that degenerative spinal conditions are largely related to the "wear and tear" they put on their spines, but genetics plays a much bigger role. As we often tell our patients, "Blame your parents, not your job, for the condition of your spine."

Degenerative disc disease

Degenerative disc disease is a medical condition typically brought on by the aging process, as we explain in the previous section. Over time, one or more intraverte-bral discs can lose water and height, just like an old seat cushion. With less cushion between them, vertebral bodies can suffer more wear and tear, and they can begin to press down on nerve roots.

Bulging or herniated disc

A *bulging disc* occurs when the outer layer of a disc protrudes but remains intact, as shown in Figure 3-8. A *herniation* (rupture) occurs when the gel-like center of the disc (nucleus pulposus) pushes out through a tear in the outer layer of the disc (the annulus fibrosus). In either case, the disc or the gel-like substance can press against the spinal cord or a nerve root, causing irritation and pain. In addition, a herniated disc loses its cushioning capacity and may lose height, causing the adjacent vertebral bodies to "pinch" the nerve root and possibly suffer additional wear and tear.

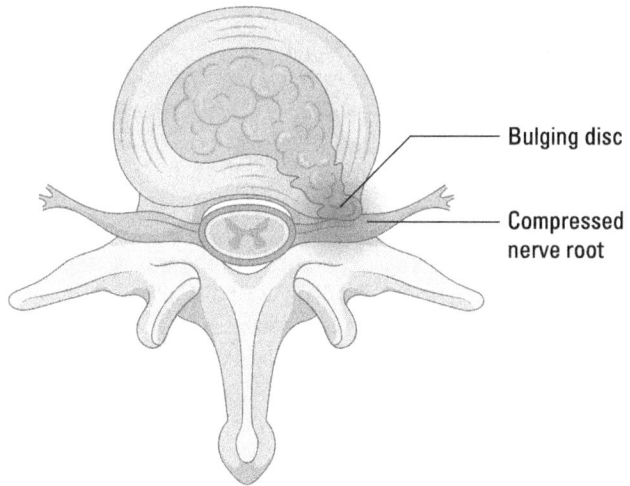

Bulging disc

Compressed
nerve root

FIGURE 3-8:
A bulging disc can
press on a
nerve root.

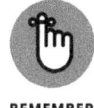

REMEMBER

Bulging and herniation most commonly occur in the lower back (lumbar spine) and neck (cervical spine), but they can happen anywhere along the spine. Treatment often begins with conservative measures such as physical therapy and pain medications, but in the case of a herniation, surgery may be required to repair or remove the disc. Although rest was the prescribed treatment for decades, the current recommendation is for patients to do their best to get up and walk around, even when they're in pain.

Bulging discs can also be a part of the natural aging process and may not be the pain generator they may appear to be on medical imaging. As you age, one or more discs may shrink, collapse, or bulge to some degree with or without causing pain. Be careful not to assume that a bulging disc is the cause of your back pain.

Osteoporosis

Osteoporosis is a condition that causes the bones to become weak and brittle, making them more susceptible to fractures. It occurs when the body loses too much bone mass, doesn't produce enough new bone, or both. This leads to a decrease in bone density and strength, increasing the risk of bone fractures, even from minor falls or normal daily activities. The condition is most common in older adults, especially postmenopausal women, but it can affect both men and women.

When it affects the spine, osteoporosis can become a major source of back pain. It increases the risk of compression fractures, as we discuss in the later section "Spinal fracture," and these fractures can cause spinal deformities, such as *kyphosis* (a forward curvature of the spine — a hunched back). Compression fractures can also lead to a gradual loss of height leading to additional strain on the back muscles, ligaments, and tendons, contributing to pain and discomfort.

Infection

When infection affects the spine or surrounding structures, it can inflame tissues, which can press on nerves, resulting in pain. This pain can be persistent and severe and worsen with movement, and it may radiate, causing numbness, tingling, or weakness, especially in the arms or legs. Fever, chills, or sweating may also occur as the body fights the infection. Spinal infections that commonly cause back pain include the following:

>> **Osteomyelitis:** Infection of the bones, which can include the vertebrae. It may be caused by bacteria or fungi that enter the body through the bloodstream or following surgery or trauma. When it impacts the spine, it can trigger an immune response that causes fever and inflammation, which can lead to back pain. In severe cases, the infection can weaken the bones, making them more susceptible to fractures.

Spinal infections can also cause *abscesses* (collections of pus that form around the spinal cord, in the epidural space around it). An abscess can press against the spinal cord or nerve roots, causing back pain, weakness, numbness, and, in some cases, loss of bowel or bladder control. Spinal abscesses are a medical emergency requiring immediate treatment, often involving antibiotics or requiring surgery to drain the abscess.

>> **Discitis:** Discitis is inflammation of one or more intravertebral discs, which may result from bacterial, fungal, or viral infection. In some cases, the infection can spread to surrounding bones, causing osteomyelitis. Infection of the discs or vertebral bones is rare.

Spinal fracture

A spinal fracture is a break or crack in a vertebral body. Such fractures can vary in severity from minor cracks (compression fractures) to more significant breaks that can damage the spinal cord or surrounding structures. Types of spinal fractures include the following:

>> **Compression fracture:** A break in the bone (often a load-bearing bone such as a vertebra) caused by pressure. Compression fractures, shown in Figure 3-9, are the most common type of spinal fracture. They're typically the

result of trauma but are more prevalent in patients who have *osteoporosis* (a weakening of the bone structure). Compression fractures can cause a vertebra to collapse, stressing the spinal cord and surrounding nerves.

>> **Burst fracture:** This type of fracture occurs when a vertebra is crushed and the bone fragments spread out, potentially damaging the spinal cord or nerves. Burst fractures typically result from high-impact trauma, such as an auto accident or a fall. They may require emergency treatment due to the risk of nerve damage or paralysis.

>> **Fracture-dislocation:** This type of fracture occurs when the vertebra is not only damaged but also displaced from its normal position, which can put pressure on the spinal cord or nearby nerves. Like a burst fracture, it's often the result of a high-impact trauma, such as an auto accident or fall.

>> **Stress fracture:** A tiny crack that develops in the vertebrae over time, typically as a result of repetitive motion or overuse. The pain associated with stress fractures is often dull and may worsen with activity. Athletes who participate in high-impact sports are more susceptible to experiencing stress fractures of the spine.

>> **Spinous process pain:** The *spinous process* is the bony protrusion you can feel along your back. Fractures of this part of the vertebrae are rare and are the result of trauma. When they do occur, they're usually less severe than other spinal fractures because of their distance from the spinal canal and nerves. More commonly, spinous process pain is the result of the spinous processes rubbing against each other.

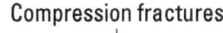

Compression fractures

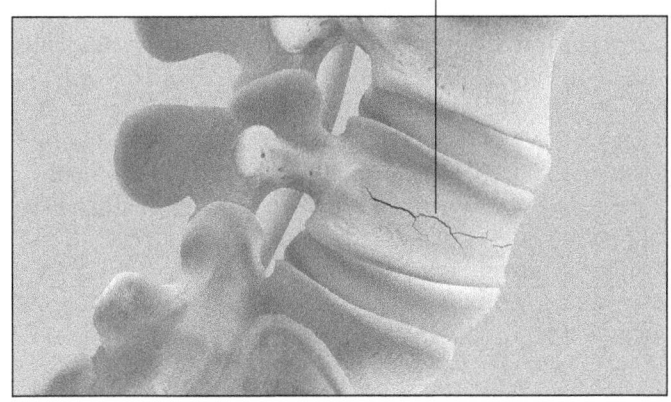

FIGURE 3-9: Compression fractures can cause a vertebra to collapse.

VISUALPOINT/Adobe Systems Incoprated

Spinal stenosis

Spinal stenosis is a condition in which the spaces within the spine narrow, leading to increased pressure on the spinal cord and the nerve roots, most commonly in the lower back (lumbar spine) and neck (cervical spine). Spinal stenosis can be caused by degeneration, age-related changes to the spine, or trauma, and it can lead to a range of symptoms. Some people are born with smaller spinal canals, making them more susceptible to age-related changes *(congenital spinal stenosis)*. Back pain typically worsens with standing or walking for long periods and often improves when sitting or bending forward, which relieves pressure on the nerves. Pain can range from mild to severe and is often described as a dull ache, a sharp pain, or a burning sensation. Stenosis in the lumbar spine can cause *neurogenic claudication* — a term used to describe leg pain, weakness, or cramping when walking.

To alleviate the pain, especially in the lower back, people with stenosis may adopt abnormal postures such as bending forward or walking in a hunched position. Improvement is so commonly noted with bending over a shopping cart that it has been called, "the shopping cart sign." Although such postures can alleviate pressure on the nerves, they can lead to muscle imbalances that can cause additional harm. Spinal stenosis is always slowly progressive. As the spinal canal continues to narrow, the pain may increase in both frequency and intensity. Other conditions, such as osteoporosis and bulging or herniated discs, can exacerbate the pain.

Spondylolisthesis

Spondylolisthesis occurs when a vertebra shifts out of its proper position and moves forward or backward over the vertebra below it (see Figure 3-10). This misalignment most commonly happens in the lower back (lumbar spine), and it can lead to back pain and a variety of other symptoms, depending on the severity of the shift and its impact on the spinal cord or, more commonly, nearby nerve roots. This shift is the result of either a stress fracture of a part of the spine called the pars interarticularis or a weakening of the facet joint and disc that stabilize the two vertebral bodies. Symptoms often include low back pain, muscle weakness, postural changes, and restricted mobility. Spondylolisthesis can also trigger pain, numbness, or tingling in the buttocks and the legs, especially in the thighs or feet, if the nerves are compressed. Medical imaging (X-ray, CT scan, or MRI) can help diagnose the condition and reveal the magnitude of the shift and any nerve compression.

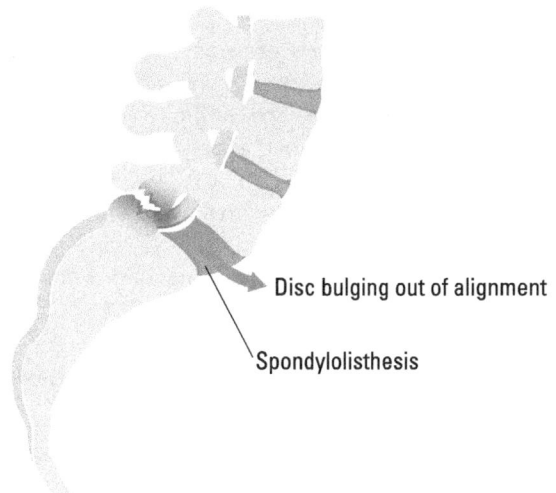

Disc bulging out of alignment

Spondylolisthesis

Pepermpron/Adobe Systems Incoprated

FIGURE 3-10:
Spondylolisthesis
occurs when a
vertebra shifts
out of alignment.

Sacroiliac pain

Sacroiliac pain has many of the same symptoms as facet pain. Symptoms are typically most prominent with standing. Techniques have been developed to diagnose it as part of a physical exam, but these are unreliable. For some time, the gold standard of diagnosis was the elimination of pain with a sacroiliac anesthetic block. We prefer the use of a single photon emission computed tomography (SPECT) scan to evaluate for sacroiliac anomalies rather than the physical exam to make a diagnosis. (See Chapter 13 for details about the SPECT scan and other medical imaging technologies.)

Examining Non-Spinal Conditions Associated with Back Pain

Back pain isn't always *back* pain; that is, it doesn't always signal a problem with the spine or the nerve roots, muscles, tendons, or ligaments related to the spine. "Back pain" can come from organs within the *peritoneum* (the membrane that lines the abdominal cavity), including the stomach, pancreas, gall bladder, and bowels. It can also come from structures within the abdomen that are outside the peritoneum, including the kidneys and ureter and the ligaments that suspend the uterus, ovaries, and prostate.

Don't assume or let your healthcare provider assume that your back pain has something to do with your spine, especially when the pain is present at all times and in all positions. Pain that changes in relation to your position is more likely to be related to the spine. If the pain is persistent, regardless of whether you're sitting, standing, lying down, walking, or engaging in other activities, consider the possibility that another condition (not related to the spine) is the cause.

In this section, we explore non-spinal conditions that commonly cause back pain.

Abdominal processes

Many diverse processes and conditions involving organs in the abdomen or pelvis can refer pain to the back, including the following:

- >> **Urinary tract infections (UTIs):** Although UTIs primarily cause lower abdominal discomfort, they can lead to back pain if the infection spreads to the kidneys. Kidney infections *(pyelonephritis)* can cause dull, aching pain in the lower back and are often accompanied by fever, nausea, and painful urination.

- >> **Kidney stones:** Kidney stones can cause intense pain in the lower back.

- >> **Pancreatitis:** Inflammation of the pancreas, which typically causes pain in the upper abdomen, can also radiate pain to the back.

- >> **Gallbladder disease:** Conditions such as gallstones and *cholecystitis* (inflammation of the gallbladder) typically cause pain on the right side of the upper abdomen, but this pain can radiate to the back, especially the right shoulder blade.

- >> **Gastrointestinal issues:** Constipation, gastritis, ulcers, irritable bowel syndrome (IBS), and other gastrointestinal issues can refer pain to the back.

- >> **Endometriosis:** In women, abnormal tissue growth inside the uterus can cause pelvic and lower back pain.

- >> **Hernia:** A *hernia* occurs when an organ pushes through a gap in the abdominal wall, causing discomfort or pain, which can radiate to the back. Some hernias produce a noticeable bulge, in which case the pain isn't likely to be mistakenly attributed to the spine, but hernias aren't always detectable during a physical exam.

- >> **Pelvic and related infections:** *Pelvic inflammatory disease (PID)* — inflection of the female reproductive organs (uterus, fallopian tubes, or ovaries) — can radiate pain to the lower back.

- >> **Uterine settling:** Women who've had babies occasionally have back pain from the uterus drooping in the pelvis and putting tension on the supporting ligaments.

Cholesterol medication

Cholesterol-lowering medications, such as statins, are commonly prescribed to reduce the risk of heart attack and stroke, but like all medications, they can produce negative side effects, one of which is muscular pain, which can present as back pain. If you're taking a statin and experiencing back pain, talk to your doctor about the possibility of switching medications or stopping the medication temporarily to see whether it's contributing to your back pain.

REMEMBER

Although we aren't opposed to medication, we advocate building health through a more natural approach — healthy diet and lifestyle choices along with exercise. Building health and fitness makes you less reliant on medications such as statins. See Part 2 for guidance on building health and fitness naturally.

Inflammation

Many chronic health conditions, including back pain, are the result of inflammation. Inflammation isn't all bad. In fact, it's a natural part of the body's immune response and its self-healing mechanisms. If you sprain your ankle, for example, your body pumps more blood to the injured area, delivering more oxygen, nutrients, and white blood cells to the area to start the healing process and flush out any debris or damaged cells. You experience some painful swelling, but that's just part of the healing process.

However, inflammation can also be caused by a variety of other factors, including autoimmune disorders, toxins, food allergies or sensitivities, and lifestyle factors such as obesity, smoking, and chronic stress. If the inflammation affects the spine or anything related to the spine (nerves or supporting muscles, ligaments, or tendons), it can cause back pain.

TIP

Many of the suggestions we provide in Part 2 can help reduce inflammation, but if you're still struggling to control it, consider consulting a doctor with training in functional and integrative medicine who can help you identify and address the root causes. You may have a hidden infection, an imbalance in gut bacteria, a food sensitivity, a nutrient deficiency, or other conditions that conventional medical practitioners don't look for and aren't equipped to treat effectively. I (Pat) tend to use imaging to look for common causes and add integrative medicine in cases where the investigation doesn't reveal a definitive cause.

Shoulder and hip pain

Your body isn't a machine made up of distinct and separate parts; it's an organic whole. What happens with one part of your body can affect other parts. Even a painful toe can throw off your gait, translating to pain in your knee, hip, and back.

So, it should be no surprise that shoulder pain and hip pain can translate to back pain. These areas of the body are all interconnected through muscle, joint, and nerve pathways. Specifically, they can affect one another in the following ways:

>> **Postural compensation and alignment:** The spine, shoulders, and hips all play vital roles in maintaining proper posture and alignment. If you have pain or dysfunction in the shoulder or hip, you may subconsciously adjust your posture to avoid discomfort. This postural compensation can result in muscle imbalances that stress your spine, especially the lower back (if you're experiencing hip issues) or the upper back (if you're experiencing shoulder issues).

>> **Overcompensation leading to muscle imbalances:** When you're experiencing hip or shoulder pain or weakness, your back muscles may overcompensate. For example, if you have a rotator cuff injury (in the shoulder), your upper back and neck muscles may try to pick up the slack, which can create imbalances that strain the vertebrae.

>> **Referred pain:** Pain originating in the spine can often radiate to the arms or legs, but that's a two-way street — shoulder or hip pain may be felt in the back, as well.

>> **Muscle tightness and fascial connections:** Tension in the hip or shoulder can cause tightness or restriction in nearby muscles and fascia, which can lead to discomfort or pain in the back.

Looking into General Diagnoses Associated with Back Pain

Specific diagnoses related to back pain typically focus on the location and nature of the injury, such as identifying a specific disc that has ruptured or a vertebra that has a compression fracture. However, you may encounter other general back pain diagnoses, such as "railway spine" and "tech neck." Here, we explain those diagnostic labels, so that you have a clear understanding of what they mean.

Whiplash

Whiplash is a neck injury caused by sudden back-and-forth movement of the head, like the cracking of a whip. It's often the result of a car accident or other traumatic event. Whiplash can lead to pain, stiffness, and other symptoms, which usually resolve on their own over weeks or months. The cause of whiplash is rarely evident on an MRI. Whatever is causing the damage is likely a combination of an initial injury and superimposed changes related to the way a patient manages the pain physically and mentally.

Railway spine

Railway spine is an outdated term used to describe a collection of physical and psychological symptoms resulting from railway commuting. Symptoms include chronic back pain, headaches, fatigue, and other musculoskeletal issues, along with nervous disorders — anxiety, depression, insomnia, and hypersensitivity to stress.

The significance of the syndrome is that simply naming the condition and suggesting that it was related to the bouncing and shaking on a train resulted in its prevalence increasing dramatically. As soon as the train ride *etiology* (origin of symptoms) was debunked, the prevalence declined precipitously. This phenomenon is sometimes referred to as the "chameleon effect" — patients taking on the characteristics of the diagnosis they're given.

Tech neck

Tech neck is a term that describes the pain and discomfort resulting from staring down at a computer or smartphone screen for prolonged periods. It's a postural strain that affects the joints, muscles, and ligaments of the cervical spine (the neck).

REMEMBER

To prevent tech neck, position your screen or book or whatever you're looking down at in front of you at about eye level so that you're not hunched over it. Turn to Chapter 9 for exercises that can help you strengthen and restore balance to your neck muscles.

Fibromyalgia

Fibromyalgia is a chronic condition characterized by widespread pain, tenderness, and other symptoms that affect the muscles, ligaments, and tendons throughout the body. It's also associated with fatigue, poor sleep, and cognitive difficulties (brain fog).

Fibromyalgia is thought by some to be caused by *systemic* (whole-body) inflammation. See the earlier section "Inflammation" for details about possible causes of and treatments for systemic inflammation. We similarly believe that fibromyalgia is a systemic disorder, but we believe that the cause is related to a reduced pain threshold involving the way the patient manages the pain both physically and mentally, similar to the way patients respond to whiplash.

IN THIS CHAPTER

» Changing how you think about pain

» Using the power of suggestion to your advantage

» Taking a holistic approach with embodied cognition

» Setting process instead of outcome goals

» Taking charge of the pain so it doesn't take charge of you

Chapter **4**

Using Your Brain to Manage Your Pain: The Mind-Body Relationship

Despite how some doctors may make you feel, your back pain isn't all in your head, but you can certainly use your head to drive the process necessary to resolve your back pain and reclaim your life. We're not suggesting hypnosis or other quick-fix mind-control techniques that target the brain's pain-processing functions, although such techniques may be effective in alleviating back pain to some degree for some period of time. What we're suggesting in this chapter is that you engage your brain in every possible way to lessen the pain and build a better back. Here, you discover how to shift the way you think about pain so it's not so debilitating while using your brain as the command-and-control center to devise and execute your personalized back health and fitness recovery program.

In the process, something very interesting happens — your body begins to change your thoughts and emotions in ways that can profoundly affect how you experience pain. Yes, your mind and body are one. What impacts one impacts the other. And in this chapter, you discover how to use that phenomenon to your advantage — using your brain to manage your pain and your body to positively influence the way your brain processes pain impulses.

Taking Control of Your Thoughts and Moods: Mindset and Mindfulness

To a great extent, you are a product of what you think. Your thoughts are the impetus for your decisions, choices, and actions. And those decisions, choices, and actions produce the conditions and circumstances in your life. You are not so much a victim of circumstances as a master of them.

Yes, many conditions in life are outside your control, but you are largely responsible for the situation you're in right now, including your overall health, relationship happiness, success at school or work, and overall satisfaction. If something in your life is a source of distress, you have four choices: accept it, complain about it, change it, or change the way you think about it.

The same is true of back pain. You can accept it (not something we recommend), complain about it (which does no good), change it (do something about it), or change the way you contextualize it. The fact that you're reading this book shows that you chose those last two options — good for you! Now, you're ready to start making changes to improve your condition, and that process begins with changing the way you think.

Adopting an empowerment mindset

Mindset is attitude. An "empowerment mindset" is a can-do attitude. We encourage you to approach the process of eliminating back pain with an empowerment mindset. As Stephen Covey advises in his bestselling book *The Seven Habits of Highly Effective People,* "Start with the end in mind." Imagine what your life will be like when your back pain is improved. Then, commit yourself to doing whatever's necessary to bring that condition to fruition in your life.

TIP

Discover your *driver* — your internal motivator. What do you value most about having a stronger, more mobile back and less back pain that you'll do anything to achieve? Is it simply having the pain be more manageable? Is it being able to return to a sport or activity you're passionate about? Is it a desire to spend quality time with friends and family members doing the things you love? Your drivers enable you to power through when you're sore, bored, or exhausted.

MOTIVATION VERSUS DRIVE

We encourage drive over motivation because drive is more internal and persistent than motivation. Motivation may start one's engine, but drive is what carries the person through to their destination. Motivation is like a reward that encourages desired behavior; as soon as the reward has been received, the impetus is gone. Drive is more like a value that governs a person's behavior from within. It continues to influence behavior even when one is no longer rewarded for it — even, in fact, when it's inconvenient or uncomfortable to behave in accordance with that value.

Building a strong, resilient back and maintaining it isn't easy; it often requires hard work, determination, and attention to detail. People with chronic back pain often need to make difficult changes to the way they've become accustomed to living over the course of decades. They have to break bad habits that have become deeply ingrained. Motivation may not be enough. It takes *drive*.

Leveraging the power of mindfulness

Mindfulness is a state of awareness focused entirely on the present moment without placing any judgment on thoughts, emotions, sensations, or external circumstances. When you're mindful, you're not angry or bitter about something that happened in the past or worried or anxious about something that may happen in the future. Your mind is focused on what you're experiencing right now. In addition, you have no personal interest in what you're thinking or feeling. You're a disinterested observer, watching your thoughts and feelings float by like clouds on a breezy day.

Mindfulness can be a powerful state of mind for coping with pain. In a mindful state, the pain is merely a sensation, neither positive nor negative. It is just something you're experiencing. When used to manage back pain, mindfulness offers the following benefits:

>> **Reduces pain sensitivity:** Emotions such as fear, frustration, and anger intensify the perception of pain. Mindfulness separates the physical sensation from the emotional response, thereby dialing back the brain's response to pain.

>> **Improves pain tolerance:** Mindfulness facilitates the brain's ability to accept pain without trying to avoid or escape it, enabling you to cope more effectively with the sensation of pain.

>> **Reduces stress and promotes relaxation:** Pain often triggers stress, anxiety, and muscle tension, all of which can amplify the pain. Mindfulness relaxes both mind and body.

>> **Improves body awareness and posture:** Mindfulness increases awareness of tensions and misalignments in the body, which can help you improve your posture and the way you move.

>> **Improves sleep:** Pain often disrupts sleep, which can, in turn, exacerbate pain, stress, and muscle tension and impair healing. Mindfulness techniques, particularly those focused on relaxation, improve sleep quality by reducing anxiety and helping you relax before bedtime. Better sleep relaxes muscles and promotes healing.

You can practice mindfulness anywhere, anytime, by focusing your attention on what you're experiencing right now. Here's a simple mindfulness exercise called the 5-4-3-2-1 Grounding Exercise, which engages all five senses to reconnect you to the present moment:

5. Look around and notice five things you see.

4. Listen carefully and identify four things you can hear.

3. Notice three physical sensations.

2. Identify two things you can smell.

1. Notice one thing you can taste.

By focusing your mind on what you're experiencing right now, you leave no space for negative emotions, such as anger, regret, or worry, which can make you tense and amplify your pain.

For more about mindfulness, check out *Mindfulness For Dummies* by Shamash Alidina (Wiley).

REMEMBER

Becoming more mindful and building mental resilience can be a tall order, and many people struggle trying to do so on their own. Everyone is different. Don't hesitate to seek help from a close friend or relative or from a personal trainer, life coach, therapist, or psychiatrist. See Chapter 19 for more about professionals who may be able to help you overcome mental or emotional challenges.

Appreciating the Power of Your Expectations: Placebos and Nocebos

A *placebo* is an inert substance or treatment often used in clinical studies to test the effectiveness of a medication or other medical treatment or procedure. The word is also used to describe something that's prescribed to patients more to provide mental relief than any physical healing. A *nocebo* is a negative effect that a substance or treatment can have resulting from a patient's expectations of it occurring; for example, a researcher tells a study participant that a certain pill the participant is taking (which, in fact, contains none of the medication being studied) can cause weight gain, and the patient gains 20 pounds over the course of the six-week study.

What may surprise you is that the placebo and nocebo represent much more than mental relief; they alter physiologic processes. For example, in one study, maids who were told that their job was also good for exercise, lost weight when compared to maids who were not given that information. The altered mindset was the cause of their weight loss, as there were no other differences. What you believe about your body can change your body.

Placebos and nocebos provide evidence to support the concept of the *placebo effect* — the benefits that a patient experiences from their own positive expectations of a treatment's effects instead of from its actual therapeutic effect. Although the placebo effect often applies in the context of medication, it applies as well to medical procedures, including surgeries, and to doctors and other healthcare providers. For example, patients often experience better outcomes when they believe that their doctors are highly skilled.

REMEMBER

If it starts in the head, it can end in the head. Only you have the power to change your thoughts and emotions. If you let back pain get you down, if you let it control your thoughts and emotions, it will keep you down. To get better, you need to believe that you will get better. Don't give up. Don't let back pain win. Far too many people live in the jails of their own minds and never realize their amazing human potential. Adopting a proper mindset goes a long way toward restoring and maintaining physical and mental health.

IS IT ALL IN MY HEAD?

Can the mind alone heal the back? Some people seem to think so, and some evidence suggests they may be right. During the late 1700s and early 1800s, German physician Franz Mesmer earned quite a reputation for himself healing people with what he claimed was his "animal magnetism." Around the same time in the U.S., Phineas Quimby, influenced by Mesmer, cured people suffering from a wide range of debilitating ailments, including back pain, through hypnosis and later spiritual healings. He healed himself of consumption by driving his horse and carriage up and down hills and finally back to his stable, at which point he felt "strong as he ever did." Sounds like our approach to eliminating back pain!

(continued)

(continued)

More recently, the late Dr. John Sarno proposed that 80 percent or more of back pain results from psychological and emotional factors rather than structural issues, such as herniated discs or pinched nerves. According to Dr. Sarno, negative thoughts and emotions create physical tension in the muscles and restrict blood flow to certain areas of the body, triggering back pain. He conjectured that the mind often produces pain as a distraction to prevent it from having to deal with psychological pain and stressful situations. He helped his patients overcome their back pain by identifying and addressing the source of their emotional and psychological stress.

The mind triggers hormones that stimulate the body to release the body's own painkillers. The mind can also block the transmission of pain as it ascends through the spinal cord. Theoretically, this physiological response eliminates the pain, and in some cases, it seems to actually cure the patient! Some studies report patients being cured of certain ailments when taking only the placebo! Imagine how powerful the proper mindset can be! Of course, genetics may play a role as well. Thanks to a certain gene variant, some people are more prone to experiencing the placebo effect; the variant codes for a higher level of dopamine release.

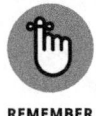

REMEMBER

The power of thought is a double-edged sword. If your thoughts and emotions are powerful enough to make you physically healthy, they're powerful enough to make you physically ill. Redirect your thoughts and emotions to maintain a positive attitude. Your body will thank you for it.

Using Embodied Cognition to Your Advantage

Just as the placebo and nocebo represent the mind's capacity to ignite physical changes in the body, the body has its own capacity to affect the mind. *Embodied cognition* is the concept that physical states, movements, and experiences shape a person's thoughts, emotions, and mental processes. That may not strike you as a ground-breaking concept; everyone knows that the body sends sensory information to the brain that influences thoughts and emotions. However, embodied cognition is more subtle. For example, someone who's on the heavy side may perceive a hill as steeper than they would perceive it if they were lighter. Here's another example: Standing erect can make you feel more confident. In the context of using your mind to overcome back pain, embodied cognition comes into play when you start building your core, for example. As you increase back strength and mobility, your brain factors that into its mental processing, so as you feel stronger and more physically fit, you feel less (or no) pain.

MENS SANA IN CORPRE SANO

Mens sana in corpre sano is a Latin phrase that means "a sound mind in a sound body." It's a phrase commonly used by athletes and trainers to stress the impact that having a strong body and a strong mind have on performance. Strength in mind and body establishes a synergy that drives the further development of both.

As your mind and body become stronger, expect to become more confident in facing and dealing with pain without needing (or wanting) to use prescription medication to dull the pain. You're likely to reach a point, if you're not already there, of refusing to be a slave to your pain or to the medication often used to manage it.

The take-home message is that whether you do it yourself or seek help for your back pain, your focus must be to change both your mind and your body. The remarkable synergy between the two creates a powerful and sustainable effect — with or without help from the medical profession. Similarly, the medical profession needs to change itself. Rather than peddle extensive quick fixes, the medical profession needs to invest in each patient's capacity to change both mind and body.

You can understand that embodied cognition is the mind extending beyond the brain and encompassing the body in such a way that the mind responds to changes in the body, and the body responds to changes in the mind. *Neuroplasticity* — the brain's ability to repurpose neurons and create new neural networks in response to changes in the body — may also play a role. Embodied cognition can also be related to *epigenetics* — the ability of the body to turn certain genes on or off in response to environmental factors, lifestyle, or experiences without changing the DNA so that genes are expressed differently. In the context of back pain, epigenetic factors may influence everything from a person's pain tolerance to their body's ability to repair damaged tissues, such as muscles, tendons, and discs.

REMEMBER

Nike's slogan "Just Do It!" can be a powerful reminder of the power of embodied cognition to overcome back pain. Increasing your physical activity and engaging in strenuous exercise can trigger changes in the brain that boost drive as well as changes in genetic expression that enhance tissue repair, build muscle, drive weight loss, and build back strength and mobility, eliminating pain or significantly reducing it and making you feel healthier and stronger overall.

Getting comfortable being uncomfortable

Imagine life without pain, hunger, sadness, anger, and other sensations and emotions that we generally think of as distressing. At first thought, such a life may seem like a dream come true, but if you had to live it, you would discover it to be a nightmare. You may suffer malnutrition because you forgot to eat, you may bleed to death from an injury you never felt, or you may remain in an abusive relationship because it never made you sad or angry enough to do anything about it. Sensations like hunger and pain and emotions like sadness and frustration have a purpose. They serve as an early warning sign and an impetus to action. In addition, pain triggers the body's self-repair and self-healing mechanisms, which can make you healthier, stronger, and more resilient.

Pleasure and pain are both great motivators of human behavior. As humans, we seek the sensation of pleasure and the avoidance of pain. This comes with a price. Unfortunately, many have fallen victim to the notion of "painless" living and have traveled the path of least resistance, which far too often leads to a dependence on pharmaceutical medication, intrusive and expensive medical procedures, and, in some cases, illicit drugs. To be fair, medication and certain medical procedures are necessary and can be very helpful in alleviating pain and restoring mobility. However, these solutions are overused and, in a large majority of cases, unnecessary.

Start with the premise that pain is a warning sign. It's a signal that indicates a problem. It doesn't point to the solution. It doesn't tell you whether you need to see a doctor, need to change your posture at work, or you're hurt and simply need to be patient as your body works things out. All it does is wave a red flag. It's up to you to decide how to interpret and act on that warning.

REMEMBER

Realize that you "feel" the sensation of pain in your brain and that you can alter your perception and interpretation of it by changing the way your brain processes incoming signals from pain receptors. For example, the United States Marine Corps used to instill in its recruits the credo that "Pain is weakness leaving the body!" Marines who embraced this credo welcomed the pain they experienced during their rigorous training. It didn't lessen the sensation of pain, but it did change their perception of it. In their brains, pain was no longer associated with fear, worry, and discouragement; it became associated with pride and courage.

We're not suggesting that you become a masochist (a pain junkie) or even a Marine, but subjecting your body to uncomfortable conditions can be good for you. Fasting, working up a sweat, pushing your body till your muscles ache, taking a cold shower or an ice bath — all these self-inflicted stresses on the body can trigger positive transformations in both mind and body:

>> **Mind:** You become more confident, determined, tenacious, psychologically resilient, and emotionally stable.

>> **Body:** Your body becomes more physically fit and better conditioned to heal itself, which shortens your recovery times. When you regularly test your bones, muscles, tendons, and ligaments by subjecting them to minor trauma (impact, strain, exhaustion), you stimulate the body's healing mechanisms, which strengthen all those tissues.

CALLOUSING THE BODY

Practitioners of various martial arts often engage in a process called "callousing the body," which involves voluntarily subjecting one or more parts of the body to trauma. You may have seen boxing movies in which a boxer in training is repeatedly punched in the gut while doing sit-ups, or a student of karate spends weeks on end punching sand or gravel. These are examples of callousing the body, and they're methods used to stimulate the body's healing processes.

People who haven't conditioned their bodies by subjecting them to muscle strain, exhaustion, impact, and other challenging conditions are often more prone to injuries. They may bruise more easily than normal or be more susceptible to bone fractures. As a result, they're not "hardened" against the physical traumas of everyday life. In contrast, you see carpenters with massive fingers, broad hands, and thick wrists; weight-lifters with callouses on their hands; and gymnasts with abnormally high bone density. They're built to handle the bumps, falls, cuts, and bruises of everyday life.

The medical term for this adaptation is *symmorphosis* — an adaptive response to stress at a cellular level that cumulatively leads to adaptations of our bodies. This is the basis of one of the major underlying themes of this book: People need to view themselves as adaptable rather than vulnerable when properly stressed.

The take-home message here is that conditioning (gently callousing) the body makes it stronger. Just be sure to do it gradually so you don't injure yourself.

WARNING

Pushing through the pain isn't always the best course of action, and it may be unsafe in certain situations, such as when back pain is caused by liver or kidney dysfunction or a serious spinal injury. If you're in pain and you've done some (or all) of the movements we present in Chapters 8 and 9, you should start to feel some relief in a matter of a few days. However, if you can't do simple movements without experiencing excruciating pain or you've been doing the exercises for two weeks and the pain isn't subsiding or is increasing, seek professional help, as we discuss in Part 3.

Developing self-efficacy

Self-efficacy is the belief that you can accomplish what you set out to do. It increases as your proficiency and consistency in performance improve. In other words, the more you do something and the better you get at it, the greater your self-efficacy. Additionally, as you develop self-efficacy, you begin to enjoy what you're doing that much more because you're becoming better and better at doing it. Trainers love to see clients develop self-efficacy because it turbocharges their progress.

What the clients do on their own builds on what they do with the trainer, enabling the clients to achieve higher and higher levels of success.

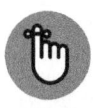

REMEMBER

Self-efficacy is an independent determinant of health. All things otherwise being equal, people who are confident in their ability to overcome health predicaments will enjoy better health. This is why people who hold jobs where they are in charge enjoy better health, on average, than those who are told what to do.

TIP

To build self-efficacy, focus on gradual progression. Avoid the temptation to push too hard too fast, which increases the risk of injury or just giving up. Also important is that you buy into the program and methods you're adopting so that you'll "stick with it." Keep in mind that you typically need to stick with a program for at least 90 days to instill it as a new habit — that's three months of doing all the right things.

Stick-to-it-iveness is especially important when you're combatting chronic back pain because it's not something that develops overnight. Chronic pain is usually the product of years and sometimes decades of poor diet, poor posture, sedentary living, and/or other bad habits. Those ruts run deep, and you not only need to get out of them but also to wear new tracks along healthier paths. Having a clear and consistent program for building a strong back is essential to success.

Setting Goals and Being SMART(ER) About Goal Setting

Desire is one of the greatest drivers of human action. Wanting to be, do, or have something is what drives accomplishment and innovation. If you want to be wealthy, you work harder, you learn a new skill, you look for a better job, or you start a business. If you want to be healthy, you improve your diet, stop smoking, avoid alcohol, exercise, figure out how to manage your stress, and get enough sleep. If you want to improve your interpersonal relationships, you develop your communication skills, cultivate your emotional intelligence (EQ), and take an interest in others.

The object of your desire is a goal. It's *what* you want to be, do, or have. Without goals, people tend to wander aimlessly through life without a sense of purpose, accomplish little, if anything, and fall short of achieving their incredible human potential. In the case of back pain, they continue to suffer unnecessarily, mistakenly believing they can't do anything about it.

In this section, we encourage you to set goals and explain how to make them SMART(ER), so you can begin to crystallize in your own mind your personal back pain management goal.

Setting your sights on an outcome, committing to a process, or both

When most people set goals, they set their sights on an outcome — to retire at 50, run a 10K, quit smoking/vaping, earn their MBA, whatever. In the context of back pain, maybe you decide you want to be pain-free by the end of the month. That's fine. The only trouble with outcome goals is that you're not entirely in control of the outcome. Unforeseen events outside your control can derail your plans. If that happens, you fall short of your goal and can end up feeling as though you failed, which can deplete your enthusiasm.

We prefer setting *process goals* — specific actions you're going to do to improve some aspect of your life. For example, instead of setting your sights on being pain-free by the end of the month, you commit to engaging in 15 minutes of strenuous physical activity daily and increasing that by 5 minutes a week until you're doing 30 minutes a day. Or, you commit to doing the broomstick and joint-limbering movements we present in Chapter 8 every day shortly after waking up. These are goals you have more control over.

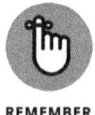

REMEMBER

Outcome and process goals aren't mutually exclusive. In fact, you can set an outcome goal and then set process goals that empower you to achieve the desired outcome. Using the two in tandem results in a more traditional framework that breaks down goals into objectives and tasks:

>> **Goal:** What you hope to achieve; for example, bring your back pain to a level at which you can fully function at home and work.

>> **Objective:** Measurable, realistic milestones that you must achieve to meet your goal; for example, lose one pound a week, decrease pain intensity by 2 points (on a 10-point scale) over the course of a month, walk a mile in 20 minutes without feeling out of breath by the end of the month.

>> **Task:** Specific actions you take to achieve objectives; for example, walk 30 minutes every other day, do four sets of 10 plans and three sets of 10 crunches daily (see Chapter 8), and fast from dinner to the next day's breakfast. Tasks are what we call *process goals*.

Simply put, you need to have a clear idea of *what* you want to accomplish and *how* you're going to accomplish it. For example, because you're reading this book, we can safely assume that you want to reduce or eliminate your back pain. *How* you're going to do it is by following our guidance as set forth in this book.

Making your goals SMART and SMARTER

To be effective, goals must be SMART — Specific, Measurable, Achievable, Relevant, and Time-bound:

>> **Specific:** Make sure that the desired outcome or process is clearly defined. For example, a goal to become physically fit is too general. A more specific goal would be to run a seven-minute mile or bench press 150 pounds.

>> **Measurable:** The goal should be something you can verify by objective evaluation. For example, overall physical fitness is difficult to measure, but if you set a goal to achieve a body mass index (BMI) of 22, that's a specific metric.

   To calculate your BMI, divide your weight (in kilograms) by the square of your height (in meters). Or you can just google your weight and height in whatever units you want to use; for example, googling "What's my BMI if I'm 5'11" and 170 pounds" returns the answer 'If you are 5'11" and weigh 170 pounds, your BMI is approximately 25.5 which is considered overweight according to the standard BMI chart."

>> **Achievable:** Make sure the goal is realistic for you. If a goal is overly ambitious, you're likely to fall short, feel as though you failed, and lose enthusiasm. Goals should be challenging but achievable.

>> **Relevant:** Align your goals with something you value in life — health, fitness, family, self-reliance. Don't set random goals that just give you something to do.

>> **Time-bound:** Set a deadline. A goal without a time limit is just a pipe dream.

Here's a sample process goal for managing back pain: Within 30 days, I will be doing 30 minutes of back-building activities from Chapters 8 and 9 of this book every day. This goal meets all the SMART criteria:

>> **Specific:** The goal is crystal clear; for example, "I will proactively, on a daily basis, engage in an exercise regiment that will strengthen my back and improve my mobility."

>> **Measurable:** You can time your 30-minute sessions and mark a calendar to indicate the days you performed your workouts.

>> **Achievable:** Thirty minutes a day is doable for most people. Note that the goal doesn't state that you'll be doing 30 minutes a day starting Day 1. You may start out doing 10–15 minutes a day and gradually increase the amount of time.

>> **Relevant:** This goal is relevant for managing back pain, which is also aligned with higher values such as becoming self-reliant, being able to perform better at work, and being able to enjoy time with friends and family.

>> **Time-bound:** The deadline is clear — you have 30 days.

Here's another example of sustainable weight loss, which is a top priority for many people who suffer from chronic back pain:

>> **Specific:** I want to lose 20 pounds.

>> **Measurable:** I will check my weight on the scale weekly to chart my progress.

>> **Attainable:** Based on my height, weight, body mass index, and personal observation, I'm carrying an excess of 40 pounds of fat. (If you determine that you're carrying 40 pounds of excess fat, losing 20 pounds is realistic.)

REMEMBER

BMI is a good starting point, but it's not always an accurate measure of proper weight because it doesn't account for muscle mass. Muscle tissue is approximately 15 percent denser than fat tissue. If you're muscular, your BMI may indicate that you're overweight when you're really not.

>> **Relevant:** Carrying less weight will enable me to become more active and energetic, improve my appearance, reduce joint pain, and boost my confidence. (Here, you want to have a compelling reason for investing the time, effort, and other resources required to achieve your goal.)

>> **Time-based:** I'm going to achieve my goal in a year. (Be careful not to get too aggressive here, especially when dealing with weight loss. People who lose weight too quickly often gain it back. Sustainable weight loss is usually accomplished through long-term changes to diet and lifestyle.)

To make your goals SMARTER, just add "ER" to the end of SMART:

>> **Evaluate:** When you reach your deadline, determine whether you achieved your goal. Learn from your success or failure. Look at what went well and what could have been done differently. Was your goal too aggressive? Was it aggressive enough? Were you lacking anything that could have helped you be more successful?

>> **Readjust:** Make any changes that you determine will improve your future success. Keep in mind that readjustment may be helpful regardless of whether you achieved the goal.

REMEMBER

Goals are powerful ways to begin to change habits, but more powerful than goals are processes. For example, a goal may be to lose 20 pounds. The more sustainable process is to eat more healthfully rather than to simply lose 20 pounds. The most powerful way to sustain a habit is with a change in identity. Rather than lose 20 pounds or eat healthfully, you become a healthy eater. (See Chapter 6 for more about changing your identity and becoming a healthy eater.)

This circles back to harnessing the powerful mind/body synergy. Identity change leads to body change, which fortifies identity change . . . and the cycle persists, driving continuous improvement.

IN THIS CHAPTER

» Calming your mind as you decide
what action to take

» Telling the difference between acute
and chronic back pain

» Deciding whether to seek
professional help or go it alone

» Using worry and bother as your
guideposts

Chapter **5**

Knowing Where to Start: Do It Yourself or See a Doctor?

One morning, you wake up and attempt to get out of bed, only to discover a significant pain in your lower back. This may be the first time, but more likely, this has happened before. Chances are, your first thought is, "This is going to take forever to go away!" or "What the heck did I do to my back?" Maybe you know what happened — you were helping your brother move into his new apartment, and the two of you were lugging a king-size mattress up the stairs, or you were shaking out the rugs. (It's *rarely* something enjoyable like playing pickleball or having sex.)

Now you're wondering, "What should I do? Should I rest and hope it goes away? Should I tough it out? Should I call my doctor?" This chapter aims to help you answer questions like those, so that you can determine the best course of action considering the state of your back pain.

Adopting a Rational Frame of Mind

The most valuable tool you have for managing your back pain is your mind. It empowers you to make well-educated decisions, enables you to alleviate muscle tension, and rallies your body's self-healing mechanisms in ways that science is just beginning to understand. So, before you do anything else, take the following steps to calm your mind:

1. **Bear in mind that back pain is extremely common.** At any given time, 20 percent of the population is experiencing back pain. You're not alone.

2. **Remind yourself that your body is well equipped to heal itself.** A large percentage of back pain resolves on its own over time.

3. **Substitute any fear, worry, or panic with calming equanimity.** Make yourself as comfortable as possible, and use controlled breathing to calm yourself (see Chapter 11 for details.)

   REMEMBER

   Fear, angst, and panic exacerbate back pain.

4. **Tell yourself that back pain is like a headache or a common cold.** It's something that's a normal part of life, something that comes and goes.

5. **Start to make sense of the pain with the information and insight we provide throughout this chapter.**

Conducting a Preliminary Self-Assessment

Most people's knee-jerk reaction to back pain is to call their doctor. That's understandable, but it can be a mistake for two reasons:

>> **Calling a doctor first thing sends your mind a subtle message that you're unable to manage your back pain on your own.** Unfortunately, if your mind believes you, that will be true.

>> **The doctor (or other professional you consult) will likely tell you that you need whatever they've been trained to provide — medicine, surgery, a spinal adjustment, whatever.** What they advise can put you on a path that's not the most conducive to your long-term health and fitness.

We believe that each patient is best equipped to manage their own back pain, and that begins at the very beginning — with an accurate assessment or diagnosis.

You may need or want professional help at some point, maybe even very early on, but we encourage you to take the leadership position on your treatment team. Start with a preliminary self-assessment.

Distinguishing between acute and chronic back pain

The first determination to make regarding your back pain is whether it's acute or chronic. In their most basic definitions, *acute* means short-term (lasting up to three months), and *chronic* means long-term (lasting over three months). Acute pain may be the result of an injury, such as lifting something heavy, twisting your back beyond its usual range of motion, or just being extremely tense, but frequently, it simply appears without a definitive origin. In contrast, chronic back pain typically results from degenerative diseases such as arthritis, spinal deformities, poor posture, poor diet, sedentary lifestyle, and so on. Chronic conditions generally take a long time to develop and a long time to resolve. Chronic pain is a baseline pain with possible periodic exacerbations.

REMEMBER

Although "chronic" typically refers to pain over a longer duration, in the context of back pain, chronic suggests not only a long duration but something that may be counterintuitive: The pain mysteriously persists despite the original insult/injury having healed or having had enough time to heal. The fact that the pain can persist after the apparent cause has been addressed can be very frustrating for people who are unlucky enough to have chronic pain. These folks are often disappointed by the current medical system and feel as though they're being brushed off as "crazy" or just trying to get drugs.

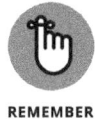

REMEMBER

The term "acute" also has some nuances in its meaning. Acute pain rarely resolves completely, and it tends to recur, so although it may last for only short periods at a time, it can share many of the same characteristics as chronic pain.

Gauging your pain: Red and yellow flags

One way to perform a quick self-assessment that can help you decide whether you need professional help is to assign your pain a red or yellow flag. A red flag indicates that you should be more cautious and probably consult a medical professional. A yellow flag indicates that you can probably manage your back pain effectively with a do-it-yourself (DIY) approach.

REMEMBER

Red and yellow flags aren't mutually exclusive. Many people who experience back pain have both and respond best to an approach that includes both DIY and professional interventions such as pain management, deep-tissue massage, and exercise, or surgery, pain management, and exercise. Sometimes, professional physical interventions are optional, but DIY interventions, including exercise, are always an essential component.

Red flags

WARNING

Red flags indicate an increased risk of underlying medical conditions that may require treatment before you embark on any self-help solutions. If any of the following conditions accompanies your back pain, consult your primary care physician for evaluation and possible referral to a specialist:

>> **Back pain lasting longer than six weeks:** Pain that isn't resolving on its own is more likely to be related to an underlying physical cause that may need medical attention.

>> **Age under 18 or over 50 years:** Typical low back pain is unusual in children and may reflect a more serious origin. New back pain in the elderly is often associated with osteoporotic fractures, spinal stenosis, and arthritis.

>> **History of cancer:** If you or other family members have had cancer, you want to consider it as a possible source of back pain. An onset of cancer may manifest itself in the form of back or neck pain. Patients who have esophageal cancer often experience neck pain well prior to the diagnosis of cancer.

>> **History of weight loss:** Weight loss may indicate a nutritional deficiency or other underlying medical condition that could be causing or contributing to your back pain. If a person loses weight too rapidly or with the aid of prescription weight loss drugs, they may suffer a reduction of muscle tissue, thus lessening the support of the spine, which can result in back pain.

>> **History of fever:** A history of fever may be a sign of underlying infection, which could affect the spine, nerves, or supporting tissues. The fever may be indicative of an infection. For example, an infection of the kidneys will result in a fever and back pain.

>> **History of physical trauma:** If you've had a serious fall or an accident (car, motorcycle, bicycle, sports injury, or something similar), your spine or its supporting structures may have been damaged and failed to heal properly. The weakened muscles and misalignment of the structure would result in pain and discomfort while moving. A compensatory gait due to loss of motion, strength, and misalignment may result in back pain as well.

>> **Arm or leg weakness:** Muscle weakness may be an indication of nerve damage or pressure on a nerve. If the pathways of the nerves are impinged,

the signal will not reach the extremities, possibly resulting in lost or impaired function.

>> **Bowel of bladder dysfunction:** Bowel or bladder dysfunction may indicate an issue affecting the nerves or an underlying condition, such as kidney stones or urinary infection, which can cause back pain. Pinched nerves, spinal cord injury, herniated and bulging discs, and spinal stenosis can lead to bowel and bladder control issues as well.

Yellow flags for back pain

Yellow flags have more to do with your mindset and beliefs (conscious or subconscious). Yes, what you think can have a tremendous impact on how you experience back pain. Your thoughts and emotions serve as fairly accurate predictors of whether acute back pain will become persistent or develop into chronic pain. If you notice any of the following yellow flags, you're a good candidate for a DIY approach to managing your back pain:

>> **Fear or avoidance of activities:** If you're afraid of exercising or other physical activity, thinking it could make your back pain worse or cause physical damage, you're probably avoiding exactly what you need to do to improve your back pain — mobility and strength training.

>> **Belief that the pain stems from an injury that needs to be addressed prior to restoration of activity:** This belief is a common misconception that often becomes an obstacle to a person's healing. Unless you have irrefutable evidence of spinal injury, the best approach to managing back pain is to increase physical activity, not decrease it.

>> **Catastrophizing personality:** If you're more of a pessimist than an optimist, you're going to suffer for that physically. Optimism promotes health and helps to alleviate pain. See Chapter 4 for more about the mind-body connection.

>> **Depression or anxiety disorder:** Just as a pessimistic outlook on life can impact your biological health and function, so too can your mental state. Taking a DIY approach to managing your back pain can help improve both your physical and mental states. However, you may also benefit from some professional help in this area; see Chapter 19 for details.

Categorizing your back pain

Categorizing your back pain can help you establish the right mindset and make educated decisions on how to manage your back pain effectively. In this section, we describe three general back pain categories and provide guidance on the approach that's most appropriate for each.

New acute low back pain

New acute back pain rarely reflects a serious underlying condition, and low back pain typically resolves over a brief period of time, but keep the following two caveats in mind:

>> **The relief is often incomplete.** That is, you may continue to feel pain after the intense pain subsides.

>> **The pain tends to recur.** In other words, it tends to come and go.

Assuming no red flags are present, here's our recommendation for responding to new acute low back pain:

>> **Don't panic.** New acute low back pain rarely reflects a serious underlying condition, and it generally resolves on its own.

>> **Be proactive.** Follow our self-help guidance in Part 2 to minimize any residual pain and the chance of the pain recurring.

>> **Don't just ignore the pain.** Even if it goes away, follow the advice in Part 2 to build resiliency. If you don't, the pain is more likely to return.

WARNING

>> **Rest only as necessary.** Bed rest is often necessary if the pain is incapacitating, but prolonged bed rest is counterproductive. Until recently, doctors routinely prescribed bed rest, but current research shows that bed rest is not only unhelpful but can also be harmful. The sooner you can get up and move around, the better, even if you have a significant amount of pain.

The most typical consequence of overdoing it is an exacerbation of the pain, not something worse, such as injury or damage.

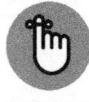

REMEMBER

Intermittent exacerbations of chronic low back pain

Most of the time, those who experience intermittent exacerbations (worsening) of low back pain have adopted a "do not exacerbate" mindset. They go through life trying to be careful and avoid activities that will "throw their back out."

Intermittent exacerbations of chronic low back pain are often yellow-flag scenarios that respond best to a change in mindset and an increase in physical activity. We recommend the following approach:

>> **Change your perspective:** Transition from a "vulnerable" mindset to an "adaptable" mindset. An *adaptable mindset* means believing that you'll progress slowly and surely with the expectation that when your body is stressed properly, sometimes referred to as *eustress* (healthy stress), it will adapt and get stronger.

>> **Be physically active:** Get back on your feet as soon as possible, even if you're still in some pain. A brief period of bed rest may be necessary, but lengthy bed rest is detrimental. As soon as you're on your feet, begin the movements and exercises we recommend in Chapter 8.

Acute back pain almost always makes people think that something is very wrong — perhaps a serious injury. Those who suffer chronic recurrences of intense acute back pain are often afraid of doing too much. This fear is often unfounded and has the potential to worsen the condition in several ways, including the following:

>> You may adopt a certain posture that provides short-term relief of the pain but causes long-term musculoskeletal imbalances that become pain generators in and of themselves.

>> You may "baby" your back, leading to weaknesses in the muscles and other tissues that support the spine.

REMEMBER

Almost regardless of what's causing the pain, strengthening the muscles that stabilize and protect the portion of the spine that's giving rise to the pain helps to alleviate the pain. Doctors used to routinely prescribe rest for inflamed joints, but doctors now know (or should know) that strengthening the muscles that subserve and protect the inflamed joint is better for the pain over time and better than rest.

OWNING YOUR PAIN

Quick fixes, such as medications and manipulations, may be tempting and may be helpful in some cases to provide short-term relief. However, we strongly recommend that if you pursue these options, you do so only for the purpose of enabling you to exercise and increase your physical activity overall. Otherwise, your back isn't going to get any better, and you're likely to become more and more reliant on quick fixes.

For long-term pain management, *you* must take responsibility for strengthening your core and shielding the pain generator (building the muscles around the part of the spine responsible for the pain). Taking responsibility (owning your pain) involves making educated and carefully thought-out treatment decisions (instead of letting others make the decisions for you), making healthy diet and lifestyle choices, engaging in challenging physical activity, managing emotional and mental stress in your life, and even building healthy social relationships. Everything in your life contributes to your physical and mental health and well-being. It's not only about your spine.

Acute back pain with leg pain

Pain in both the back and leg may indicate that a nerve is involved, in which case, we recommend proceeding a little more cautiously. Although this combination of symptoms may be considered a worse scenario than back pain alone, it has an upside — the origin of the back pain is easier to trace, and treatment is more predictably successful. Based on where the pain radiates to most distally on your leg (the farthest point where you feel the pain), your doctor can deduce which nerve is involved. (See Chapter 3 for more about this topic.) You also need to know whether the nerve is injured or merely irritated, which you can determine by evaluating for leg weakness.

TIP

You can test for leg weakness yourself by performing the following steps:

1. **Walk on your toes, trying your best to keep your heels off of the ground.**

2. **Walk on your heels, trying your best to keep your toes off the ground.**

3. **Do a partial one-legged squat with each leg and judge for symmetry of ease performing the move.**

   If you complete the first two steps successfully and can do one-legged squats equally easily with either leg, you are likely experiencing only nerve irritation, not nerve injury. With these simple moves, you just screened for the majority of types of weakness from nerve injury.

If you have weakness in one of your legs, you are in a category similar to having one of the red flag scenarios we discuss in the earlier section "Gauging your pain: Red and yellow flags." In such a case, we generally recommend consulting a medical professional.

Using Worry and Bother to Determine Your Approach to Back Pain

Over the years, we've encouraged our patients to consider whether the back pain they're experiencing is more *worrying* them or *bothering* them. You would be surprised how often the worry part is the more significant of the two. A patient who's more worried than bothered is likely to say, "If I knew that nothing was broken, I could live with the pain." In contrast, a patient who's more bothered than worried is likely to say, "I should take some definitive steps to make my pain better and improve my function."

How much the pain bothers you versus how much it worries you is an important distinction, because if your issue is mostly worry, recognizing that you'll very likely improve with time really helps. If you're more bothered by the pain, remember that your focus should be not on ridding yourself of the pain but on maximizing your function. Reestablishing some degree of function, even if you're still experiencing some pain, is almost always attainable and is compatible with a full and enjoyable life. And if the pain subsides, which certainly happens on occasion, you can consider it a fringe benefit of becoming more functional.

REMEMBER

Another key distinction is the difference between *having* back pain and *suffering* from back pain. At any given time, nearly 20 percent of the population, anywhere in the world, *has back pain*. However, the percentage of the population *suffering from back pain* varies enormously from culture to culture. This evidence reveals that although pain may never be eliminated, much can be done to diminish the suffering and disability associated with it, and the solution often doesn't require quick fixes, such as medication and manipulations.

TIP

A good rule of thumb is to do more than you think you're capable of doing. Forcing yourself to get up and move around leads to better, quicker outcomes. We've found that most back pain sufferers are far more likely to err on the side of caution than on the side of reckless abandon.

PLAYING IT SAFE

Conventional medicine in the U.S. has not fully evolved to embrace the idea of treating back pain by getting up and doing one's best to get around. Although most doctors no longer prescribe bed rest, they still tend to err on the side of caution. In the doctor's mind, caution is safer because it protects the doctor from a perceived liability. However, being overly cautious is not doing their patients any favors. Not only is bed rest unhelpful, it's harmful. The medical literature demonstrates that placing healthy young male subjects on bed rest for a couple of weeks creates back pain that's indistinguishable from an injury to the back. Doctors should view caution as a liability, and so should you.

Think of it this way: Playing it safe isn't safe at all; it's harmful. Your back won't get any healthier or stronger, and you won't become more mobile. In fact, your back is likely to get weaker the more you rest it, and you'll lose mobility. Being *less cautious* is actually the *safer* option.

2

Taking a Do-It-Yourself Approach to Back Pain

Improving your overall health with diet, lifestyle choices, better sleep, stress management, and increased physical activity and social interaction.

Learning common-sense home and work strategies to avoid subjecting your back to unhealthy stressors such as poor posture.

Harnessing the power of your hidden core to relieve back pain.

Building back strength, mobility, and resilience with dozens of gentle movements and more challenging exercises.

Employing home remedies to loosen up your back and relieve the pain.

Mastering deep-breathing techniques that can relieve your pain and oxygenate your spine, muscles, and other tissues.

Chapter **6**

Starting with Everyday Changes

When you're experiencing back pain, you have plenty of options to help relieve it, ranging from over-the-counter pain relievers to pharmaceutical medications, self-help to medical intervention, conventional approaches to alternative treatments, and all sorts of specialized furniture and back-soothing gadgets like heating pads, massage chairs, and inversion tables.

We cover many of your treatment options in this book, and you're free to skip around and choose the ones you think are best for you in your current situation. However, you may want to start with some everyday changes that people often overlook — things like diet, exercise, sleep, and stress management, the chair you sit in all day, the mattress you sleep on all night, and your posture at work. Sometimes, a few adjustments to what you're currently doing are enough to get you back on your feet and make your pain more manageable, if not relieve it entirely.

In this chapter, we start you out slowly on the path to restoring back health by introducing you to everyday changes you can make at home and at work or school to improve your overall health, avoid doing things that may be causing your back pain, and start doing things that can help make it go away.

REMEMBER

Making everyday changes isn't necessarily easier or less important than other steps we recommend in this book. Diet, physical activity, sleep, and stress management are fundamental to your overall physical and mental health. They impact back health and function as much as they do the health and function of other systems, organs, and tissues that make up your body. And what you do at home and at work (and how you do it) can play a huge role in your recovery.

Improving Your Overall Health

Conventional medicine takes a somewhat mechanical approach to health, as though human beings are nothing more than robots made up of a collection of parts. Cardiologists specialize in treating the circulatory system, orthopedic doctors focus on bones and joints, gastroenterologists treat digestive dysfunction, neurologists care for the brain and nerves, pulmonologists deal with the lungs, and so on. However, your body is an organic whole — everything works together — and the health of every cell in your body relies on what you provide it — food, air, water, physical and mental activity, social engagement, and everything else it needs to thrive, physically and mentally.

When your body doesn't get what it needs or is exposed to something harmful, it experiences some degree of distress, which degrades its health. Optimizing health essentially boils down to giving your body and mind what they need and avoiding or limiting anything that degrades their health, such as processed foods, smoking/vaping, alcohol, chronic emotional stress, a sedentary life, social isolation, or other harmful substances or conditions.

WHAT IS HEALTH?

The World Health Organization defines *health* as a state of complete physical, mental, and social well-being and not merely the absence of disease or infirmity. What's critical in this definition is that your health is not just physical. It includes both mental health and social well-being.

The second point to remember is that health is not defined as an absence of illness but rather as something that can be built. Modern healthcare would love you to believe that it can make you healthy by removing disease, but being healthy requires much more than just not being sick. The good news is that you have an incredible amount of control over just how healthy you are.

Adjusting your diet

The standard American diet (SAD) is characterized by high consumption of processed foods, refined sugars and other simple carbohydrates, unhealthy fats and oils, and red and processed meats (such as bacon, sausages, and cold cuts), along with a scarcity of vegetables, nuts, seeds, whole grains, fruits, and legumes (beans). This diet, which is common in industrialized nations, is linked to a host of serious chronic health conditions, including obesity, diabetes, arthritis, heart disease, cancer, and dementia. It's especially prevalent in the U.S., which does a lousy job of regulating the country's food supply and food manufacturing processes and chemicals.

Here are some suggestions for improving your diet:

>> Eat whole foods, mostly plants — vegetables, nuts, seeds, whole grains, fruits, and legumes.

>> Drink mostly water. Avoid sweet drinks, including those that include artificial sweeteners. Unsweetened tea and coffee without creamer are fine.

>> Don't eat too much. See the later section, "Curbing your calorie consumption," for suggestions on how to eat less without feeling hungry.

>> Eat healthy proteins, such as fish, free-range chicken, and grass-fed beef, and eat leaner cuts of red meat in moderation. Eggs are fine (organic are best), but consume them in moderation as well. Generally, look for sources of protein that are lower in saturated fat.

>> Avoid sugar, sweets, baked goods, and starchy foods, such as pasta, white rice, potatoes, bread, cereals, and chips. These simple carbohydrates, when consumed in excess, are converted to fat for storage. Most foods made from wheat flour also contain gluten, which is highly inflammatory for many people.

>> Be careful with dairy products, such as milk, cheese, yogurt, and ice cream (more because of the sugar than the dairy). Many people are sensitive to dairy products. You may want to try to eliminate it from your diet for a couple of weeks and see whether you feel better without it. If you don't have a sensitivity to dairy, good for you — enjoy!

>> Eat healthier fats, and by fats, we mean oils. Limit saturated fats, such as those in red meat, butter, and high-fat dairy products, and avoid seed oils (such as vegetable, soybean, and canola). Healthy oils include extra virgin olive oil and avocado oil from trusted manufacturers. Top water fish, such as salmon and tuna, as well as oily fish, like sardines and anchovies, are also great sources of healthy fats. Among freshwater fish, rainbow trout is one of the best sources of healthy fats.

>> Drink alcohol sparingly, if at all.

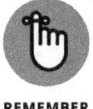

REMEMBER

Dietary fat doesn't make you fat. A diet high in sugar and other simple carbohydrates is what makes people fat. The body converts sugar and simple carbs into body fat to store for when you go hungry, and in industrial societies, that rarely happens, so people just keep packing on the pounds.

These are *general* dietary guidelines. Keep in mind that everybody is different, and *every body* is different. Not everyone processes the same foods the same way. However, you're not going to suffer by eating healthier.

HOW TO CREATE AN OBESITY EPIDEMIC

As a modern society, we couldn't have done a better job of creating an obesity epidemic had we tried. Here's how you do it:

1. Convince people that fat is unhealthy. Don't distinguish between healthy and unhealthy fats.

2. Promote low-fat foods that are high in sugar and simple carbohydrates as alternatives to fat.

3. Add chemicals to foods that make people hungrier so that they want to eat more of those foods.

4. Make great movies and television shows and comfortable furniture to watch them from.

5. Make kids afraid to play outside. Give them video games for entertainment and smartphones so they can interact with one another without going anywhere.

6. Create search engines and artificial intelligence (AI) so people don't have to learn anything or even think much.

7. Automate everything so people no longer have to do anything physical.

8. Popularize fast-food restaurants and biggie-size everything on the menu.

9. Overprescribe antibiotics to upset the sensitive balance of beneficial bacteria in the gut that help manage appetite and food cravings.

We could probably extend this list, but it's a good start. The point is that modern living is geared to make us sick, not healthy. As a society, we've done it to ourselves, and as a society and individuals within that society, we have the power to reverse this unhealthy trend and reclaim our health. We just need to start making healthier choices.

TIP

Don't buy it. Don't buy sweets, baked goods, processed foods, sweet drinks, fast food, junk food, or anything else that's unhealthy. If you buy it, you will bring it into your home, and you and your family will consume it. If it's not in your home, you won't eat it, drink it, or smoke it. It is that simple. Exercise self-control at the grocery store. Once you get that stuff home, it's a lot harder.

In the following sections, we delve more deeply into a few key topics related to diet and eating.

Breaking a sugar addiction

Sugar is one of the most addictive substances on the planet, and the food industry is well aware of that fact. Sugar and other simple carbs trigger the brain to release *dopamine,* a "feel good" neurotransmitter associated with pleasure and reward. This is similar to the way the brain responds to addictive substances such as nicotine. Over time, repeated sugar consumption can lead to a sort of chemical dependency, in which the body craves increasing amounts of sugar to experience the same pleasurable response.

Grocery stores are packed with "comfort foods," which consist, in large part, of high-processed sugar, flour, and dairy — candy bars, cookies, donuts, macaroni and cheese, pizza, crackers, chips, ice cream, and more. These items may provide you with short-term comfort, but the temporary burst in energy and awareness is typically soon followed by a crash as your body releases insulin to process all that glucose, and your blood sugar level drops precipitously. Here are a couple of suggestions to keep that from happening and to start breaking any sugar addiction you may have:

>> Satisfy your craving with a healthier snack, such as a handful of nuts, some berries, a raw carrot, a rib of celery, or a small apple.

>> Tell yourself that you'll have it later, and then take a short walk or drop to the floor and do some planks or crunches until the craving passes — anything to get your mind off food.

TIP

To fine-tune or ramp up your approach to limiting consumption of sugar and other low-carb foods and beverages, consider each item's glycemic index. The *glycemic index (GI)* is a number from 0 to 100 assigned to a food that represents the relative rise in blood glucose level it produces two hours after it's consumed. Sweets and baked goods typically have a high GI, whereas green leafy vegetables, nuts, whole grains, and legumes generally have a low GI. However, some vegetables, fruits, and whole grains have a relatively high glycemic index, including potatoes, cooked carrots, canned veggies, beets, white rice, peaches, and pineapple. You can find charts online that show the glycemic index of many common foods.

REMEMBER

If you're in menopause or andropause, you have diminished levels of estrogen and testosterone, making you more susceptible to *fat deposition* — the process by which the body converts sugar into fat and stores it in the body (usually in areas you don't want it). Foods that have a high glycemic index increase blood glucose, which triggers the release of *insulin* — the fat deposition hormone, which is unopposed by estrogen and testosterone when they are diminished.

Addressing food sensitivities

Many people have food allergies or sensitivities. A *food allergy* is an abnormal immune response to eating a food; it produces mild to severe symptoms such as itching, hives, diarrhea, vomiting, swelling, trouble breathing, and, in some cases, a drop in blood pressure or even death. A *food sensitivity* (or *intolerance*), on the other hand, involves difficulty digesting or breaking down certain components of food, such as gluten or lactose. Reactions are typically delayed and less dramatic than those of an allergic reaction and may include bloating, gas, stomach cramps, fatigue, and headache. Both food allergies and sensitivities can trigger an inflammatory response that can cause or contribute to back pain and a host of other health issues.

TIP

If you have a chronic health condition that your doctors cannot trace to any other cause, consider trying an *elimination diet* — exclude certain foods or food groups from your diet for a couple of weeks and monitor how you feel. Then, reintroduce the foods gradually while monitoring for any adverse symptoms. Many people have sensitivities to dairy and wheat (specifically gluten, which is a component of wheat), so start there. We've found that eliminating gluten and lactose has helped many of our patients/clients reduce their back pain. You may also be sensitive to certain chemicals in foods, such as sulfites. Identifying a problem food or food group can be a complex and time-consuming process. Be patient and persistent. Keep a food journal.

Supporting gut health and function

The ancient Greek physician Hippocrates was onto something when he wrote, "All disease begins in the gut." A growing body of research links the gut not only to its role in extracting nutrients from food and making them available to every cell in the body but also to the immune system and the brain. And it's not just your anatomical gut that's such a crucial component to your overall health but also the trillions (yes, trillions) of beneficial bacteria and other microorganisms that reside within it.

Various factors can upset the healthy balance of microorganisms living in the gut, including C-section (versus vaginal) birth; overuse of antibiotics, acid blockers, and other medications; stress; smoking; alcohol consumption; and exposure to environmental toxins. Such an imbalance can trigger a chain reaction of events leading to chronic inflammation; for example, an imbalance that damages the protective lining of the gut may allow chemicals that should stay inside the gut to leak out, triggering an immune response, resulting in an inflammatory state.

Treatment involves addressing whatever triggered the imbalance in the first place, repairing the gut lining, and restoring balance to the gut's *microbiome* — the community of microorganisms that reside in the gut. Treatment is beyond the scope of this book, but addressing any food sensitivities and adopting a healthier diet go a long way toward restoring gut health and function.

Consuming whole and organic foods

Ideally, everyone should be eating whole foods (because that's what real food is) and organic foods, which are richer in nutrients and lower in pesticides and other potentially harmful chemicals. If, for whatever reason, you can't or won't eat organic foods, at least eat whole foods.

TIP

An easy way to focus on whole foods is to shop along the periphery of the grocery store, where you'll find produce, meats, eggs, and dairy. Generally, the boxed, bagged, and canned goods in the middle aisles are processed, but you may need to visit certain aisles in the middle for whole grains, rice, and beans. Definitely steer clear of the aisles with chips and crackers, breakfast cereals, pasta, and bread and desserts. Frozen veggies and fruits are great, but ignore the ice cream and frozen meal items.

REMEMBER

Whole and organic foods may be more expensive, but as experts in nutrition often say, "You can pay the farmer now or pay the pharmacist later," or as Hippocrates wrote, "Let food be thy medicine, and medicine be thy food." Understandably, eating all organic may be cost-prohibitive; what's more important is that you avoid consuming excessive amounts of highly processed foods.

Curbing your calorie consumption

If you're trying to lose weight, try curbing your calorie consumption. Here are a few strategies that can help:

>> **Eat when you're hungry.** Before eating, ask whether you're really hungry or just want to eat out of boredom, stress, or habit.

>> **Use portion control to your advantage.** Consume smaller portions. Use a smaller plate and a smaller glass or cup if that helps, and don't go back for seconds. Don't eat out of a box or bag; serve a portion on a plate or in a bowl instead, and don't go back for seconds.

- » **Slow down and pay attention.** Eat mindfully, not while you're watching TV or scrolling on your phone or tablet. Take your time to chew and savor each bite. Eating slowly and mindfully enables your body to sense fullness, which can prevent you from eating more than you need.

- » **Eat fiber and protein with most meals.** Fiber-rich foods slow digestion and keep you feeling full longer, and protein helps increase feelings of fullness and satisfaction.

TIP

Fill up on low-calorie, nutrient-dense foods like leafy green vegetables, cucumbers, and broccoli so you can eat more bulk while consuming fewer calories.

- » **Get enough sleep.** Lack of sleep can increase cravings for high-calorie foods.

- » **Try healthier snack alternatives.** If you're craving something sweet, eat fresh fruit. If you're craving something salty, eat some air-popped popcorn or a few salted nuts.

Avoid smoking and vaping

Everyone knows that smoking and vaping are unhealthy, so we're not going to subject you to a lengthy lecture. We do feel compelled, however, to mention that smoking and vaping are closely associated with back pain and with *osteoporosis* — bone deterioration — which is a significant trigger for back pain, especially in older adults. If you smoke or vape, you know you should quit. Here are some suggestions that may help:

- » **Try nicotine replacement (gum, lozenges, or patches) to gradually wean yourself off nicotine.**

- » **Identify and avoid your triggers — bars, parties, drinking, hanging out with other smokers.**

- » **Delay it.** If you feel the urge to smoke or vape, tell yourself, "I'll do it later" or "Wait for 10 or 15 minutes," and then do something to keep your mind off it.

- » **Chew on something — gum, a raw carrot, a licorice root, a straw — to satisfy your oral fixation.**

- » **Don't let yourself have "just one."** That never works.

- » **When the craving hits, drop to the floor and bang out some push-ups or crunches or go for a walk.** Exercise helps curb the craving.

- » **Don't buy cigarettes.** At least if you have to bum one to smoke one, that's a hurdle you have to clear.

- » **Perform deep-breathing exercises as suggested in Chapter 11.**

VAPING VERSUS SMOKING

The vape industry touts vaping as a healthier alternative to smoking. It may be less harmful, but to describe it as healthier is misleading. Vaping poses a number of health risks, including the following:

- **Nicotine addiction:** Nicotine can have a negative impact on brain development, especially among young people, and it can increase the risk of heart disease and high blood pressure.

- **Respiratory problems:** Vaping has been linked to lung injury. The steaming vapor entering the lungs destroys the *alveoli* — the sacs in the lungs where oxygen is transferred to the bloodstream. When these sacs are destroyed, they never recover. Every single puff from an e-cigarette results in irreversible lung damage.

- **Exposure to toxins:** Although vaping produces fewer toxins than smoking, it can still expose users to potentially harmful chemicals, including *formaldehyde* (a carcinogen) and *diacetyl,* a substance linked to "popcorn lung" (bronchiolitis obliterans), a severe lung disease.

- **Popcorn lung:** Vaping causes popcorn lung, according to data provided by the American Lung Association. Popcorn lung damages the bronchioles and alveoli. There is no known cure or method to reverse the damage.

- **Unknown long-term effects:** Additional long-term health impacts of vaping are still being studied.

Bottom line: Although vaping may be less harmful than smoking, it still poses a significant health risk.

The American Cancer Society offers a free guide called "How to Quit Using Tobacco," which you can find at `https://www.cancer.org/cancer/risk-prevention/tobacco/guide-quitting-smoking.html`.

Getting the sleep you need

Sleep is essential for maintaining physical health and mental well-being. It supports the body's repair and restoration processes, boosts brain function, regulates hormones, and reduces the risk of chronic illnesses. If you're an adult, you should be getting about 7–9 hours of sleep per day. Younger people generally need more sleep because their brains and bodies are still developing.

If you're not sleeping at least six hours a day or you're feeling tired soon after waking, your sleep quantity or quality is suffering. Here are some suggestions for improving both:

>> **Invest in a comfortable mattress and pillows.** Theoretically, firm mattresses are better for herniated discs, whereas softer mattresses are better for arthritic conditions, but trying out different mattresses is the best approach. Try to find a local mattress dealer that allows you to try before you buy.

>> **Try to structure your sleep schedule by going to bed at the same time each day/night and waking up at about the same time each day/night.**

>> **If you nap during the day, limit your nap time to an hour or so and nap at least six hours before your usual bedtime.**

>> **Keep your bedroom cool, dark, and quiet.** White noise, such as from a fan, is okay if that works for you.

>> **Don't eat or drink anything that's likely to prevent you from falling asleep or staying asleep.** Avoid caffeine 4–6 hours before bedtime, avoid heavy meals and spicy foods, and limit consumption of alcohol and other fluids, which can disrupt sleep.

REMEMBER

Caffeine has a half-life of five hours, so if you consume an eight-ounce cup of coffee that has 95 milligrams of caffeine at 5 p.m., you'll still have 43 milligrams of caffeine in your system at 10 p.m.

>> **Establish a relaxing bedtime routine.** Stop any stimulating activities 30–60 minutes before bed. No TV, computer, game console, or smartphone; blue light from screens can suppress melatonin production, impairing your ability to fall asleep. Do a deep breathing or other relaxation exercise for 5–10 minutes as you lie in bed to let any tension leave your body.

We'd love to tell you that you'll get instant results from a soothing night-time routine, but you may need to give it a few weeks before you begin to notice a difference.

Experiment to find the sweet spot between too little and too much sleep. Consider journaling your sleep habits to find out what works best for you. You may find that less sleep makes you feel more invigorated and productive. However, if you're routinely getting less than six hours of sleep daily, you may be subjecting yourself to unhealthy levels of sleep deprivation.

TIP

Exercising

When your back is killing you, exercising may seem counterintuitive, but that's exactly what you should do.

REMEMBER

The belief that the best treatment for a sore back is rest is a fallacy that's reinforced by the fact that rest usually makes it feel better at first. The problem is that it ends up making most people feel worse over the long term. You can usually start exercising sooner after an injury than you think, and you will be rewarded for it with a stronger, healthier back that feels better, too! Decades ago, doctors recommended rest for a painful joint. Experts now know that strengthening the muscles that support and protect the joints works far better. The back is no exception.

When you're experiencing significant acute back pain, settling down your back with a brief period of rest, heat, massage, and/or pain relievers (pills or topical analgesics) can be helpful for the first 24 hours or so. Chiropractic can also be helpful. Then, engage in some gentle back movements, nothing too aggressive. If the pain is severe, radiating down an arm or leg, and is accompanied by weakness (for example, partial drop foot), consult a medical professional before engaging in any strenuous exercise. (See Chapter 5 for more guidance on when to see a doctor.)

Chapters 8 and 9 are packed with physical movements and exercises to increase back strength, mobility, and flexibility. Chapter 8 includes some very gentle movements to start with. At this point, just be aware that physical movement and exercise are not only acceptable but are actually what we prescribe for addressing back pain. Here are some additional important insights pertaining to exercise and back pain:

>> **Your body isn't fragile unless you treat it as such.** In fact, the more you challenge it, the more durable and resilient it gets. Properly and progressively stress the back and body to make them stronger. Rather than manage your vulnerable back, make it more durable.

>> **To build back strength and mobility, combine strengthening exercises with aerobic fitness (higher reps with lower weights/resistance), emphasizing endurance over strength.** We've found this approach most effective and built it into the exercises we present in Chapters 8 and 9.

>> **Prioritize strength over flexibility.** Although many doctors and therapists promote stretching for back pain (and we agree that it's important), focus first on building strength and mobility. In general, a muscle should be strengthened prior to being stretched. Muscles serve the purpose of stabilizing joints. Almost regardless of what the cause of pain is, stabilizing the back joints reduces pain.

REMEMBER

>> **Prioritize the muscles behind you (back, butt, and hamstrings) over the muscles in front of you (chest, abs, and thighs).** Most people have a stronger *anterior chain* (frontside core) than a *posterior chain* (backside core), which creates an imbalance. By over-emphasizing the backside muscles, you restore balance.

Don't be fooled by what you see in the mirror. Looking like a bodybuilder from the front doesn't mean you have a structurally sound back. It can indicate the opposite — that you have a structural imbalance that's stressing your back . . . and not in a good way.

In addition to the back-building exercises we present in Chapters 8 and 9, consider engaging in other forms of exercise, such as walking, yoga, Pilates, tai chi, or qi gong. Pilates is exceptional for building core strength — front, back, and sides. Yoga is great for increasing range of motion and flexibility. And tai chi and qigong are excellent disciplines for improving posture. All of these systems promote overall physical and mental health and well-being.

Building mental health and social well-being

The mind-body relationship is closer than most people realize. A growing body of evidence suggests that what people think and feel has a direct impact on their bodies. In fact, thoughts and emotions may even change the way your body functions through *epigenetics* — turning genes on or off without changing your DNA. For example, chronic stress can flip a genetic switch, telling your body that instead of burning that donut you're eating for energy, it should store it as fat just in case there's a famine next week.

The take-home message here is this: It's not only true that "you are what you eat," but also that "you are what you think." Your thoughts, emotions, and overall attitude can impact everything from how you experience back pain to how your body responds to changes in diet and exercise. It may even influence how long you live. Here are a couple of studies that provide evidence of the mind's influence on the body's physical function:

>> **The milkshake study:** Participants were given milkshakes. Some were told they were drinking diet shakes, while others were told they were drinking high-calorie shakes. Each participant's satiety after consuming the milkshake was checked by looking at a protein called gremlin. Even though the milkshakes were all the same, those who were told they were drinking high-calorie shakes were more satiated; they had higher gremlin levels.

>> **The Harvard longitudinal study:** (A *longitudinal study* is a research design that involves repeated observations of the same variables over long periods of time.)

In 1938, researchers started keeping track of groups of Harvard graduates until they died and tried to make sense of which factors had the greatest influence on how long they lived. (John F. Kennedy was among the initial participants). They concluded that positive relationships had a greater impact on longevity than exercise, not smoking, career achievement, and financial success.

In the following sections, we share practical advice on how to improve your mind-set and your overall psychological and emotional well-being.

Nurturing a positive attitude

As you embark on your personal back-improvement program, we encourage you to do so with a positive attitude. If you're thinking, "Ugh, I still have to get my workout in today," it's not going to be as enjoyable and beneficial as if you approached it thinking, "Man, I can't wait till I'm off work, and get to play pickleball with Joni!" Here are a few quick tips for boosting your mood and outlook (we provide additional guidance in Chapter 4):

» **Take three deep breaths prior to engaging in exercise or a difficult undertaking** to help prepare your mind and body for the task ahead.

» **Focus on the present** so that you can approach the task unencumbered by anything in the past (which you can't change) or worry about the future (which you can't possibly know).

» **Shed the dread.** View what you're about to do as an opportunity instead of as a burden.

» **Be the hero, not the coward.** In a threatening situation, both are subject to the same sensations, but differences in how they perceive the situation determine how they think, feel, and act, usually resulting in dramatically different outcomes.

» **Don't look for excuses or someone to blame.** Look for ways to succeed and people who can help.

» **Don't fear failure.** You are better off trying and failing than sitting idly by making no progress. Failure is an opportunity for growth.

Following the PERMA model for mental and social well-being

Just as physical health requires attention to various aspects of one's life (diet, exercise, lifestyle, and so on), so does mental health and well-being. But what exactly do you need to attend to? The PERMA (positive emotions engagement, relationships, meaning, and achievement) model, which is a product of the positive psychology movement, seeks to answer that question. Here's what you need to feel mentally and socially complete:

>> **P = Positive emotions:** Positive emotions include happiness, enthusiasm, gratitude, optimism, pride, serenity, and many others. Sometimes, just repeating the words that describe these emotions can shift your emotional state in a positive direction.

>> **E = Engagement:** Engagement means being fully immersed in whatever you're doing right now. You're not thinking about something that happened in the past or looking forward to or worrying about something that may happen in the future. And you're certainly not thinking about back pain.

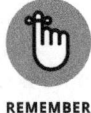

REMEMBER

Researchers have discovered that many people are actually happier at work than they are on weekends and holidays. This "work paradox" may be due to the fact that work provides structure, social interaction, and a sense of purpose that many people don't have in their personal lives. Some people also feel guilty when they're not productive.

>> **R = Relationships:** Humans are generally social animals. They need to interact with others to feel a sense of belonging and feel that they're loved and appreciated. Put some effort into meeting people and nurturing relationships with friends, family members, coworkers, neighbors, and others. Social isolation can contribute significantly to poor physical health.

>> **M = Meaning:** Having a sense of purpose is key to happiness. If you feel you're in a dead-end job or a loveless relationship or that your life is meaningless, your physical health will suffer. When you have a sense of purpose, your primary objective becomes your focal point, and everything else — including any back pain you may feel — becomes a peripheral concern.

>> **A = Achievement:** "Achievement" refers to productivity or progress. To achieve personal fulfillment, people need to see that they're contributing something of value or moving forward. If you're frustrated or feel that you're losing ground, you won't have that sense of accomplishment that is so crucial.

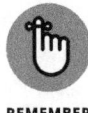

REMEMBER

Go with the flow. According to psychologist Mihaly Csikszentmihalyi (try pronouncing *that* name), flow is the ultimate form of engagement. He associates it with optimal wellness. Think of flow as being "in the zone." When you're engaged, you're acting instinctively with no awareness of yourself as a separate being.

Managing stress

Stress is complex. It can be positive or negative, healthy or unhealthy, depending on numerous factors, including the source and nature of the stress, its intensity and duration, the amount of stress (collectively) you're dealing with at any given time, your stress tolerance, and how you view and deal with it. In this section, we present a few key insights into stress, along with some guidance and a tool to enable you to manage it more effectively.

Bad stress, good stress, and how you look at it

Stress has gotten a bad reputation. You've probably heard people say, "Stress kills." That's true, but it also builds strength and resilience. As German philosopher Friedrich Nietzsche once said, "What doesn't kill me makes me stronger." Stress can be negative or positive:

>> **Distress** is negative. It typically causes anxiety and can trigger mental or physical illness, and it can overwhelm a person's ability to manage it.

>> **Eustress** is positive. It's exciting, motivating, and challenging without being overwhelming. Eustress is the kind of stress you feel when you're taking on a big project, preparing for an event, or facing a challenge.

The mind and body respond to eustress with the *specific adaptation to imposed demand (SAID)*; they become stronger and more resilient. Distress, on the other hand, can deplete your energy and make your body less resilient.

REMEMBER

Whether stress is positive or negative may have something to do with how you view it. In a study into the power of mindset, some subjects were educated on the upside of stress while others were educated on its downside. The subjects were then stressed, and their physiologic responses were measured by testing their levels of stress hormones. Subjects who were educated on the upside of stress had lower levels of stress hormones.

Keeping your stress cup from filling up

You can view stress as filling your cup and the capacity of your cup as your stress tolerance (see Figure 6-1). Stressors can be physical (such as lack of sleep, poor diet, sedentary life, infection) or emotional/psychological (relationship conflict, a financial setback, a job change). These stressors and others drip, drip, drip into your cup, and if you don't find a way to manage them effectively, they can eventually overwhelm your mind and body.

The stress cup reveals ways to start emptying it — improve sleep, adopt a healthy diet, lose weight, exercise, fix or end emotionally draining relationships, pursue a more rewarding career, and so on. You target each stressor (distressor) and then take positive action to fix it.

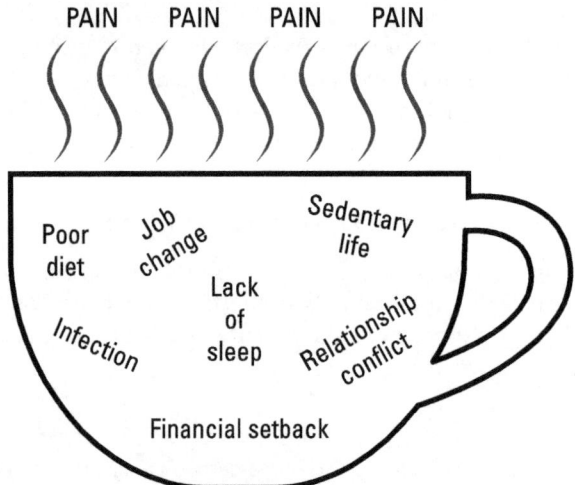

PAIN PAIN PAIN PAIN

Poor diet
Job change
Sedentary life
Lack of sleep
Infection
Relationship conflict
Financial setback

FIGURE 6-1: Stress fills your cup.

Prioritizing tasks

An effective way to manage stress is to prioritize tasks, address the ones that matter, and let the little stuff go. You can use the Eisenhower Matrix, as shown in Figure 6-2, to assign tasks to the following four categories:

>> **Important/Urgent (Do):** Tasks that have a significant upside or potential downside and a deadline are your top priority, such as responding to a complaint from one of your business's best customers or studying for an upcoming exam. These are tasks you need to do right away or very soon.

>> **Important/Not Urgent (Schedule):** Essential tasks that you can do later, such as earning your MBA so you can pursue that management position you've always wanted. This is the quadrant you should strive to operate in, because by identifying these tasks early enough, you have plenty of time to plan and implement your plan without feeling overwhelmed.

>> **Not Important/Urgent (Delegate or Delay):** Tasks that have little or no consequence whether you do them or not but have a sense of urgency attached to them in your mind, such as feeling as though you need to reply to Tik Tok video or Instagram post immediately.

>> **Not Important/Not Urgent (Drop/Delete):** Busywork. Regardless of whether you complete the task, it won't have much impact on your life; for example, you buy a boat that's in bad shape, thinking you'll fix it up someday, and it becomes a constant reminder that you're always too busy to work on it.

To figure out which quadrant a task belongs in, ask yourself the following questions:

>> Why is this task on my list?

>> What will I gain by doing this? What will I lose if I don't do it?

>> Can I make better use of my time?

>> Is this something I can delegate?

>> Can I push this out to a later date or time?

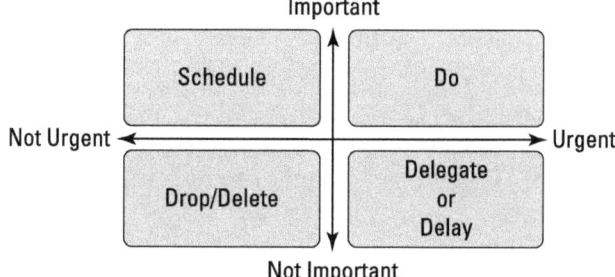

FIGURE 6-2:
The Eisenhower
Matrix.

Prioritizing can help you dramatically reduce your stress. When you have a better sense of what requires your energy (and what can fall away), you reduce your stress by reducing your tasks. You make more time for the important things and give yourself more time for the things you enjoy.

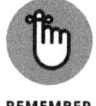

REMEMBER

Do what you can about what matters to you, and let everything else go. You can't control everything.

THE ORIGIN OF THE EISENHOWER MATRIX

The Eisenhower Matrix is the brainchild of Stephen Covey, author of *The 7 Habits of Highly Effective People*. Covey was inspired by something President Dwight D. Eisenhower said in a 1954 speech. Eisenhower quoted an unnamed university president who told him, "I have two kinds of problems, the urgent and the important. The urgent are not important, and the important are never urgent."

Carefully evaluate everything you do based on its importance and urgency. Chances are good that much of what you do and even more of what you worry about is neither important nor urgent.

Making diet and lifestyle changes

Making lasting diet and lifestyle changes can be challenging. Over many years and sometimes decades, habits become deeply ingrained. Over time, you may even develop a chemical or psychological dependency. The good news is that you developed these habits, so you have the power to replace them with healthier habits. To do so, follow this three-step process:

1. **Believe you can change.** We've seen people undergo incredible mental and physical transformations. We know it isn't always easy, but we see it happen every day in our work. You can do it, too.

2. **Understand how to change.** This chapter offers practical guidance on how to make a variety of diet and lifestyle changes to improve your overall health, and throughout this book, we provide advice on how to restore back health and function — proven ways to reduce back pain.

3. **Take ownership of the change.** This is on you. Only you can make the choice and the commitment to improve your physical and mental health. Only you can make the tough choices and invest the time and effort to implement change.

REMEMBER

As James Clear points out in his book *Atomic Habits*, habit formation occurs at three levels:

1. **Outcome:** An outcome is a single, often transitory result, such as losing 20 pounds. Unless the actions taken to achieve that outcome have been instilled, the outcome will not be sustained.

2. **Process:** This is a more powerful approach and a higher level of habit formation. In this case, the goal may be to eat healthier or to buy only healthy foods. Having a process or a system in place makes forming a habit easier and ensures consistent and repeatable outcomes.

3. **Identity:** Changing one's identity is the most powerful approach and the highest level of habit formation. You may still set goals and develop processes for achieving them, but now you're developing habits aligned with your values. For example, you may identify yourself as someone who takes charge of your own health, in which case, you're committed to giving your mind and body everything they need to maintain optimum health — healthy food, pure water, strenuous physical activity, mental challenges, social engagement, and so on.

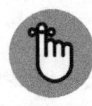
REMEMBER

Taking care of yourself overall is an important way to manage your back pain. When you do well with the basics, you can expect health improvements of all kinds.

Adding Movement to Your Day

Physical movement is essential for optimal health, including back health. However, most people with back pain believe deeply that exercise, or any physical movement for that matter, will exacerbate their pain. A growing body of evidence suggests the opposite — physical movement reduces back pain.

We strongly recommend that you make a concerted effort to integrate physical movement into your daily routine. In Chapters 8 and 9, we provide movements and exercises that target the back specifically, but any physical movement you can add to your day can help. Here are some ways you can be more physically active throughout the day:

>> **Use exercise as a snack.** Take a short walk (5–10 minutes) or do some of the back-strengthening and mobilization movements in Chapter 8 several times throughout the day. Drop to the floor and do some push-ups, planks, or crunches. You can set a timer on your smartphone to remind you to move.

>> **Use the stairs instead of the elevator or escalator.** If you have a choice, taking the stairs is the healthier option. It boosts your heart rate and strengthens your legs.

>> **Walk or ride your bike to work or when you run errands.** If neither of those options is feasible, park farther away from wherever you're going or get off the bus or train at an earlier stop and walk the rest of the way.

>> **Do household chores.** Sweeping, vacuuming, washing dishes, dusting, cleaning windows, and getting organized all engage the body while giving you a sense of accomplishment, not to mention a cleaner, less-cluttered living space.

>> **Do yard work.** Gardening, mowing (especially with a push mower), raking, sweeping the sidewalks or driveway, and pruning trees all engage the body while exposing you to fresh air and sunshine. They also have the potential to increase your engagement with the neighbors for some healthy social interaction.

>> **Use TV time to get physical.** There's no law stating that you have to sit on a sofa to watch TV. Replace your recliner with a treadmill, rowing machine, or stationary bicycle, or clear a space on the floor to jump rope or do yoga, Pilates, or some of the back-building movements in Chapters 8 and 9 while you binge-watch your favorite TV series.

>> **Dance.** Fire up your playlist and dance around your home or apartment, around your yard, or even through your neighborhood. Dancing is fun, energizing, and a great way to get your whole body moving.

Making Changes at Home and Work

In addition to the general guidelines we provide in this chapter to improve health through diet, exercise, and lifestyle, you can make a few everyday changes at home and work to support your back health and build a stronger, more resilient back. Here are a few suggestions to start with that apply to both home and work:

>> **Maintain a neutral spine all the time.** To avoid subjecting your spine to excessive strain, be mindful of your spinal alignment at all times. See Chapter 7 for more about what a "neutral spine" is and why it's so important.

>> **Stay hydrated.** Proper hydration helps maintain the elasticity and health of your spinal discs, reducing the risk of disc-related pain.

>> **Stay relaxed.** Stress makes you tight all over, which makes your muscles, tendons, and ligaments more susceptible to injury. Find a relaxation technique that works for you. See the earlier section, "Building mental health and social well-being," for suggestions.

>> **Do what you love, and love what you do.** Enjoying what you do at home and at work is one of the most effective ways to promote back health and reduce back pain.

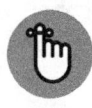

REMEMBER

Most people think back pain interferes with their ability to enjoy life, but the converse is also true — not enjoying life can be a major trigger for back pain.

In the following sections, we take a closer look at steps you can take, specifically at home and at work, to protect and strengthen your back.

Making changes at home

If you're like most people, you spend a good part of every day at home. Here are a few suggestions that can make that time more back-friendly:

>> **Invest in a comfortable mattress.** See the earlier section, "Getting the sleep you need," for details on selecting a mattress.

>> **Buy a comfortable pillow.** The limited science suggests that larger pillows that produce neck flection are good for arthritic conditions, and cervical pillows (which go behind your neck, not your ear) are better for disc herniations, but trial and error is the best approach for choosing pillows.

>> **Sleep on your back.** You can sleep on your side but put a pillow between your knees to help maintain your spinal alignment and a pillow in front of your chest to support your upper arm and prevent your thoracic spine from

twisting to the side. Avoid sleeping on your stomach, which strains your neck and spine.

>> **When you sit, do it on a physioball (yoga ball).** Sitting on a physioball increases your core strength, improves your posture, and stimulates the flow of spinal fluid, increasing blood flow and promoting healing along the spinal column. In addition to sitting on your physioball, use it to build your core; you can find plenty of core-building workout videos online that incorporate the use of a physioball.

>> **Maintain a neutral spine all the time.** Yes, we know we're repeating ourselves, but when you're doing little things around your home, this rule is easy to forget. When you're doing anything around the house — opening or closing a window, sweeping, vacuuming, shaking out rugs, dusting, rearranging furniture, making a bed, whatever — you can twist your body (and back) into unstable configurations that make it more susceptible to injury, even when you're not doing any heavy lifting.

>> **Supplement your diet with vitamin D and collagen peptides.** You can find plenty of supplements for helping with back pain, including turmeric (curcumin), omega-3 fatty acids, glucosamine and chondroitin, and magnesium, but we've found vitamin D and collagen peptides to be the most beneficial.

Making changes at work

We don't know what you do for a living, so we can't give you any specific suggestions to change what you're doing at work or how you're doing it, but we can offer some general advice. Here's the single most effective "change" you can make to reduce back pain.

Do work you love or find a way to love the work you do.

Job satisfaction is the single factor that has the greatest impact on back pain in the workplace and the most research to back it up. Finding ways to enjoy work is probably the most important and effective worker-initiated intervention.

Other changes you may be able to make at work fall under the rubric of *ergonomics* — design factors for the workplace intended to maximize productivity by minimizing worker fatigue, discomfort, and injury. Feel free to experiment with ergonomic factors as much as you can in your workplace to find out what works best for you:

>> **Modifying the workstation.** Modifications include using a lordotic chair if you sit for a long time, adjusting your keyboard height so your elbows bend

at a 90-degree angle, setting up the monitor so that your neck is either slightly flexed or extended, using headphones so you can talk on the phone hands-free, and using an adjustable desk that you can sit or stand at.

>> **Enhancing your physical capabilities.** You or your employer may have equipment or techniques that enable you to perform physical tasks easier and with less risk of injury. Strengthening your body also falls in this category.

>> **Adjusting the frequency and/or duration of a physical activity.** Modifying the time or intensity of an activity, taking frequent breaks, or rotating job responsibilities can all help to support back health and may be especially helpful in preventing repetitive stress injuries.

WARNING

Be careful about putting your trust in any generic ergonomic solutions. What's effective for one person may not be as effective for another. Solutions need to account for the following factors:

>> **Back anatomy:** Everybody is built a little differently.

>> **History of back trauma:** Whether a person has had back trauma and the nature of that trauma are instrumental in determining which modifications, if any, are likely to be most effective.

>> **Genetic susceptibilities:** A tendency for discs to desiccate (dry up) or a particular facet shape can make a person more vulnerable to suffering back strain when performing a certain task or performing it in a certain way.

Unfortunately, modern medicine and ergonomics haven't yet reached a level at which they can offer solutions that are effective for all or most people suffering from back pain. In fact, that may never happen. The solutions that hold the most promise are personalized and account not only for each individual's anatomy, genetics, and history of back trauma but also their mindset and their willingness to engage in a rigorous back–strengthening regimen.

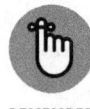

REMEMBER

We understand that not all employers will allow their workers to experiment with getting up from their desks every hour or tempering the frequency or duration of more strenuous or repetitive activities in a work week. However, if you've found that something at work is associated with your back pain, we encourage you to initiate a conversation with your supervisor to explore remedies. Although your employer has some responsibility to ensure workplace health and safety, it's your responsibility to communicate your needs and take the initiative to find solutions.

Replacing R.I.C.E. with M.E.A.T.

When back pain visits, as it will for approximately 80 percent of the population, treat it as a natural occurrence, a normal part of life. The newest and most successful form of physical therapy is called M.E.A.T. (movement, exercise, analgesics, and treatment). M.E.A.T. is an active treatment protocol for injuries affecting the joints, muscles, and tendons. This treatment protocol consists of the following four components:

>> **Movement:** The movement of the joint creates an environment that promotes tissue growth and repair by increasing the flow of nutrient-rich blood to the injury site. Movements should be gradual and controlled to minimize pain and avoid further injury. Most people increase movement gradually under the guidance and supervision of a physical therapist, but you can do it on your own. Start with the gentle movements we present in Chapter 8.

>> **Exercise:** As soon as the pain is manageable, you can begin to exercise the injured limb or joint, gradually increasing movement and load. Exercise further increases the flow of nutrient-rich blood to the injury site while increasing strength and mobility. Again, you can start exercising under the guidance and supervision of a physical therapist or on your own. (See Chapters 8 and 9 for movements and exercises.)

>> **Analgesics:** "Analgesic" is a fancy word for "pain reliever." It can be a medication, such as acetaminophen or ibuprofen; a physical treatment, such as ice or pressure; a natural supplement, such as turmeric, ginger, capsicum, or magnesium; or a topical ointment or cream, such as Arnica or the Chinese liniment dit da jow. See Chapter 15 for more about pain relief.

>> **Treatment:** Treatment consists of any medical intervention, such as acupuncture, Active Release Technique (ART), chiropractic adjustments, myofascial release, massage, red light therapy, electrical stimulation, surgery, and others.

The M.E.A.T. protocol has taken favor over its predecessors, R.I.C.E. (rest, ice, compression, and elevation) and P.R.I.C.E. (protect, rest, ice, compression, and elevation). Why? As we explain throughout this book, the body wants to heal itself, and the key, particularly when it comes to back pain, is movement. So, if you consider R.I.C.E. and P.R.I.C.E., there's ice involved and rest. That protocol contains nothing to stimulate movement and blood flow. The only real use of the ice is as an analgesic for pain relief, which is in the M.E.A.T. protocol but *after* movement and exercise. M.E.A.T. has proven itself to be more effective than its predecessors and has demonstrated quicker recovery times, especially for treating soft-tissue injuries. Obviously, with a fracture or compound fracture, exercise and movement are *not* recommended until the bone has healed.

Chapter 7

Building Your Core and Hidden Core

At its most basic, your body is a torso (core) with a neck, head, and four appendages. Back pain usually originates in the torso or neck, specifically along the spine. Likewise, the treatment for back pain (and the key to preventing its recurrence) typically focuses on the torso and neck — specifically, the spine, along with the muscles, tendons, and ligaments that support it.

Almost regardless of what's triggering your back pain, strengthening the muscles that support the spine and enable its mobility is often the best approach to managing the pain. In short, you want to strengthen your core (your torso), especially, your *hidden core* — certain back muscles that are often neglected.

In this chapter, we introduce you to the basics of building a strong core and hidden core and provide guidance on posture that's essential to healthy and safe movement.

What (and Where) Is Your Hidden Core?

Our patients and clients consistently tap their bellies when saying they need to improve their core strength, but the core is a cylindrical wall of connected muscles that extend around the entire upper body. It consists of front, side, and back muscles that are interconnected by *fascia* (thin, tough tissue that encases and binds body parts). This interconnectedness enables the contraction of all of the muscles to squeeze the abdominal contents and act as a "hydraulic amplifier" that stiffens the spine (in a good way).

The cylindrical core has an outer and inner component, as shown in Figure 7-1. The outer component, consisting of the abdominals, obliques, and lower back extensors, is responsible for flexing, extending, and bending from side to side, while the inner component, consisting of the diaphragm, multifidus, transversus abdominis, and pelvic floor muscles, acts more as a spine stabilizer. In addition to the two layers around the abdomen, the cylindrical structure of the core attaches upward to the pectorals, lats, and serratus muscles and downward to the psoas, quadriceps, and gluteal muscles (see Figure 7-2). These latter connections are essential for connecting and stabilizing the spine with the pelvis.

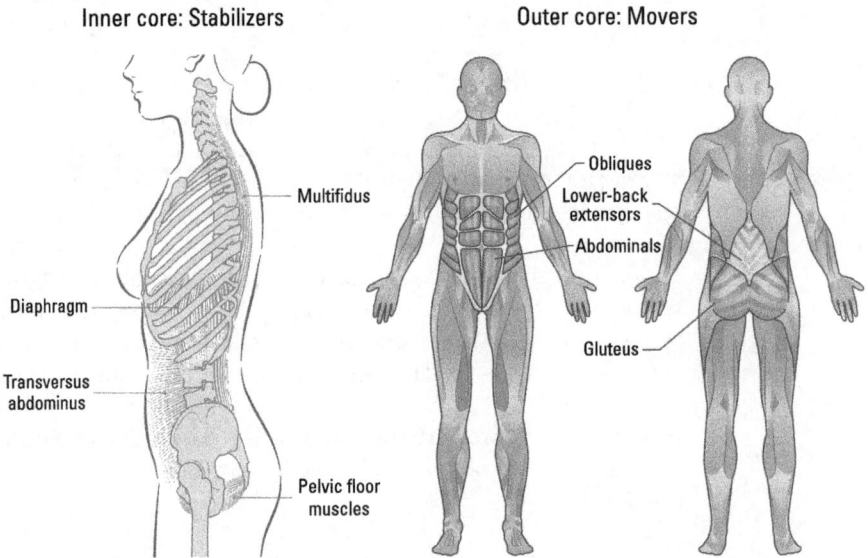

Inner core: Stabilizers

Multifidus

Diaphragm

Transversus abdominus

Pelvic floor muscles

からだ・けんこうサポーター/*Adobe Systems Incoprated*

Outer core: Movers

Obliques

Lower-back extensors

Abdominals

Gluteus

VectorMine/*Adobe Systems Incoprated*

FIGURE 7-1: The cylindrical core has an outer and inner component.

One hundred years ago, Pilates conceptualized and extolled the virtues of the *transversalis muscle*, the main contributor to the inner-front part of the core — the *anterior core*. It's incredibly important and deserves the attention Pilates gives it. We aim to do the same for the *posterior core*, in particular, the *multifidus muscles*, which we call the "hidden core."

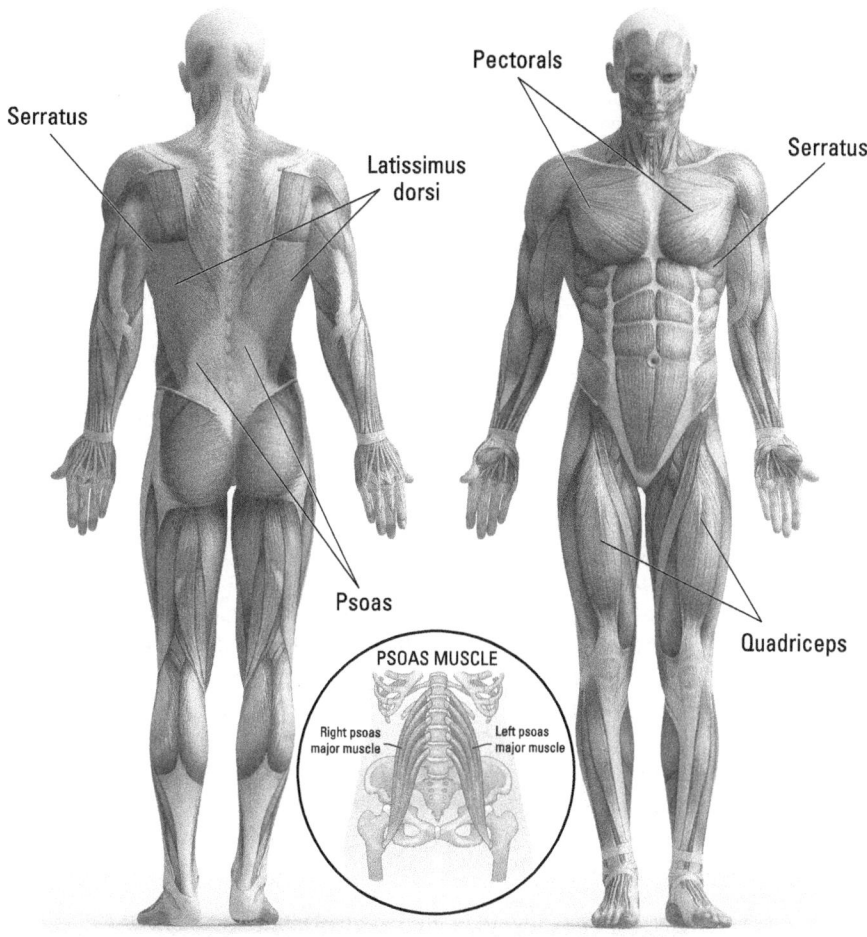

Serratus

Pectorals

Latissimus dorsi

Serratus

Psoas

Quadriceps

PSOAS MUSCLE

Right psoas major muscle

Left psoas major muscle

FIGURE 7-2:
The core attaches upward to the pectorals, lats, and serratus muscles and downward to the psoas, quadriceps, and gluteal muscles.

adimas/Adobe Systems Incoprated

VectorMine/Adobe Systems Incoprated

By "hidden," we mean both anatomically and metaphorically. Ever since the discovery of mirrors, people have paid more attention to their front sides. Because the anterior core is easier to see, people give it more focus, but the posterior core is equally important, especially in the management of back pain.

The posterior core has an outer layer, the erector spine muscles, and the inner layer, the multifidus muscles. The multifidus muscles are special because they provide *inter segmental movement* (each vertebral body can be moved individually) so that they can together move the entire spine or separately move individual vertebrae.

REMEMBER

Together, this posterior chain of muscles is the "hidden core" and the key to back health. Strengthening these muscles enables you to properly hip-hinge (keep your back straight when reaching down), and strengthening these muscles reduces back pain. After surgery, these muscles can atrophy and be a source of back pain.

This can be seen on an MRI of the spine. Strengthening these muscles reverses the atrophy and alleviates the back pain.

TIP

Focus less on developing the muscles that you can see when you look in a mirror and more on developing the muscles you can't see — the muscles of your hidden core. Even a person who carries very little body fat and is "ripped" will not see these support muscles, which are essential to spine health. Strengthening your hidden core will do far more to alleviate back pain and improve your appearance (by improving your posture) than having a six-pack.

Mastering Core Fundamentals

In Chapters 8 and 9, we provide exercises for strengthening the core, including the hidden core. However, before subjecting your back to any sort of weight-bearing or resistance exercise, focus on ensuring that your spine is structurally sound with respect to your posture. You wouldn't stand on a ladder that's leaning to the left or right or set a heavy stack of books on a table or chair that's teetering to one side, so don't subject your spine to any sort of load, including your own bodyweight, without proper spinal alignment and support.

In this section, we present five techniques for ensuring proper spinal alignment and support. You can think of them as five best practices for maintaining good posture.

Maintaining a neutral spine

Maintaining a neutral spine means assuming a posture that conforms to the natural curves of your spine — the *kyphotic curve* (the gentle forward "hunch" to the upper back (thoracic spine) and the *lordotic curves* at the neck (cervical spine) and lower back (lumbar spine) in the opposite direction (see Figure 7-3). Remind yourself throughout the day, whether you're sitting, standing, or crouching down, "Neutral spine all the time!" Make it your mantra.

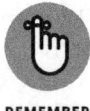

REMEMBER

Assuming and maintaining a neutral spine is essential for proper posture and preventing injury, especially when you're lifting or sitting or standing for long periods of time.

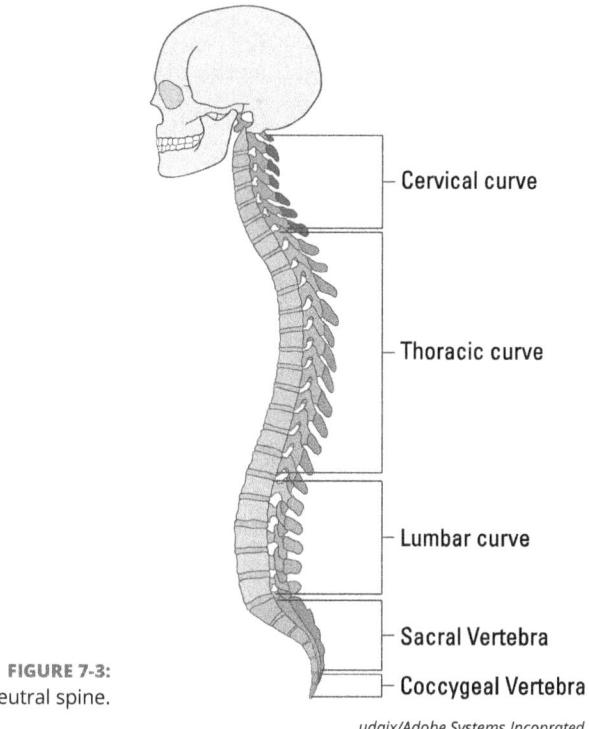

Neutral spine.

Cervical curve

Thoracic curve

Lumbar curve

Sacral Vertebra

Coccygeal Vertebra

udaix/Adobe Systems Incoprated

To physically understand and reinforce the concept of a neutral spine, practice the following exercise:

1. **Stand tall with your feet aligned with your hips, knees slightly bent (not locked), and your weight evenly distributed (not leaning back or forward).**

2. **Engage your abdominals just enough to support your spine while maintaining your ribcage alignment (not pushing it out or letting it collapse inward).**

3. **Shift your pelvis as necessary to a neutral position.** To find neutral, arch your lower back and then round your lower back; neutral is the comfortable position between those two extremes.

4. **Maintain the natural curve of your lower back toward the front of your body (your lower back's lordotic curve; refer to Figure 7-2).** Don't try to flatten it.

5. **Keep your upper back in a natural position without thrusting your chest outward or rounding your shoulders forward.** Your shoulder blades should be slightly pulled back and down (see the later section, "Packing your shoulders").

CHAPTER 7 **Building Your Core and Hidden Core** 111

6. **Align your head with your spine, eliminating any tilt up, down, or to either side. Imagine a straight line extending from the crown of your head down to your spine.** Your neck should be curved slightly, and you should be looking straight ahead.

Here are a few tips for maintaining a neutral spine when you assume different body positions:

>> **Standing:** Stand straight, not stiff. Imagine a string attached to the top of your head gently pulling you upward as you look straight ahead.

>> **Sitting:** Keep your feet flat on the floor, legs and knees bent at about 90 degrees, hips slightly higher than your knees. Sit in a chair or use a lumbar support that helps you maintain the natural curvature of your lower back.

>> **Lying down:** When lying on your back, place a rolled-up towel or small pillow under your knees to maintain your lower back's natural curve. When lying on your side, place a pillow between your knees.

>> **Crouching/lifting:** Bend at your knees while keeping your torso erect (not leaning forward just enough to maintain your balance) — see the later section, "Getting hip to the hip-hinge" for details.

Packing your shoulders

When we tell you to pack your shoulders, we're advising you to hold them back, pull them down toward your waist, and make your neck as long as possible. These movements immediately put you in the "Head up, chest out, and shoulders back position." We also refer to these movements collectively as *scapular retraction*; you're essentially pulling your *scapulae* (shoulder blades) together, as shown in Figure 7-4.

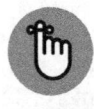

The shoulders are built for mobility over stability, which makes them vulnerable to injury. For stability, they rely on several muscles, especially these three:

>> *Trapezius* is the large triangular muscle that spans the upper back and neck. It helps to ensure the shoulder blades move correctly and remain stable during arm movements, such as lifting, pulling, and pushing.

>> *Rhomboids*, which are located between the shoulder blades, help to stabilize the scapulae (shoulder blades) and keep the shoulders from rounding forward.

>> *Latissimus dorsi* (lats) is a large muscle that runs from the lower back to the upper arm and is primarily responsible for shoulder extension, *adduction* (moving the arm toward the body), and internal rotation.

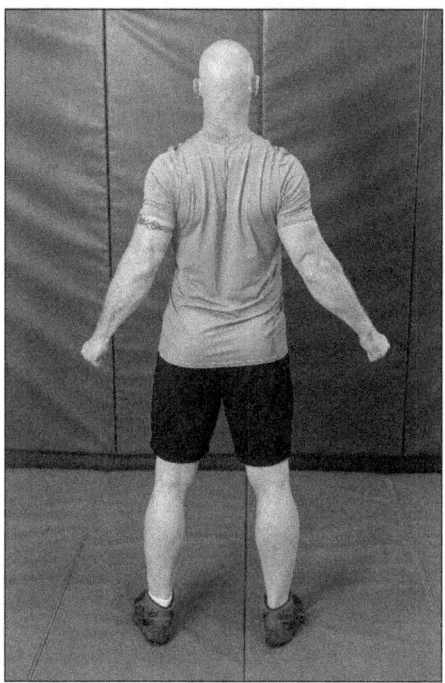

FIGURE 7-4:
Scapular
retraction.

Strengthening these muscles can improve shoulder stability and movement, prevent injury, and reduce any shoulder or upper back pain. The exercises in Chapters 8 and 9 help to develop these and other shoulder and back muscles.

Tightening your butt and gut

In addition to constantly reminding yourself to maintain a neutral spine, remind yourself to tighten your butt and your gut. When you tighten your butt and gut, you're drawing your hips forward while engaging your abdominal muscles, thus forming a protective "cylinder" around the hips and spine. This cylinder ensures that the weight you're carrying above your hips is transferred straight down to your legs.

REMEMBER

By maintaining a neutral spine, packing your shoulders, engaging your lats, and tightening your butt and gut, you create a solid, cylindrical structure that can bear an incredible amount of weight and carry much of the burden that would otherwise be transferred to the spine.

Getting hip to the hip-hinge

We often advise people not to bend their backs to pick something up. Almost invariably, they get a bewildered look on their face, as if we had just told them to bend over without bending over. However, you can reach down without bending your spine by squatting slightly and hip-hinging. Here's how:

1. **Stand erect, feet about shoulder-width apart.**

   Maintain a neutral spine as you perform the next step.

2. **Bend your knees while thrusting your butt back and hinging your torso forward at the waist.** Pretend that you're trying to sit on a chair that's too far behind you.

   Your feet should be planted firmly on the ground, knees bent slightly, spine neutral, butt back, your back at about the 10 o'clock position, and your tailbone at about the 4 o'clock position (see Figure 7-5). If your hamstrings are very flexible, you may be able to hip-hinge down so that your back is nearly parallel to the ground.

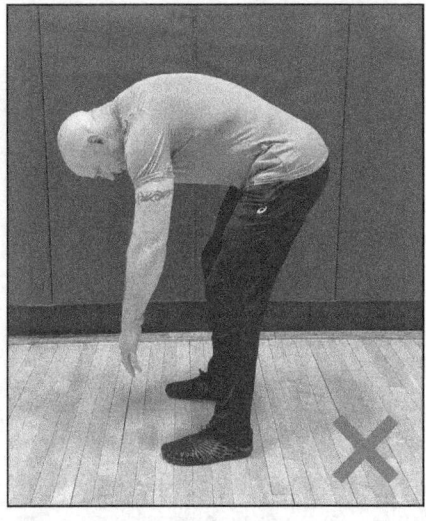 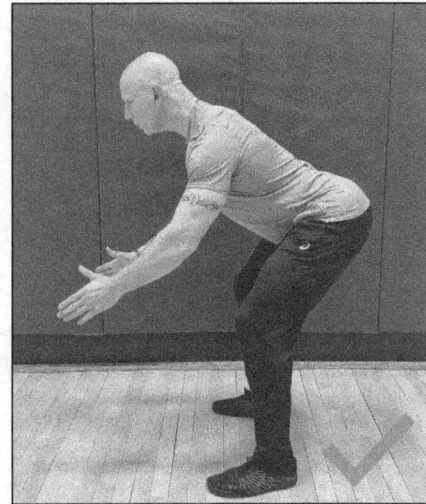

FIGURE 7-5:
Hip-hinge. The curved back (left) is incorrect. The neutral spine on the right is correct.

TIP

Proper form is essential. If you're rounding your back, you're doing it wrong. Here are a few tips that may help:

>> **Squeeze your shoulder blades together (scapular retraction) to prime your back before hip-hinging.** Packing your shoulders keeps the spine neutral.

>> **If trying to sit on a chair that's too far behind you doesn't work for you, imagine you have a big tiger tail, and someone is pulling it back.** If that doesn't work, try karate-chopping your hips; chop your hands simultaneously into your hip flexors (the fronts of your hips where you hinge at the waist).

> » Team up with a partner to observe and critique your form, or use your smartphone to record yourself so you can be sure you're not rounding your back.

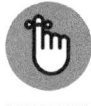

REMEMBER

Not everyone can hip-hinge correctly right off the bat. I (Phil) was teaching a kettlebell certification course, and one of the strongest students in the class just wasn't getting it. The other 60 students in the class got it, and we had to move forward, but I needed him to get it, too. Out of frustration, I feigned a kick to his groin. Driven by a strong self-preservation instinct, he pulled his groin back and thrust his butt back behind himself, performing a perfect hip-hinge. I'm not recommending this as a teaching method; I'm just pointing out that given the proper instruction (and, in some cases, motivation), everyone eventually can figure out how to do it.

Breathing behind the shield

"Breathing behind the shield" involves maintaining tension in the core and compression in the lungs to brace the spine, especially when picking up an object or hoisting it overhead. What you're doing is filling your lungs with air while tensing your core muscles to create a solid air-filled structure like an air mattress or a car tire — in this case, a pneumatic pillar. This structure carries much of the load that would otherwise be transferred to your spine.

REMEMBER

You don't need to take a deep breath. You only need to fill your lungs with enough air to maintain compression through the duration of the movement.

Your hidden core needs a certain measure of strength to execute this technique. If the hidden core is weak, you won't be able to maintain the required degree of tension. Build your core strength gradually by starting with the movements and exercises in Chapter 8. When you're comfortable performing those movements and exercises, proceed to Chapter 9.

Paying Attention to Your Upper Back and Neck

Although the lower and middle sections of the core get all the press coverage, we think of the core, especially the hidden core, as extending up through the upper back and neck. The upper back and neck muscles are crucial to back health and function, and we would be remiss not to stress their importance in a book about managing back pain.

Many strong and healthy individuals who do a very good job developing their core muscles, along with the muscles in their arms and legs, neglect their neck muscles. Even worse, many of the trainers we talk to openly admit that they don't spend any time training their necks, meaning they're not encouraging their clients to train their necks either. Instructors *should* be aware of the fact that the neck is part of the spine and that the muscles of the neck are integral to back health, and they should be teaching their clients to train their necks.

REMEMBER

The neck supports the head, and a weak neck can lead to stress, pain, headaches, and even temporomandibular joint (TMJ) issues (the TMJ is the joint where the jawbone connects to the skull). The stronger and more supple your neck, the less pain and discomfort you're likely to experience.

Immediately below the neck is the upper back region. This region is home to the trapezius, deltoids, rhomboids, and a host of smaller but no less important support muscles. These muscles play a key role in shoulder stability and mobility, but they also act together to increase spinal integrity throughout the upper back and neck.

The takeaway message here is this: As you strengthen your core, don't neglect your neck and upper back. Many of the movements and exercises we present in Chapters 8 and 9 engage these muscles, and a few of the movements and exercises target them specifically.

IN THIS CHAPTER

» Focusing your efforts on strength and mobility

» Building a balanced core — front and back

» Recognizing the importance of maintaining a neutral spine

» Keeping it cheap and simple with broomstick exercises

» Getting started with basic back-building exercises — no weights!

Chapter **8**

Laying the Foundation for Optimal Back Health

To build anything in life, whether it's a physical building, a healthy body, a successful career, or something entirely different, you first need to lay a firm foundation. A building requires a solid substructure; a healthy body requires nutritious food, fresh air, and challenging physical and mental activity; a successful career requires education and training in a certain trade or field. To build a strong and healthy back, you have two foundations to attend to:

» **Physical foundation:** The physical foundation of back health is your *core* — the central part of your body, essentially your torso and your butt. Your neck, which isn't a part of your core, is also a crucial component of back health. Exercises and other movements for improving back strength and mobility focus on building your core and other muscles that support your spine.

» **Fundamentals (concepts and exercises):** Fundamentals are essential concepts and exercises that you must master before moving on to intermediate and advanced back strengthening.

In this chapter, you focus on laying a firm foundation for building a strong and healthy back by mastering fundamental concepts and exercises that specifically target your core.

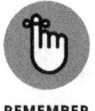

REMEMBER

Master the fundamentals and focus on core strength and mobility first. These components lay the foundation on which intermediate and advanced techniques rest.

Prioritizing Strength and Mobility Over Flexibility

Fitness gurus and instructional materials often recommend focusing on flexibility before strength and stretching before strengthening. Many recommend stretching for several minutes *before* beginning any exercise. We recommend getting your body in motion first. Here's the sequence we recommend that you follow for every exercise session (we also recommend that you focus on increasing strength and mobility for days or weeks before incorporating stretching into your routine):

1. **Mobilize and warm up.** Elevate your heart rate and increase your core temperature to reduce the risk and severity of injury. A good warm-up also sets the stage for higher performance during a session.

2. **Perform your strengthening exercises.** Working your muscles first increases blood flow to the muscles and joints, thereby improving mobility. Start with light exercise before getting into more strenuous movements. We cover strengthening exercises throughout this chapter and the next.

3. **Perform self-massage.** Massaging your muscles improves circulation, reduces tension, and relaxes the muscles. You can self-massage by gently kneading (squeezing and releasing) your muscles, using a massage gun or foam roller, or using other devices and techniques.

4. **Stretch your muscles.** Stretching your muscles after exercise and massage (when they're warm and relaxed) improves flexibility and range of motion over time. We're not recommending that you forgo stretching, only that you do it last.

WARNING

Don't stretch a pulled muscle. A muscle pull is a tear in the muscle. Stretching it can aggravate the tear. Imagine a towel or other fabric with a tear in it. Tugging on that towel or fabric near the tear would only make it worse. The same is true of a muscle. Decide whether you have a "hurt" (pain with little to no tissue damage) or an "injury" (significant tissue damage). If you're able to move and the damage isn't significant, movement, exercise, analgesics, and treatment (MEAT), along with gentle massage, is the best approach. If you have a more extensive injury, protect, rest, ice, compression, and elevation (PRICE) is the better approach.

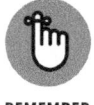

REMEMBER

Flexibility is important but less so than muscle strength and mobility. Recognize and appreciate the differences among these three qualities:

>> **Strength** is both physical power and endurance. Muscle strength is important for supporting the skeletal structure, moving the body, and getting the blood flowing.

>> **Mobility** is the ability to move through a full range of motion. It's directly attributed to both the strength and the flexibility of the muscles and joints. Several factors affect mobility, including injury to the muscles, joints, tendons, and ligaments and the formation of scar tissue. You can restore mobility through purposeful exercise focused on muscle strengthening, self-massage, and stretching.

>> **Flexibility** pertains to how far a joint can move and how much a muscle can stretch (its elasticity). Lengthening muscles improves their mobility and the power they can deliver. If you've ever held a cat, you know that its muscles are loose, but if you try to hold a cat down against its wishes at a veterinary clinic, it can practically lift you off your feet. Its muscles are long, so when it contracts those muscles, it can perform powerful movements.

When you experience back pain, the source of the pain may be unclear at first. You may not know which structure(s) are responsible for the pain — the muscles, the ligaments, the joints, or something else entirely. Starting your treatment with strengthening and self-massage prevents further injury as you build strength and circulation around the injury site. As your back strength increases and your body heals, you can add stretching to your routine.

TIP

Focus daily on increasing mobility. Mobility increases strength and flexibility while improving blood flow, which promotes healing. As mobility increases, strength and flexibility naturally increase as well, and you will feel better overall. Your body will love you for it!

Building Strength and Endurance

Strengthening muscles is about more than building biceps, triceps, quads, and calves. Muscles deliver both power and endurance. Generally, the deeper muscles that support the skeleton and promote good posture are endurance muscles. They are slow-twitch muscles, which don't *hypertrophy* (pump up) as much as the visible, powerful muscles of the arms and legs. These muscles are the most important to target for improving back health and reducing back pain. They're optimally trained for endurance rather than strength, which enables you to engage in an activity for a sustained period of time without succumbing to fatigue. Endurance makes exercise sessions more productive and accelerates progress. Endurance allows for sustained and improved posture. Think about the contrast between doing squats and running. Squats optimize leg strength while running optimizes leg endurance. Similarly, the core should be trained optimally with high reps of low weight to build endurance.

Traditional endurance workouts, such as running on a treadmill and training on other aerobic equipment (such as rowers or steppers), are not the only solutions. You may have more fun and better neurological engagement by dancing or boxing, doing Zumba or martial arts, or participating in other fun, stimulating, and physically intense activities.

TIP

Consider a workout that combines strength with muscular and cardiovascular endurance, such as one or more of the following:

>> **High-intensity interval training (HIIT):** Alternating short bursts of physically exhausting exercise with brief periods of rest or low activity.

>> **Circuit training:** Completing a set of physically challenging exercises that include endurance training, resistance training, and high-intensity aerobics.

>> **Hybrid calisthenics:** A form of strength training that combines weight training with exercises that use only your body weight (calisthenics).

>> **Skipping rope:** A whole-body exercise that involves jumping over a rope as it passes beneath one's feet. This old-school exercise popularized in schoolyards and classic boxing movies builds strength, endurance, and coordination.

These workouts are fun, challenging, and a heck of a lot more engaging than watching TV while running on a treadmill like a hamster on an exercise wheel.

REMEMBER

The American Heart Association recommends that adults do a minimum of 150 minutes of moderate-intensity or 75 minutes of high-intensity aerobic activity per week. If you break that down into daily workouts, it equates to five 30-minute moderate-intensity workouts or five 15-minute high-intensity sessions per week. Only about 20 percent of the adult population in the U.S. meets this recommended minimum.

Warming Up and Getting Limber

At least once every day — preferably shortly after you wake up and before any other exercise session — get your body moving with some gentle warm-ups. Make it part of your morning ritual — roll out of bed, hit the restroom, start brewing a pot of coffee, grab your broomstick or bo staff (more about that in a minute), and perform the gentle movements we present in this section.

Follow the lead of the family pet — the first thing they do when they get up from a nap is walk around slowly and stretch. You should do the same. It's a great way to start your day!

Mobilizing your back with a broomstick: Six essential movements

You can perform several essential back-building movements using a narrow rod (one inch or so thick) about as long as you are tall (or a couple of inches shorter) — a broomstick, a curtain rod, a PVC pipe, or any similar object will do the trick. If you're into martial arts, consider using a bo staff.

In the following sections, we present six essential back–building movements you can perform with a broomstick or similar object.

Maintain a neutral spine throughout these movements.

The neutral spine drill

Maintaining a neutral spine all the time is essential for improving back pain and preventing injury. The neutral spine drill helps to train neutrality into your spine. Take the following steps:

1. **Stand straight with your feet slightly farther apart than shoulder width, toes pointed slightly outward.**

   Maintain rhomboid engagement throughout these steps.

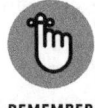

2. **Hold your staff behind you vertically along your spine, as shown in Figure 8-1. Grasp one end with your left hand above your head and the other end with your left hand just below your butt.** The staff should touch the three critical points of your spine — the back of your skull, your upper back, and the point where your lower back meets your butt.

3. **Shift your weight to your heels and stick your butt out behind you as you hinge at the hips while maintaining contact between the staff and the three critical points of your spine (see Figure 8-2).** Maintain tension throughout the back and tighten the abdominals while performing this movement.

4. **Repeat Steps 1–3 to complete about ten reps.**

Side twists

Side twists are great for toning the *obliques* — the muscles to either side of your abdominals. To do side twists, take the following steps:

1. **Stand erect, feet about shoulder-width apart, and hold your staff across the back of your shoulders, parallel to the floor, with hands spaced about 12–18 inches out from each shoulder (see Figure 8-3).**

   This is the starting position for the rest of the broomstick exercises.

2. **Tighten your gut and your butt while keeping your ribs down.**

   Tightening your gut and butt engages your "hidden core" — the core muscles you never see. This step is critical to creating a "cylinder of power," which helps to stabilize the core and create a solid base for many of these broomstick movements.

3. **Twist your torso from side to side while squeezing your obliques (see Figure 8-4).** Do ten reps on each side.

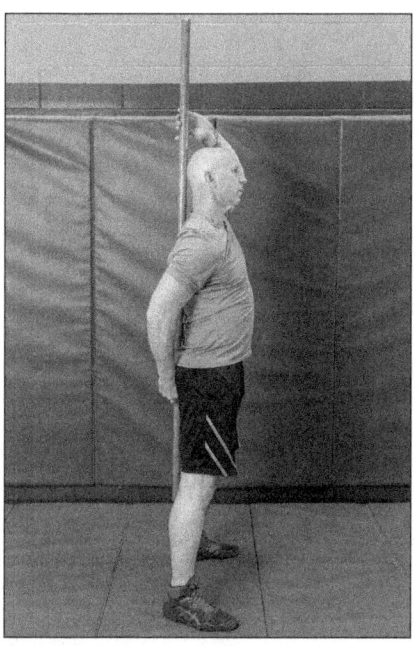

FIGURE 8-1:
Hold the staff along your spine.

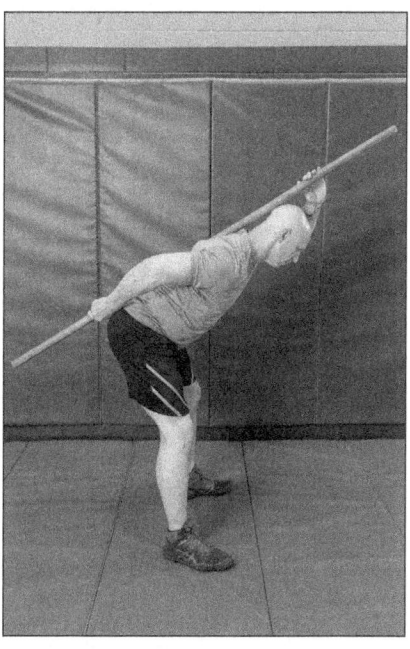

FIGURE 8-2:
Hip-hinge forward while bending your knees slightly and moving your butt back.

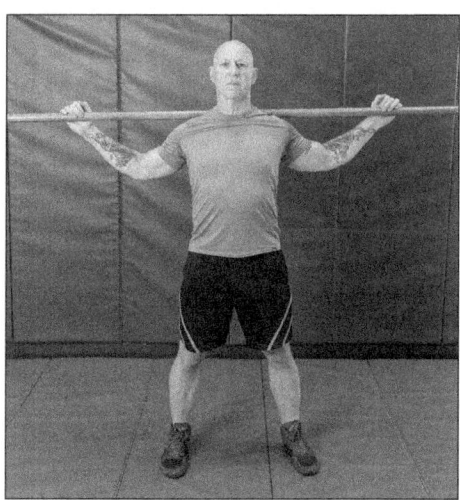

FIGURE 8-3:
Stand erect while holding your staff across the back of your shoulders.

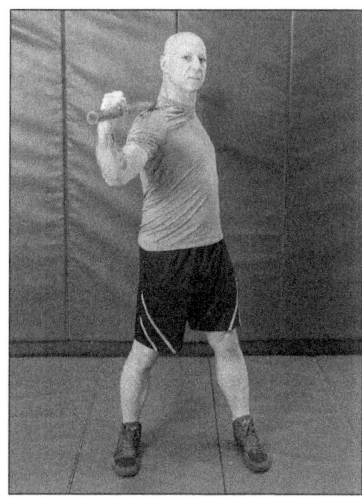

FIGURE 8-4:
Twist from side to side while squeezing your obliques.

Side bends

Side bends are great for strengthening the internal and external oblique muscles and increasing lateral (side-to-side) lumbar flexibility. To do side bends, take the following steps:

1. Stand erect, feet about shoulder-width apart, and hold your staff across the back of your shoulders, parallel to the floor, with hands spaced about 12–18 inches out from each shoulder, as shown in Figure 8-3.

2. Tighten your gut and your butt while keeping your ribs down.

3. Bend to one side while keeping your hips and shoulders along the same plane as you bring your elbow down toward your hip, as shown in Figure 8-5. Repeat this motion ten times on alternating sides.

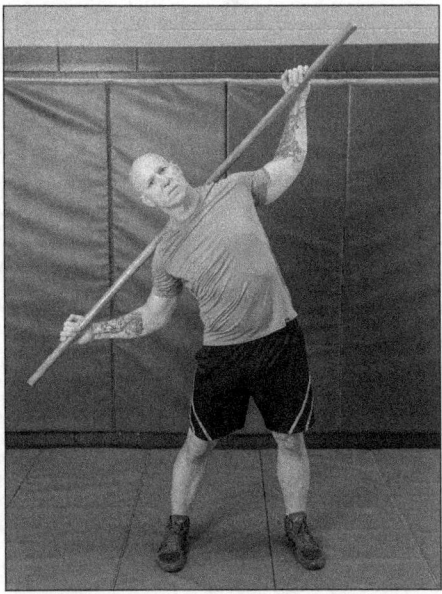

FIGURE 8-5:
Bend from side to side.

Reachbacks

Reachbacks help to tone the rhomboids. To perform reachbacks, follow these steps:

1. Stand erect, feet about shoulder-width apart, and hold your staff across the back of your shoulders, parallel to the floor, with hands spaced about 12–18 inches out from each shoulder, as shown in Figure 8-3.

2. Tighten your butt and gut while keeping your ribs down.

3. Move your elbows back and then return to a relaxed position (as if you're "flapping your wings"), repeating this motion ten times.

Bent-over twists

Bent-over twists force you to hold a hip-hinge isometrically — contracting the muscle against resistance without changing the length of the muscle (which improves back muscle endurance) — while doing a rotational range of motion of the lumbar spine and hips. Here's what you do:

1. **Stand erect, feet about shoulder-width apart, and hold your staff across the back of your shoulders, parallel to the floor, with hands spaced about 12–18 inches out from each shoulder, as shown in Figure 8-3.**

2. **Tighten your gut and your butt while keeping your ribs down.**

3. **Bend your knees slightly and hip-hinge, and lean forward slightly so that your torso is in the 10 and 4 o'clock or 9 and 3 o'clock positions.**

4. **Twist your upper body from side to side, as shown in Figure 8-6, repeating this motion ten times each way.**

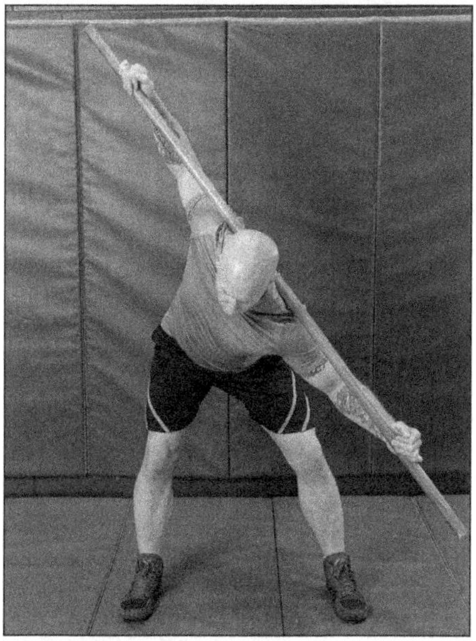

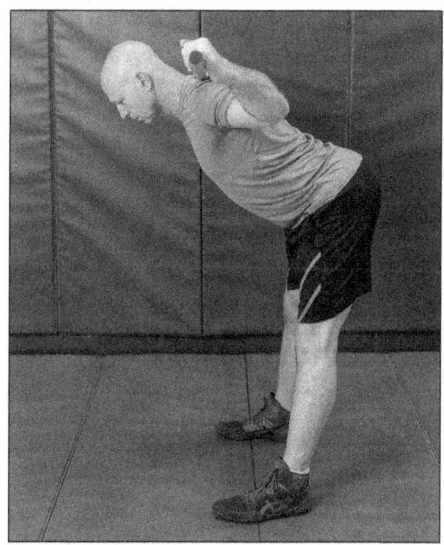

FIGURE 8-6:
The bent-over twist.

Good mornings

Good mornings are like the traditional touch-your-toes stretch but with a staff. They're great for improving lower back mobility and flexibility. To perform this movement, take the following steps:

1. **Stand erect, feet about shoulder-width apart, and hold your staff across the back of your shoulders, parallel to the floor, with hands spaced about 12–18 inches out from each shoulder, as shown in Figure 8-3.**

2. **Tighten your gut and your butt while keeping your ribs down.**

3. **Bend forward at the waist as far as possible while keeping your knees and back straight (neutral), as shown in Figure 8-7.** Do ten reps.

FIGURE 8-7:
The good morning stretch.

TIP

Always maintain good posture by holding your shoulders back and down and your head up with your spine in a neutral position.

Limbering up your joints

Your joints carry a heavy load beyond just bearing weight; they help to stabilize the body and facilitate movement. Limbering up your joints shortly after waking up and before any strenuous activity prepares them for the work they're about to do. It increases blood flow to the joints, lubes them up by stimulating the production of synovial fluid, improves flexibility and range of motion, and reduces the risk of injury. In this section, we present gentle movements for limbering up your joints from head to toe . . . well, actually, from ankle to neck.

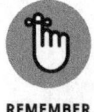

REMEMBER

Joints favor mobility or stability, but even those that favor stability need to be mobile and should be warmed up soon after waking and before performing any strenuous activities.

Ankles: Mobility

Start with ankle rotations in a standing position (neutral spine):

1. **Rest the ball of one foot on the floor and roll the ankle in all four directions.** Repeat this movement, alternating clockwise and counterclockwise, for 8–10 repetitions with each foot.

2. **Rock your feet from side to side so you're shifting weight back and forth between the insides and outsides of your feet.** Focus on using the ankles for movement and minimizing knee movement. Repeat 8–10 times.

Knees: Stability

Knees favor stability, but they need to have some degree of mobility. The following movement can help:

1. **Stand erect, bend the knees slightly, and place your hands above (not on) the kneecaps.**

2. **Rotate your knees in *very small* circles, using your hands and a slight squatting/standing motion to guide your knees.** Repeat for 8–10 repetitions in both directions.

Hips: Mobility

Plenty of dance songs testify to the fact that hips favor mobility, so get those hips in motion:

1. **Place your hands on your hips and flex your knees slightly.**

2. **Rotate your hips a full circle clockwise or counterclockwise and then in the opposite direction.** Repeat this motion 4–5 times.

Thoracic: Mobility

To mobilize your upper back (thoracic region), do the standing zombie roll:

1. **Stand erect and apply tension from your solar plexus (the bottom center of your rib cage) on down.** The area above your solar plexus should be as loose as possible.

2. **Drop your head, relax your neck, arms, and shoulders, and roll the upper section of your body around in a circle.** Do five repetitions in alternating directions.

TIP

Note that we skipped the lumbar region, which favors stability because the area gets warmed up while opening the hips (below) and performing the thoracic movements (above).

Shoulders: Stability

Shoulders, especially the *glenohumeral joint* (the ball and socket), generally favor motion, although the shoulder blades favor stability. To mobilize your shoulders, take the following steps:

1. **Extend your arms wide, palms up, and arch your chest toward the ceiling (see Figure 8-8).**

   Keep your arms relatively straight throughout the full range of this movement.

REMEMBER

2. **Bring your arms forward while rotating them inward so that your wrists touch, and bow your head, as shown in Figure 8-9.** Do five repetitions.

Elbows: Stability

Although elbows favor stability, they do a lot of bending. To warm them up, perform the following exercise:

1. **Pin your hands to your sides with your fingers and thumbs of each hand pointing straight down.**

2. **Slide your hands down as if you're putting money into your pockets, but continue down as far as you can reach.** Then, slide them back up. Repeat five times.

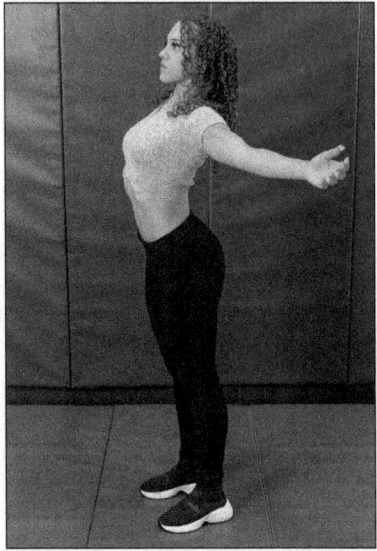

FIGURE 8-8:
Start with arms outstretched, palms up, chest up.

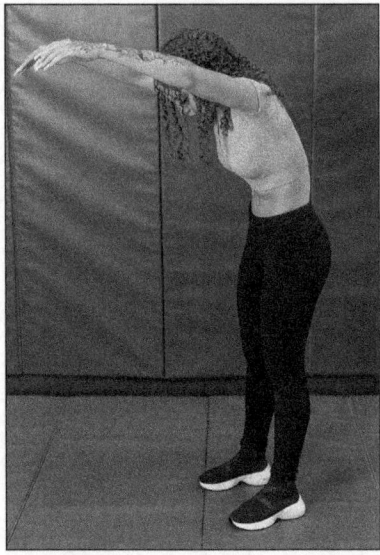

FIGURE 8-9:
End with your wrists touching, head bowed.

Wrist Rolls: Mobility

Wrists favor mobility, so be conscious of just how much you're holding them in one position throughout the day, and put them through their full range of motion several times daily. This exercise can help:

1. **Press your palms together, interlock your fingers as if you're praying, and pin your elbows to your ribs.**

2. **Roll your wrists around and around, ten times in each direction, keeping your elbows pinned to your sides as you rotate your wrists along their full range of motion.** When you go in the opposite direction, it may seem strange at first. The elbows should remain stationary.

Neck: Mobility

Keeping the neck mobile is essential to good health. You can reduce headaches and other effects of stress (and reduce stress overall) by ensuring that your neck moves freely and can maintain a neutral position. This exercise can help:

1. **Hold your wrists behind you, grabbing one wrist with the opposite hand, pull your arms down, make your neck as long as possible, and *pack your shoulders* (pull them down and back).**

   Maintain this position for the duration of the four movements that follow.

REMEMBER

2. **Perform the following four motions:**

   - **Side to side:** Rotate your head as far as possible right and then left.

   - **Ear to shoulder:** Keep the head in the same plane as the shoulders and tilt it to one side and then the other (see Figure 8-10).

   - **Down and back:** Bring the head all the way forward and all the way back (see Figure 8-11).

   - **Pendulum swing:** Tuck the chin while rotating your head clockwise and counterclockwise so that your chin follows the collarbone.

WARNING

   Do not roll your neck in a complete circle because such a movement could harm your cervical spine.

3. **Perform ten repetitions of each in each direction.**

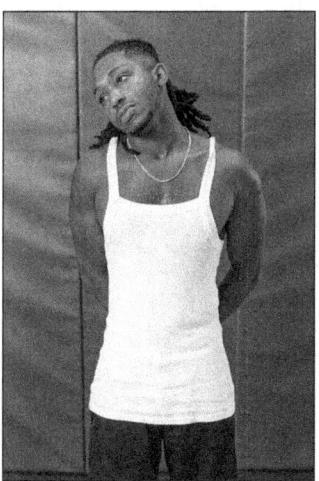

FIGURE 8-10:
Ear to shoulder.

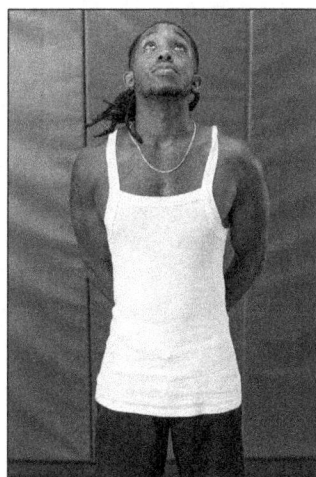

FIGURE 8-11:
Down and back.

Back-Building for Beginners: Using Only Your Bodyweight

Back-building doesn't require pumping iron, and you don't need any fancy equipment. All you need is a body — your body, that is. In this section, we present over a dozen back-building exercises that require only your body weight. These exercises can be incredibly effective at targeting all the major muscles of the back, including the latissimus dorsi, rhomboids, and trapezoids, while also helping to improve posture, mobility, stability, flexibility, and overall strength.

Do something every day to maintain your mobility, whether it's exercise, such as riding a bike, rowing, or walking on a treadmill, or a common activity, such as gardening or doing household chores. Plan to spend 5–25 minutes a day engaging in a variety of activities and/or exercises that get your body moving.

Every other day, focus on your core. In this section — and in Chapter 9 — we provide an array of core mobility and strengthening exercises to choose from. You don't have to do all of them every day; you can choose 5–10 exercises for each session and rotate them so you're not neglecting any areas or creating imbalances. We recommend dedicating 15–20 minutes three times a week to this core work. If you're doing additional strength training, do your core work at the end of your workout; you don't want to fatigue your core muscles prior to doing strenuous strength training when you need a strong core for support.

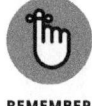

REMEMBER

In the movements below, we use the letters P, A, and T to designate which areas a movement engages:

>> **P** = Posterior chain (hidden core)

>> **A** = Anterior core (abdominals)

>> **T** = Transverse plane (contralateral movements)

Crunches, planks, rolls, and more

This section contains a hodgepodge of exercises that engage various back muscles.

Crunch (A)

Crunches are great for the abs, assuming you can tolerate them. If they're too painful to do, substitute with planks until you reach a point at which you can do crunches (see the later section "Tall Plank" for details). To perform a basic crunch, take the following steps:

1. **Lie flat on your back, knees bent and above your hips, fingers behind your ears, elbows back.** Tilt your pelvis to keep your cervical spine and head off the ground, which will keep your upper and lower abdominals engaged.

2. **Contract your abdominals, bringing your back up as high up as possible off the ground, and squeeze your abs when you reach the top of the movement.**

3. **Relax your abdominals to bring your upper body back toward the ground without letting your head or feet touch the ground.**

4. **Repeat steps 2 and 3 as many times as you can.**

Cross-elbow-to-knee crunch (A)

This variation of a basic crunch engages the obliques and helps you develop more side-to-side mobility:

1. **Lie flat on your back, knees bent, feet flat on the ground, fingers behind your ears and elbows out.**

2. **Contract your abdominals, lift one knee, and raise and twist your torso to one side to bring your opposite elbow to the raised knee, as shown in Figure 8-12.**

3. **Relax your abdominals to bring your upper body back toward the ground without letting your head touch the ground.**

4. **Repeat steps 2 and 3 as many times as you can, alternating sides.**

TIP

Twist and squeeze the abdominals and switch sides rapidly while keeping your head off the ground.

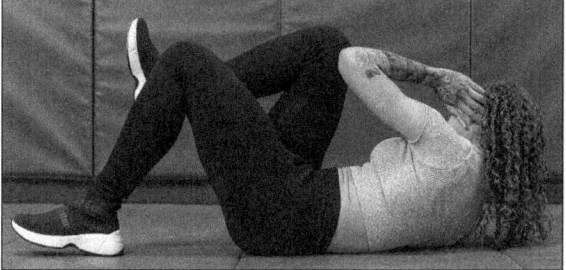

FIGURE 8-12:
The cross-elbow-to-knee crunch.

Tall plank (P, A)

Planks are the staple of core-building exercises. To perform a tall plank, take the following steps:

1. **Assume the push-up position, arms extended with your spine in the neutral position.**

2. **Tense your body by tightening your gut and butt, packing your shoulders (holding them back and down), engaging your lats, and bringing your kneecaps up into your quadriceps.**

3. **Hold this position for 15–30 seconds.** We don't recommend firing all your muscles for any longer than 30 seconds.

Pilates egg (P, A)

The Pilates egg is a back roll that engages your abdominals and back muscles. To do a Pilates egg, take the following steps:

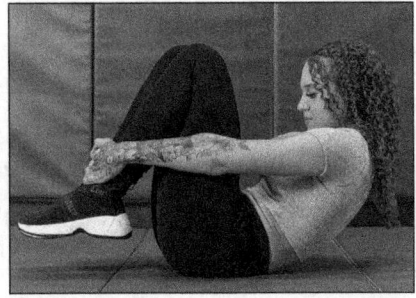

1. **Sit on the floor with a neutral spine and feet flat, and grab around your shins (see Figure 8-13).**

2. **Tuck your head and "rock" back and then forward to return to the sitting position, inhaling as you rock back and exhaling as you reach the top of the movement.**

3. **Repeat 5–10 times.**

FIGURE 8-13:
Grab your shins, tuck your head, and rock back and forth.

Bird dog (P, A, T)

The bird dog engages the hips, shoulders, abdominals, lats, knees, and more. To do the bird dog, take the following steps:

1. **Get down on all fours as though you're about to give a small child a horsey ride.**

   Keep your hips and shoulders parallel to the floor and your abdominals engaged throughout this exercise.

REMEMBER

2. **Extend your right arm and left leg as far out as possible, as shown in Figure 8-14, and hold this position for a couple of seconds.**

3. **Bring your right elbow and left knee together, as shown in Figure 8-15, hold for a second, and then extend them out again.** Repeat this movement about five times.

4. **Repeat Steps 2 and 3 with your left arm and right leg.**

5. **Repeat Steps 2–4 to complete a total of about five reps.**

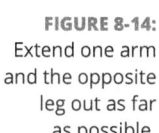
FIGURE 8-14: Extend one arm and the opposite leg out as far as possible.

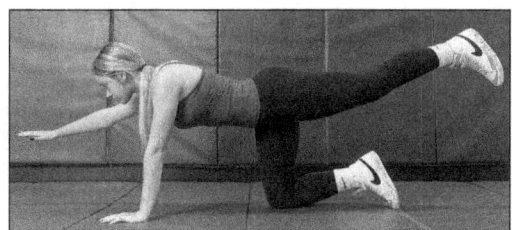

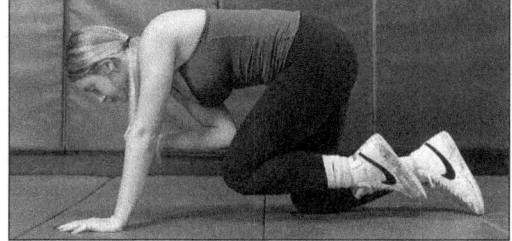

FIGURE 8-15: Bring your knee up and your elbow down.

Superman/woman (P, T)

The Superman/woman is a great movement for building core strength and reducing asymmetries. Here's what you do:

1. **Lie face down on the floor with the arms outstretched above your head, legs straight and raised above your body (see Figure 8-16).**

2. **Lift your right arm while rotating your head right and lifting your left leg off the ground.**

3. **Hold this position for a count of three seconds.**

4. **Repeat Steps 2 and 3, alternating sides for a total of ten reps per side.**

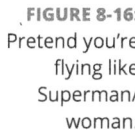
FIGURE 8-16: Pretend you're flying like Superman/woman.

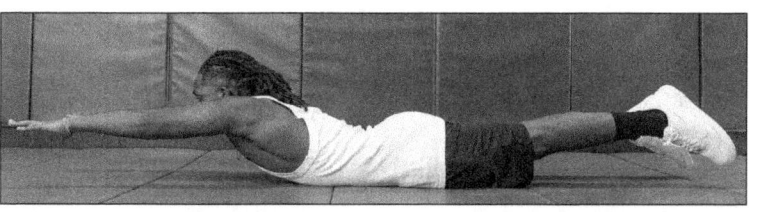

Scapular retraction (P)

Scapular retraction is great for strengthening and mobilizing the rhomboids — muscles that control and stabilize the shoulder blades (scapulae). You use these muscles in nearly every back-strengthening exercise we cover in this chapter and the next.

To do a scapular retraction, simply pull your shoulder blades down and as far back as possible (see Figure 8-17). Imagine *squeezing* a lemon between your shoulder blades. Your shoulders should go back, and your chest should push out.

REMEMBER

Scapular retraction is key to developing and maintaining good back health.

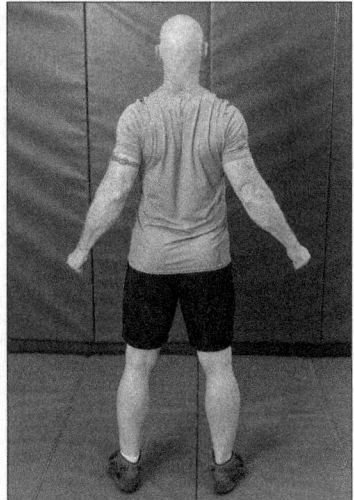

FIGURE 8-17:
Scapular retraction in action.

X-roll (P, A, T)

No, this move doesn't involve hooking up with your ex for a little tête-à-tête, but it's an excellent core-building exercise all the same. Here's how it's done:

1. **Lie face down, arch your back, stretch your arms and legs to form an X shape, arms and legs off the floor, and tighten your core (see Figure 8-18).**

2. **Roll to one side to complete one full rotation (see Figure 8-19).** You should complete this step face down.

3. **Repeat Step 2, rolling in the opposite direction, and continue rolling in alternate directions to complete a total of 3–5 reps in each direction.**

FIGURE 8-18:
Start your x-roll face down.

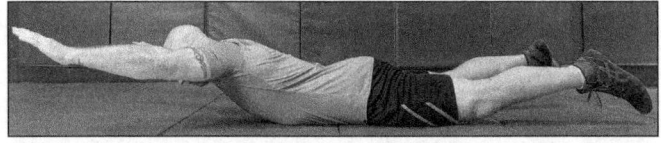

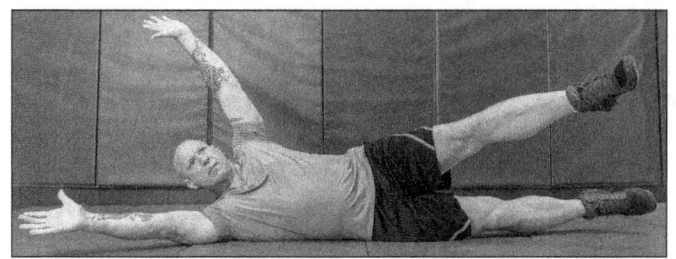

FIGURE 8-19:
Roll to one side to complete one full rotation.

Zombie roll (P, A, T)

Wanna roll like a zombie? If so, this one's for you. The Zombie roll works your upper back and shoulders and engages the core. Here's what you do:

1. **Lie on your back, arms extended out to your sides, and totally relax your lower body.**

2. **Bring your right arm up and across your body, as shown in Figure 8-20, and roll to the left as you raise your arms over your head and continue to roll onto your stomach with your arms extended straight out above your shoulders, palms down.** Your upper body does the rolling, and your lower body is dead weight that simply follows the motion of your upper body.

3. **Continue rolling by raising the left side of your torso and reaching back with your left arm, as shown in Figure 8-21, until you're flat on your back again (one full rotation).**

   Avoid any temptation to engage your glutes. Relax those butt muscles!

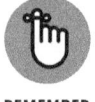

REMEMBER

4. **Repeat Steps 2 and 3, reaching across with your right arm, this time rolling in the opposite direction.** Roll five times in each direction.

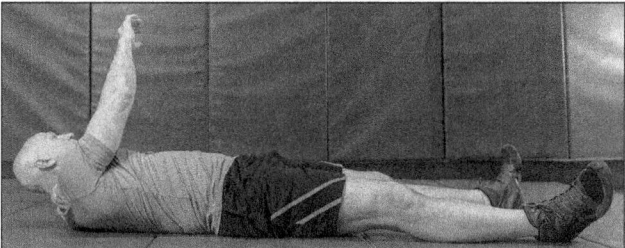

FIGURE 8-20:
Bring your right arm across your body to make it roll in that direction.

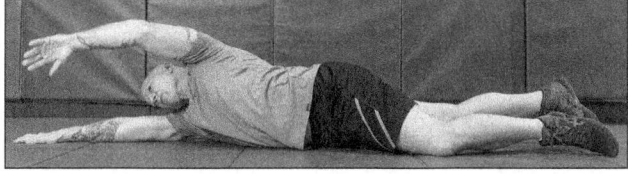

FIGURE 8-21:
Raise your left arm and reach back to continue rolling onto your back.

Cobra stretch (P)

The cobra stretch arches the lower back to increase its mobility and strengthen the support muscles of the spine. To perform a traditional cobra stretch, take the following steps:

1. **Lie face down on the floor, hands close to your shoulders, palms down, elbows pointing back as if you're about to do a push-up, the tops of your feet against the floor.** (See Figure 8-22.)

2. **Contract your glutes and your lower and upper back muscles and drive your hips into the floor while pushing your upper body off the floor and lifting your head toward the ceiling.** (See Figure 8-23.) At the top of the movement, your elbows should be locked in place.

   TIP

   Try using your abs and back muscles to do most of the lifting. In other words, try not to put too much pressure on your hands.

3. **Hold this position for 3–5 seconds and then lower yourself gently to the ground.**

4. **Repeat Steps 2 and 3 to complete 5–10 repetitions.**

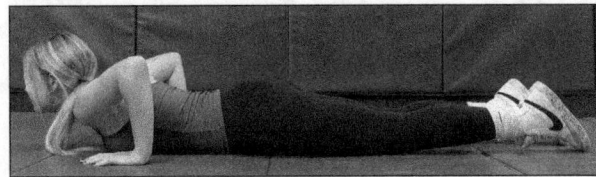

FIGURE 8-22: Lie face down on the ground in a push-up position but with the tops of your feet against the floor.

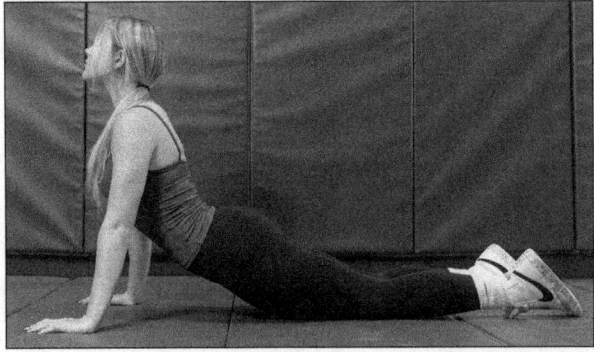

FIGURE 8-23: Push up to raise your torso off the ground.

After completing your repetitions of the cobra pose, do a child's pose, as explained in the next section, for a count of five seconds.

Child's pose (P)

The child's pose is a classic yoga position that's great for stretching and lengthening the spine and relieving muscle tension. To perform the child's pose, take the following steps:

1. **Kneel and point your toes down so the tops of your feet touch the ground.**

2. **Extend your arms above your head and bend all the way forward to bring your palms to the ground.** (See Figure 8-24.)

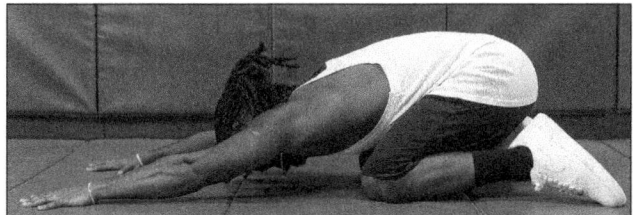

FIGURE 8-24:
Child's pose

TIP

You can do another version of the cobra by starting face down in a conventional push-up position, with palms flat on the ground a little below your shoulders. Push your upper body up while leaving your legs in contact with the floor. Keep your head level — looking forward.

Cat and cow (P)

The cat and cow is great for warming up in preparation for a back-building session, for cooling down afterward, or whenever your back is feeling tight. It's great for increasing spinal mobility, stretching the abs, and getting the spinal fluid flowing. To do the cat and cow, perform the following steps:

1. **Get down on all fours, wrists below your shoulders, and knees below your hips.**

2. **Gradually tighten your abs while arching your upper back upward, as shown in Figure 8-25, and hold this position for a few seconds.** This is the cat position.

3. **Slowly relax your abs, allowing your lower back to return to the neutral position, as shown in Figure 8-26, and hold this position for a few seconds.** This is the cow position.

4. **Repeat Steps 2 and 3 four to five times.**

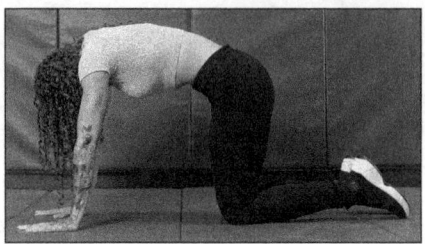

FIGURE 8-25:
Arch your back like a threatening cat.

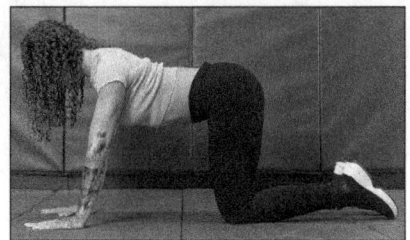

FIGURE 8-26:
Let your lower back slump like that of a cow.

Snake (P, T)

The snake, not to be confused with the cobra pose, is a great exercise for toning the core as a whole but especially the side muscles. Here's how you do it:

1. **Get down on all fours, toes bent and pressing against the ground.**

   REMEMBER

   Don't turn your head. Keep it in the same plane as your neck and back, face parallel to the ground throughout the exercise.

2. **Scrunch your body to the right, trying to bring your right ear and right hip together, as shown in Figure 8-27.**

   REMEMBER

   Perform this movement slowly and with some measure of tension through the body.

3. **Repeat Step 2 to the opposite side and continue to alternate sides for a total of ten repetitions per side.**

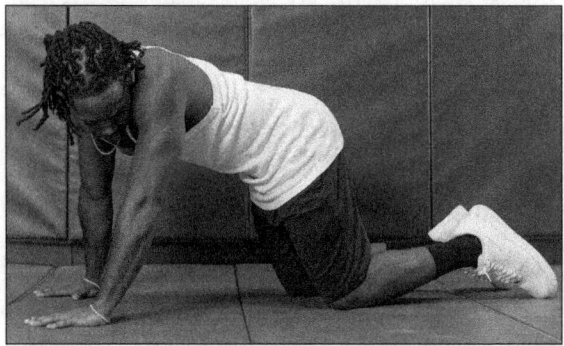

FIGURE 8-27:
Try to bring your hip to your ear.

Gelebart abs (A)

I (Phil) learned this movement in the 1980s from the late, great Raul Gelebart, a dance and fitness instructor in New York City. He laughed when I told him that I named a back-building movement after him, but what he showed me lives on. Gelebart abs are great for building core strength and mobility. Here's what you do (best done on an exercise mat):

1. Lie on your back, knees bent, feet flat on the mat, arms extended in front of you, palms up.

2. Drive your hips and lumbar spine into the mat and tense your entire body, squeezing up in the abdominal area to raise your upper body slightly off the mat and bring your hands over your knees (see Figure 8-28). Exhale slowly at the peak of the movement.

3. Repeat Step 2, but instead of reaching your hands over your knees, reach them to the outside of one knee, as shown in Figure 8-29.

4. Repeat Step 3, reaching your hands to the outside of the opposite knee.

5. Repeat Steps 2–4 until you've completed four repetitions for the center position and three repetitions to each side.

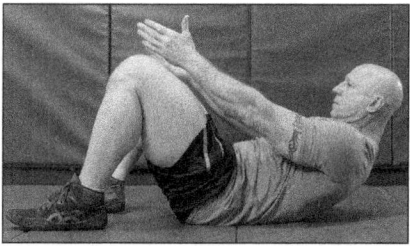

FIGURE 8-28:
Gelebart abs to center position.

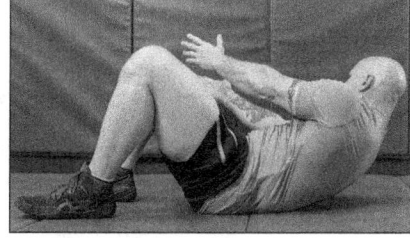

FIGURE 8-29:
Gelebart abs to the right.

Bridges

Bridges involve arching your body, which strengthens your core muscles and builds both mobility and flexibility. A bridge serves as a means of connecting two areas — in this case, the upper and lower body. Bridgework is essential for strengthening the posterior chain. The following sections guide how to perform several different bridge movements.

Glute bridge (P)

The glute bridge is the most basic and easiest to perform of all of the bridges. Take the following steps:

TIP

1. **Lie flat on your back and with your feet up as close to your butt as possible, arms at about a 45-degree angle to your body pressed to the ground, palms up (see Figure 8-30).**

   The closer the knees are together, the more difficult the bridge is to perform, so adjust the space between your knees to the desired level of difficulty.

2. **Drive through the heels and squeeze your hamstrings, lumbar muscles, and rhomboid muscles to bring the scapulae together, and raise your upper body off the mat as you exhale slowly (see Figure 8-31). Hold the peak position for 2–10 seconds.** As you become stronger and want to add variety, do your bridges for up to 30 seconds to increase your muscular endurance.

TIP

   To increase the arch of your back, you can grab your ankles. This variation enables you to create more tension by pulling on your ankles with your hands and creating a higher arch.

3. **Gradually lower your hips to the floor.**

4. **Repeat Steps 2 and 3 for ten repetitions.**

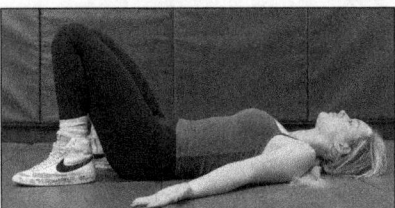

FIGURE 8-30:
Glute bridge starting position.

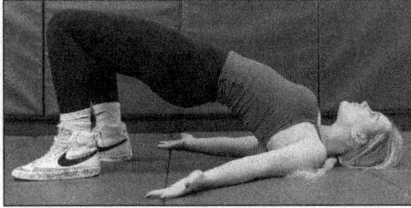

FIGURE 8-31:
Arch your back while squeezing your scapulae together and exhale slowly.

Straight leg bridge (P)

The straight leg bridge is one of the easiest to execute, but it engages and tones the entire posterior chain. To do a straight leg bridge, take the following steps:

1. **Sit on the floor with your legs together and straight out in front of you, toes pointed toward the shins, palms flat on the ground and slightly behind your butt, about shoulder-width apart, fingers pointed down toward your feet, and elbows locked, as shown in Figure 8-32.**

2. **Raise your hips upward to a neutral spine while pressing your feet together, as shown in Figure 8-33.** Hold the position at full contraction of the posterior chain (hamstrings, glutes, spinal muscles, and rhomboids) for a count of 2–5 seconds.

Avoid the common temptation to look at your feet; look up at the ceiling!

TIP

3. **Relax gradually, slowly lowering your butt to the floor.**

4. **Repeat Steps 2 and 3 for 10–15 repetitions.**

The triceps tend to get taxed a great deal during this exercise. Don't be surprised if they become sore.

REMEMBER

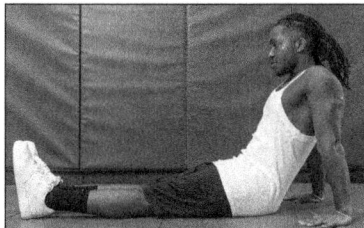

FIGURE 8-32:
Straight leg bridge starting position.

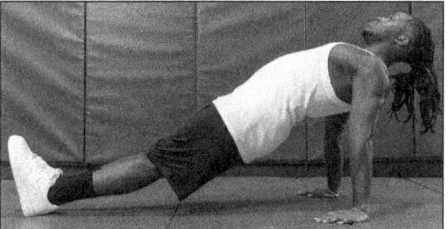

FIGURE 8-33:
Raise your hips to assume the neutral spine position.

Single leg bridge (P)

The single leg bridge requires more core strength than other bridges. Doing each side separately helps to iron out any asymmetries in strength. This movement also serves to stretch the hamstrings and increase the range of motion. Take the following steps to do a single leg bridge:

1. **Lie flat on your back, knees bent, feet flat with the heel of the left foot close to your butt, your right leg extended straight out with toes pointed up, arms at about a 45-degree angle, palms down, and lift your right leg straight up, as shown in Figure 8-34.**

2. **Squeeze the rhomboids, lumbar support muscles, and hamstrings as you elevate your hips as high toward the ceiling as possible, as shown in Figure 8-35.** Hold this position for a count of 3–5 seconds.

3. **Gradually lower yourself back down to the ground.**

4. **Repeat Steps 2 and 3 four to five times, and then repeat Steps 1–3 with your right foot close to your butt and your left foot extended straight out.** Do five reps for each leg.

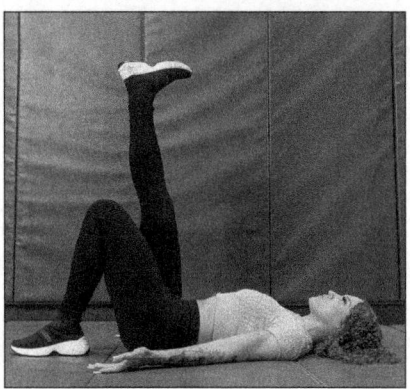

FIGURE 8-34:
Single leg bridge starting position.

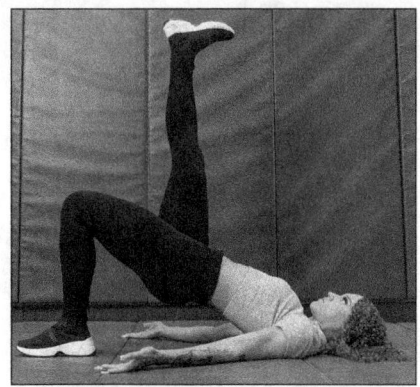

FIGURE 8-35:
Elevate your hips as high toward the ceiling as possible.

Runner's bridge (P, A)

The runner's bridge helps to mobilize your glutes and hamstrings. Dorsiflexion (raising the foot toward the shin) also engages the hip flexors. To do the runner's bridge, take the following steps:

1. **Lie flat on your back, knees bent, heels close to your butt, feet flat but toes curled upward, arms extended at about a 45-degree angle, palms up, and then lift one knee toward your chest, as shown in Figure 8-36.**

   Keep the knee as close to the chest as possible throughout the whole movement.

TIP

2. **Squeeze the rhomboids, lumbar support muscles, and hamstrings as you elevate your hips as high toward the ceiling as possible, as shown in Figure 8-37.**

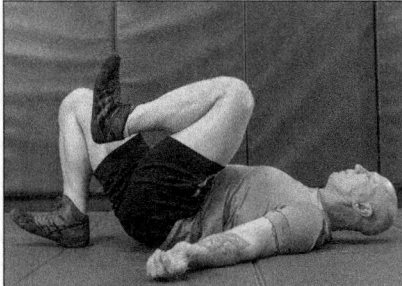

FIGURE 8-36:
Runner's bridge starting position.

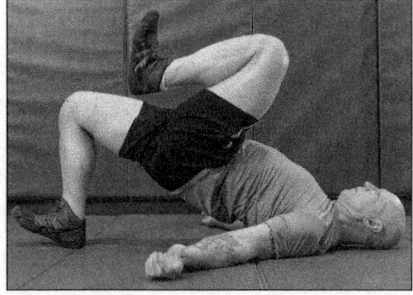

FIGURE 8-37:
Elevate your hips as high toward the ceiling as possible.

3. Hold this position for a count of 3–5 seconds.

4. Repeat Steps 1–3, alternating leg positions to perform five repetitions for each leg.

Tabletop bridge (P)

The tabletop bridge transforms your body into a coffee table, increasing core strength through sustained isometric contraction and extremity flexibility. It also benefits the shoulder girdle by increasing its strength and expanding its range of motion. To execute this movement, take the following steps:

1. Sit on the ground, knees bent slightly, feet flat, upper body leaning slightly back, arms extended behind you for support, elbows locked, palms down, fingers pointing down toward the heels of your feet, as shown in Figure 8-38.

2. Drive through the heels of the feet and the palms of your hands and bring the hips skyward as you contract your rhomboids, hamstrings, and glutes until your upper legs and torso form a flat "tabletop," as shown in Figure 8-39. Your spine should be in the neutral position. Hold this position for 3–5 seconds.

3. Gradually lower your butt to the ground and then repeat Steps 2 and 3 to perform a total of at least five reps.

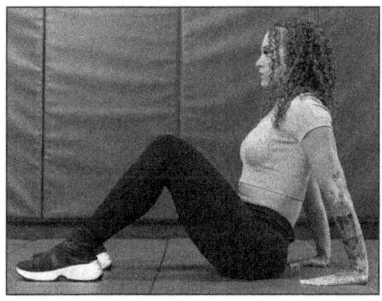

FIGURE 8-38:
Tabletop bridge starting position.

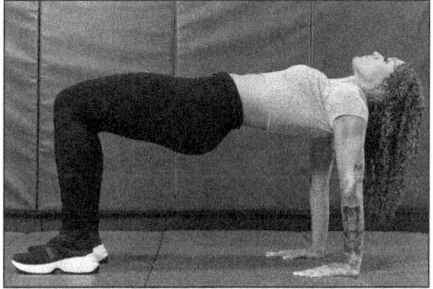

FIGURE 8-39:
Elevate your hips to the point of achieving a neutral spine.

The scale (T)

Also known as the single-leg Romanian deadlift (RDL), the scale is great for building balance as well as strength and mobility. Extending the body while supporting it on one leg requires and develops balance and strengthens the support muscles in the feet, legs, and back. To perform this movement, take the following steps:

1. **Stand tall with your spine in the neutral position, shoulders down and back, as shown in Figure 8-40.**

2. **Plant one foot into the ground, tighten your gut and butt, keep your hips in line with your shoulders, and allow your body to pivot forward from the hip of the leg that's planted, as your other leg swings back to maintain balance (see Figure 8-41).**

   REMEMBER Your body should not twist at all as your chest moves down and you swing your leg straight back.

3. **Stop pivoting and maintain your position when your chest and thigh are nearly parallel to the ground, as shown in Figure 8-42.** Hold this position for about five seconds.

4. **Repeat Steps 2 and 3, alternating leg positions until you've completed five reps for each leg.**

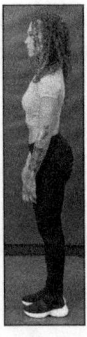
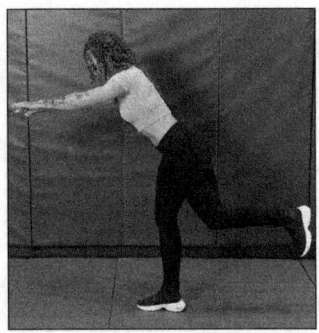
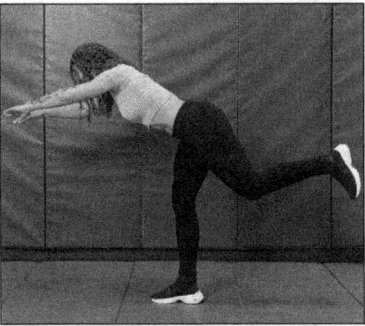

FIGURE 8-40:
Stand erect.

FIGURE 8-41:
Pivot on the hip that's set, bringing your chest down and swinging your other leg back.

FIGURE 8-42:
Hold this position for about five seconds.

Crawls

Children naturally move in ways that promote strength, mobility, flexibility, balance, and coordination. Unfortunately, as people age, they engage in many repetitive motions that are counterproductive to all these great abilities. Sometimes, returning to one's childhood can be just what the doctor ordered, so we encourage you to get back on the floor and start crawling around!

In this section, we present a few of our favorite crawls. Perform these movements forward and backward for maximum benefit.

The six-point crawl (T)

The six-point crawl is what most infants do. This is a great beginner crawling motion for beginning your floor work. This movement serves as a warm-up for the more demanding crawls and is a good one for deconditioned people to perform with little risk of injury.

1. **Get down on all fours so that your palms, knees, and balls of your feet (toes curled upward) are all in contact with the floor.**

2. **Move the hand on one side and its opposite knee forward at the same time, as shown in Figure 8-43, bring them to the ground, and then bring the other hand and its opposite knee forward and bring them to the ground.** You know how it's done! Keep alternating sides, crawling around on the ground.

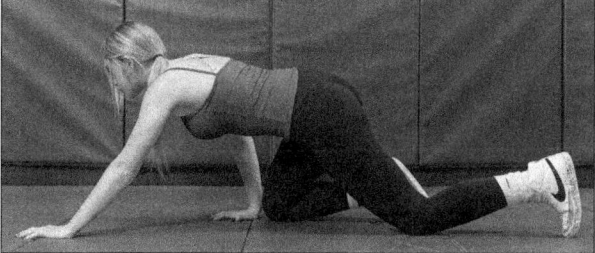

FIGURE 8-43: The six-point crawl.

The four-point crawl (T)

Do the four-point crawl just as you would do the six-point crawl, but without letting your knees touch the ground (see Figure 8-44). This crawl requires more effort and core engagement than the six-point crawl and develops more balance and strength.

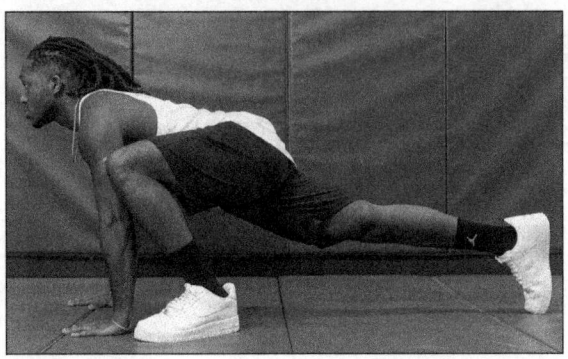

FIGURE 8-44:
The four-
point crawl.

The lizard crawl (T)

With the lizard crawl, you're lower to the ground, creating more exaggerated joint movements and putting more strain on your muscles. To do the lizard crawl, take the following steps:

1. **Get on all fours with the palms of your hands and the balls of your feet in contact with the floor, toes curled upward.**

2. **Position your body close to the floor.**

3. **Alternate moving one hand and its opposite leg forward at the same time as you drop your hips toward the ground so your rear end "wags" as you crawl in an "S" motion akin to the movement of a lizard.** As you bring your knee forward, it will ride above your elbow, as shown in Figure 8-45.

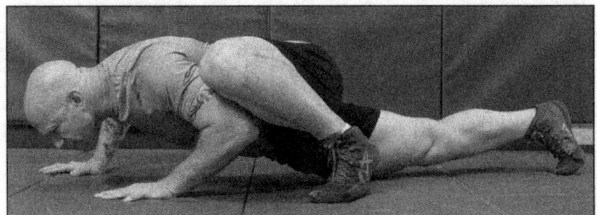

FIGURE 8-45:
The lizard crawl.

The upper-back triple-play

Three freehand exercises work wonders for developing strength and stability in the upper back, and they're relatively easy to do. The resulting improvements in strength and range of motion of the shoulder girdle and rhomboids are exceptionally beneficial to overall back health. Collectively, we refer to these three movements as the upper-back triple-play.

Perform each of these movements slowly, smoothly, and deliberately.

Pullbacks (P)

Pullbacks are great for toning the rhomboids. To do pullbacks, take the following steps:

1. **Stand erect and extend your arms straight out in front of you at shoulder level, palms down, fingers straight out (see Figure 8-46).**

2. **Bring your elbows back as far as possible while bending them to keep your fingers pointing forward, as shown in Figure 8-47.** Focus on squeezing your rhomboids together.

3. **Repeat Steps 1 and 2 for 8–10 reps.**

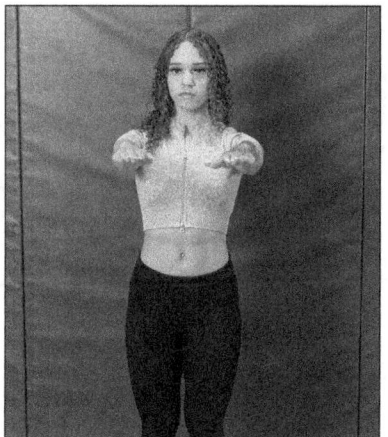

FIGURE 8-46:
Arms in front at shoulder level, palms down.

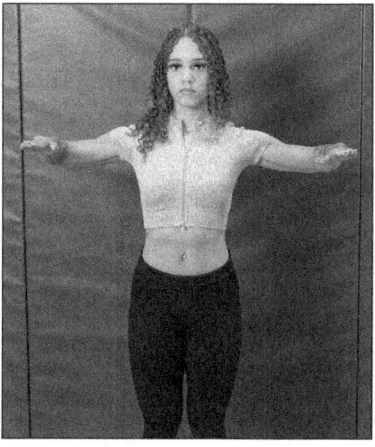

FIGURE 8-47:
Bring your elbows back as far as possible, keeping your fingers pointing forward.

Hand levers (P)

Hand levers flow naturally from pullbacks (which we cover in the previous section). They're great for developing strength and muscular endurance in the lats and the abdominals without the use of a pull-up bar. Here's what you do:

1. **Stand erect, arms raised to about shoulder height, elbows back as far as possible, hands pointing forward, palms down, as shown in Figure 8-47.** (This is the same position in which you end a pullback.)

Keep your elbows elevated and pulled back throughout the entire exercise. Except for rotating, your elbows should maintain their position.

2. **Rotate your upper arms to bring your hands down so they're pointing toward the ground, as shown in Figure 8-48.**

3. **Stick 'em up! as if a burglar were holding a gun to your back — hands up, palms forward, as shown in Figure 8-49.**

4. **Repeat Steps 1–3 to complete 8–10 reps.**

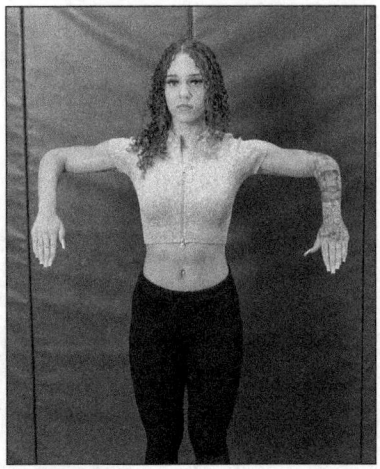

FIGURE 8-48:
Rotate your upper arms to bring your hands down.

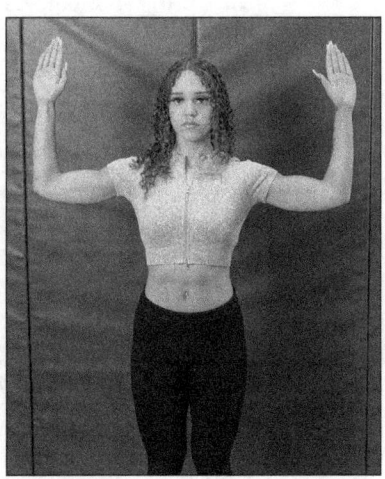

FIGURE 8-49:
Stick 'em up!

Straight arm squeeze (P)

The straight-arm squeeze is great for contracting your pectorals (chest muscles) while stretching your rhomboids. Here's what you do:

1. **Stand erect and extend your arms straight out from your shoulders, palms down, as shown in Figure 8-50.**

2. **Contract your chest muscles to bring your palms as close together as possible, as shown in Figure 8-51.** The broader your chest, the farther your hands will be apart. Don't bend your elbows or wrists to try to bring your palms together — no cheating!

3. **Repeat Steps 1 and 2 to complete 8–10 reps. When you bring your arms back, squeeze the rhomboids.**

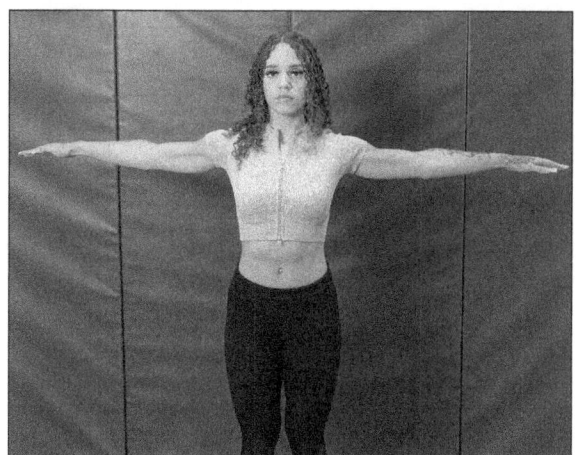

FIGURE 8-50:
Stand erect,
arms akimbo!

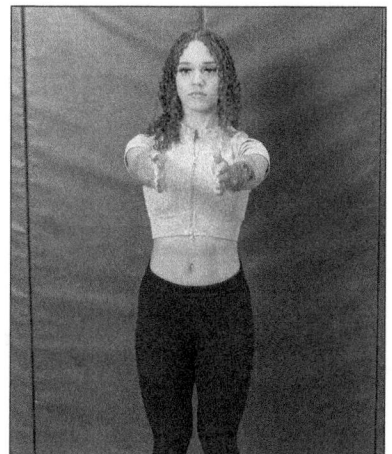

FIGURE 8-51:
Squeeze your
pecs, palms
facing
one another.

Neck-cercises: The four-way neck dynamic tension routine

The neck is an integral but often ignored component of the spine. Stretching the neck and maintaining its suppleness is a great start, but it's not enough. Strengthening the neck improves the spine's overall integrity.

WARNING

If you have an existing neck condition, proceed carefully with any neck-strengthening exercises. Start by applying only very light pressure, and then slowly and gradually increase pressure as you strengthen your neck muscles.

Here's a routine we suggest that you perform daily called the four-way neck dynamic tension routine:

1. Stand erect, neutral spine, with your feet shoulder-width apart.

   Maintain a neutral spine and stable stance for the duration of this movement.

2. **Place the palms of your hands on your forehead, fingers pointing upward, as shown in Figure 8-52.**

3. **Tilt your head back as far as comfortably possible, as shown in Figure 8-53.**

4. **Move your head forward slowly while applying counterpressure with your hands until your head is fully bowed.** Move your head forward slowly enough so that it takes about 10 seconds to move from fully back to fully forward. Apply counterpressure over the full range of motion.

5. **Move your hands to the back of your head, as shown in Figure 8-54.**

6. **Move your head back slowly while applying counterpressure with your hands until your head is as far back as comfortably possible (see Figure 8-55).** Move your head back slowly enough so that it takes about 10 seconds to move from fully forward to fully back. Apply counterpressure over the full range of motion.

7. **Move your head back to the neutral position without applying any counterpressure.**

   Keep your head and neck aligned along the same plan for the side-to-side movements in the next steps.

8. **Place your right hand on the right side of your head directly above the ear and use it to apply counterpressure as you tilt your right ear toward your right shoulder, maintaining packed shoulders (down and back) — see Figure 8-56.** Move your head/neck slowly enough so that it takes about 10 seconds to move from fully upright to as close as comfortably possible to your shoulder.

9. **Repeat Step 8 with your left hand, moving your head/neck in the opposite direction, as shown in Figure 8-57.**

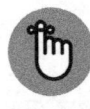

You don't need to develop a neck the size of Mike Tyson's, but having neck strength makes you far less susceptible to pain, and it serves as a "shock absorber" in the event of a motor vehicle accident or fall. Additionally, a stronger and more mobile neck reduces a great deal of stress on the entire body and can even help alleviate headaches.

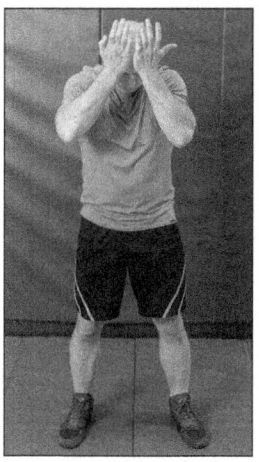

FIGURE 8-52:
Place the palms of your hands on your forehead.

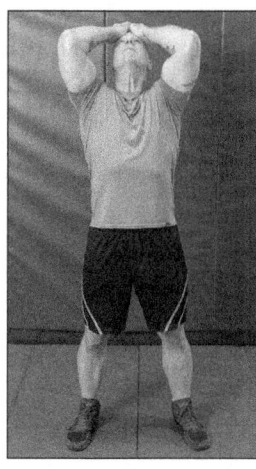

FIGURE 8-53:
Tilt your head back as far as comfortably possible.

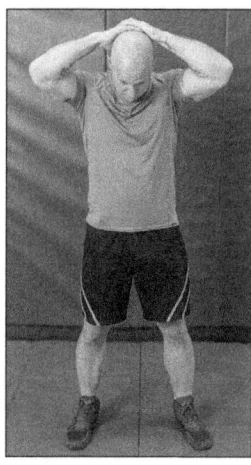

FIGURE 8-54:
Place your hands on the back of your head and bow forward.

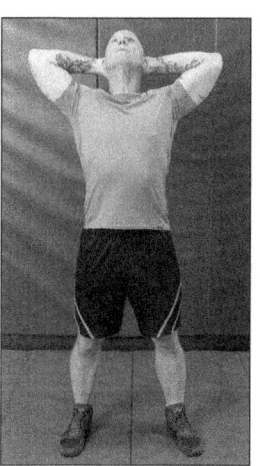

FIGURE 8-55:
Move your head back while applying counterpressure with your hands.

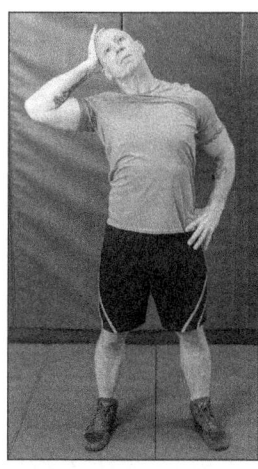

FIGURE 8-56:
Press against the right side of your head while tilting your head right.

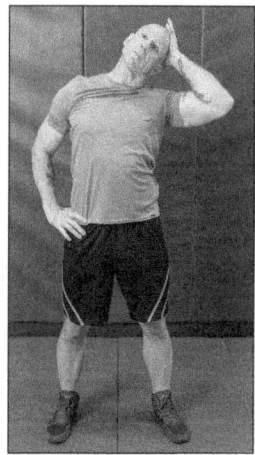

FIGURE 8-57:
Press against the left side of your head while tilting your head left.

Sample workouts

We don't expect you to do all two dozen–plus exercises we just presented. As a matter of fact, we don't recommend it. We include a variety of exercises to encourage you to move your body in different patterns to build a balanced core, stimulate the body's mechanisms for adaptation, and stave off boredom.

We recommend that you create groups of five or so movements and rotate the groups every few days or every week or so. Here, we provide three sample workouts you can add to your warm-up routine (broomstick movements and joint limbering, as presented in the earlier section "Warming Up and Getting Limber.") Feel free to construct your own workouts from the list. However, be certain to include movements that access the posterior chain (hidden core), the anterior core (abdominals), and the *transverse plane* (where your upper and lower body meet — near the top of your hip bones).

REMEMBER

In the workouts below, we use the letters P, A, T to designate which areas a movement engages: P = Posterior chain (hidden core), A = Anterior core (abdominals), and T = Transverse plane (contralateral movements). If you're initially unable to do the number of repetitions we recommend, do as many as possible with the goal of increasing the number of reps. What's important is that you have a routine you do at least once a day at least six days a week. Missing a day is okay, but try to make it a day of active rest; for example, take a long walk or leisurely ride on your bicycle.

Workout 1

1. **Tall plank:** 15–30 seconds (P, A)
2. **Bird dog:** five repetitions with a one-second hold on each side (P, A, T)
3. **Superman:** ten repetitions on each side (P, T)
4. **Gelebart abs:** 1–3 repetitions to the center and each side (A)
5. **Glute bridge:** ten repetitions with a two-second hold at the top (P)

Workout 2

1. **Six-point crawl:** ten steps forward and back (T)
2. **Four-point crawl:** ten steps forward and back (T)
3. **Straight-arm squeeze:** 8–10 reps (P)
4. **Thoracic bridge:** three repetitions each side with a five-second hold (P)
5. **Crunch:** 20–30 repetitions (A)

Workout 3

1. **Lizard crawl:** ten steps forward and back (T)
2. **Single leg bridge:** five repetitions on each side with a two-second hold at the top (P)
3. **The scale:** five repetitions each side with a two-second hold at extension (T)
4. **Cross-elbow-to-knee crunch:** 10–15 repetitions on each side (A)
5. **Cat and cow:** ten repetitions (P)

Chapter **9**

Back-Building Next Steps: The First and Second Floors

Chapter 8 provides relatively light movements and exercises for building back strength and mobility. Those exercises form the foundation upon which you can further strengthen and bullet-proof your back. (*Bullet-proofing* refers to making your back more resilient — less susceptible to pain and injury and able to recover faster after strenuous physical activity or an injury.)

This chapter moves from the foundation to the first and second floors — intermediate and advanced back-building exercises — and encourages you to continue to explore additional ways to maintain and build a strong and resilient body.

WARNING Establish a solid foundation before progressing to the first and second floors. You can usually tell when you're ready to progress to the next level — when the movements and exercises you're currently doing seem too easy or too basic, or you're craving something more challenging.

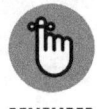

REMEMBER

Your mind and body are an organic whole. As you work out, you're empowering yourself, mentally and physically, to be healthy and strong. You're engaging your adaptation response and self-healing mechanisms as you reinforce your sense of *self-efficacy* — your belief in your ability to recover from any injury and maintain and improve your own health and vitality.

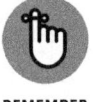

REMEMBER

The exercises in this chapter target the hidden core, the traverse plane (which divides the upper and lower body), and the abdominals. We recommend alternating bodyweight-only exercises with resistance (weight training) and mobility movements (no weight). We use the codes B, RT, and M to designate the three different exercise types:

>> **B:** Bodyweight (no external load)

>> **RT:** Resistance Training (external weight used)

>> **M:** Mobility (no weight, movement through the joint)

Intermediate Back-building: Using Your Bodyweight and Kettlebells

Success in any endeavor is a matter of gradual progression — you start with relatively easy challenges and gradually dial up the complexity, intensity, frequency, or duration to force your mind and body to adapt to increasingly difficult conditions. Through repetition and adaptation, you become gradually better at a task, and it gets easier and easier to perform.

In this section, you dial up the difficulty level of your back-building activities from the level you achieved in Chapter 8 to these intermediate activities, which will prepare you for the even higher-level challenges presented in the later section "Advanced Exercises: 'Bullet-Proofing' Your Back."

REMEMBER

Perform these movements as precisely as possible. Following proper form and technique is important both for preventing injury and for maximizing the benefit of the movement. You will improve with each session to the point at which you will be able to perform the movements without giving much thought to your posture and technique, but when you're starting out, you need to be mindful about doing them correctly.

Many of these intermediate movements and many advanced movements we present later in this chapter involve the use of a kettlebell. The images show a fairly large, heavy kettlebell, but they come in different weights. Start with the heaviest weight that feels manageable to you. You can even use a small, light dumbbell when you're getting started. If you don't have a kettlebell or dumbbell, improvise with a large can of soup or vegetables, a jug of water, or a bowling ball, or stuff a small bag full of marbles or coins.

WARNING

To avoid injury, err on the side of caution; choose a smaller/lighter weight at first and increase the weight as your proficiency improves. Here are some additional guidelines to consider when choosing a weight:

» **Choose a weight that's appropriate for your age, size, and physical condition.** Children, older adults, smaller people, and people with existing health conditions typically start with lighter weights. Healthy and fit teens and adults can generally start with heavier weights.

» **Use any previous weight-training experience you have to inform your choice. If you have little to no experience, start with lighter weights.**

» **Gauge the weight according to the movement:**

- For lower body pull movements, deadlifts, swings, and similar movements, choose a moderate to heavy weight. For example, a healthy man of 200 pounds can try starting with a 35-pound kettlebell, and a woman of 150 pounds can try starting with a 20-pound weight.

- For squats, a healthy man of 200 pounds can try starting with a 25-pound kettlebell, and a woman of 150 pounds can try starting with a 15-pound weight.

- For presses, rows, get-ups, and other movements, a healthy man of 200 pounds can try starting with a 20-pound kettlebell, and a woman of 150 pounds can try starting with a 10-pound weight.

Standard scapular push-up (B)

The standard *scapular* (shoulder blades) push-up is great for increasing your awareness of the location of your rhomboids and improving the strength and stability of your midback and upper back. To perform standard scapular push-ups, take the following steps:

1. **Assume the power plank position, as shown in Figure 9-1 — forearms on the floor, hands together, spine in the neutral position.**

REMEMBER

Keep your gut and butt tight and maintain a neutral spine throughout this exercise. (See Chapter 8 for more about what the neutral spine concept is all about.)

2. **Squeeze your shoulder blades as close together as possible (see Figure 9-2), and then spread them as far apart as possible while maintaining the power plank position.** Do ten reps.

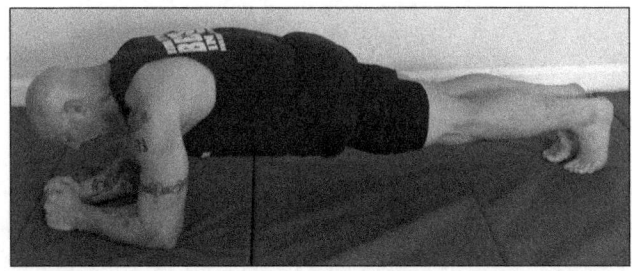

FIGURE 9-1:
Assume the power plank position.

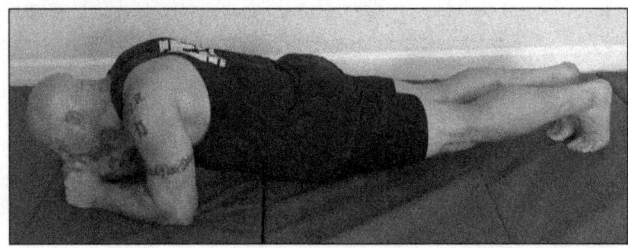

FIGURE 9-2:
Squeeze your shoulder blades together.

Squats

A *squat* is a strength exercise in which you bend your knees and flex your ankles to bring your hips down toward the ground. Squats generally promote lower body (leg) strength, but they also strengthen the core and the hidden core — the *posterior chain* (the muscles on your backside). This section presents two squats — the full squat (bodyweight only) and the goblet squat (with extra weight).

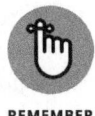

REMEMBER

Properly done squats require mastery of the hip hinge. Instead of bending your spine, you thrust your butt back as you tilt your upper body forward. See Chapter 7 for instructions on how to hip-hinge properly.

Full squat (B)

Before you try squatting with added weights, do full squats and focus on perfecting your posture and form. You want to be sure that you're doing these correctly with only body weight before bringing in additional weight. To do squats, perform the following steps:

1. **Stand erect, neural spine, palms pressed together at about stomach level (see Figure 9-3), and tighten your gut and butt.**

   Keep your heels on the ground and maintain a neutral spine throughout this movement.

REMEMBER

2. **Pull your butt down toward the ground far enough so that your hips are below your knees, as shown in Figure 9-4.** Keep your spine neutral — no tail tuck — and gaze straight ahead.

   Tail tuck occurs when you bring your butt too far forward, reducing the natural curve in your lower back (your lumbar spine); you want to maintain that curve.

3. **Drive upward, through your heels, to full extension, gripping the floor with your toes and shifting the position of your hands as necessary to maintain balance.**

4. **Tighten your gut and butt to fully lock in your position at the top.**

5. **Repeat Steps 2–4 to complete ten reps.**

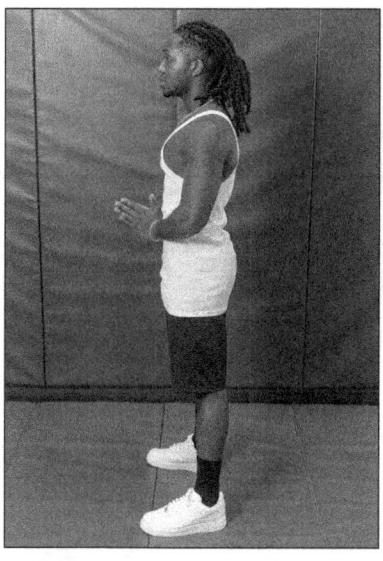

FIGURE 9-3:
Stand erect, spine in the neutral position, hands pressed together at stomach height.

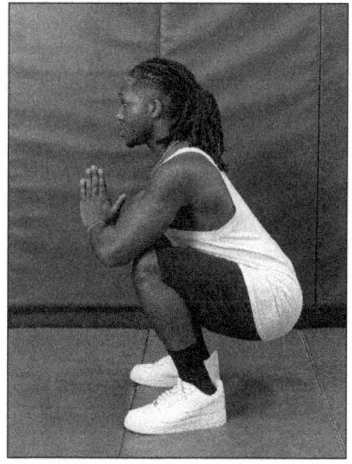

FIGURE 9-4:
Pull your butt down toward the ground.

Goblet squat (RT)

The goblet squat may be the only weighted squat you need. It strengthens the quadriceps, hamstrings, glutes, and gastrocnemius (gastroc) muscles as well as the core. It also opens up the hips and reinforces a neutral spine. Follow these steps for the goblet squat.

1. **Stand erect, arms flexed, holding the kettlebell by its horns at about chest height, feet spaced about shoulder width apart, toes pointed out at about a 15-degree angle (see Figure 9-5).**

2. **Pull your butt down toward the ground far enough so that your hips are below your knees, as shown in Figure 9-6.** Keep your spine neutral — no tail tuck.

3. **Drive upward, through your heels, to full extension, gripping the floor with your toes.**

4. **Tighten your gut and your butt to fully lock in your position at the top.**

5. **Repeat Steps 2–4 to complete five reps.**

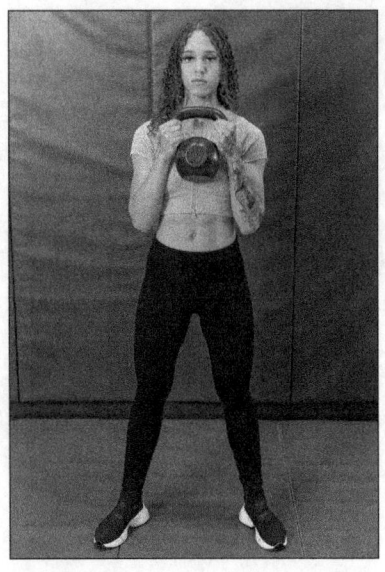

FIGURE 9-5:
Stand upright, holding the kettlebell by its horns about chest high.

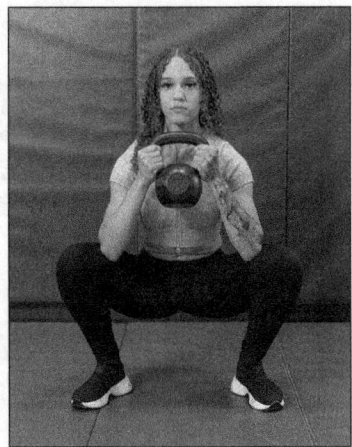

FIGURE 9-6:
Pull your butt down toward the ground.

Ab work

Engaging the abs and *obliques* (the side muscles between the bottom of the ribcage and the top of the hips) is key to developing a strong core. This group of exercises targets those muscles.

Get-up sit-up (RT, M)

The get-up sit-up involves sitting up from a prone position while punching one arm toward the ceiling, with or without a weight. This movement builds core and upper body strength and improves shoulder stability.

TIP

If you're unable to do a full get-up (standing up from a prone position while holding a weight above the head) due to injury or another constraint, the get-up sit-up is a great alternative. It's also a great way to condition your body to perform the more advanced full get-up.

To do get-up sit-ups, take the following steps:

1. Start in the fetal position with the kettlebell on the mat near your left bicep, holding the bell's handle with your left hand, your right hand wrapped over it, and your elbows close to your body, as shown in Figure 9-7.

2. Keep your arms flexed tight while rolling onto your back so that the kettlebell follows you, straighten your right leg, and press the bottom of your left foot against the mat (see Figure 9-8).

3. Raise both hands toward the ceiling, pushing the bell skyward, as shown in Figure 9-9.

4. Deliver a karate chop to the mat with your right hand, creating tension up through your back as you raise the bell straight up with your left arm, locking your wrist and elbow in place (see Figure 9-10).

5. Roll in the direction of the extended leg and onto your opposite elbow as you "punch" the bell skyward (see Figure 9-11).

6. Slowly roll down onto your back, keeping your left wrist and elbow locked in place and the bell raised high.

7. Bring the bell down to rest between your left upper arm and torso, and then roll left to bring the bell back down to the mat.

8. Repeat Steps 1–7 for a total of five reps.

9. Use two hands to slide the bell around your head (not across the chest) to the opposite side and repeat Steps 1–8 for that side, raising the bell with your right arm this time.

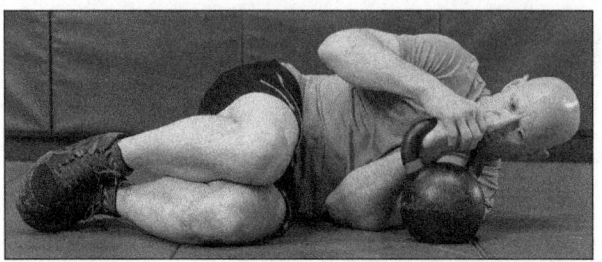

FIGURE 9-7:
Start in the
fetal position.

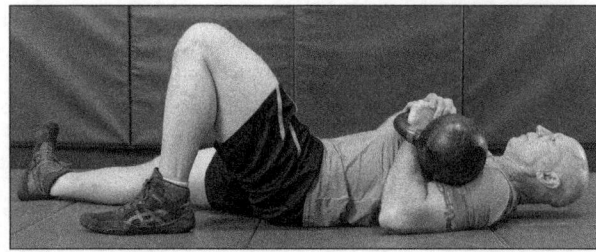

FIGURE 9-8:
Clutch the bell
to your body
as you roll.

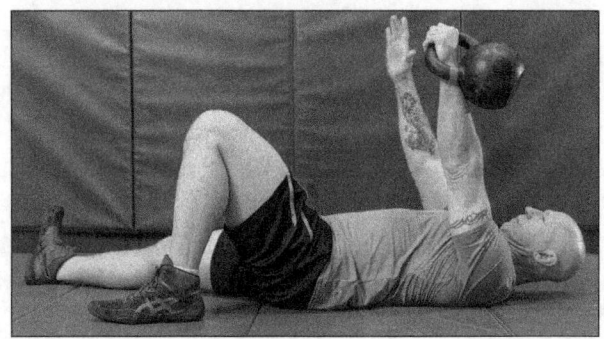

FIGURE 9-9:
Push the bell
toward
the ceiling.

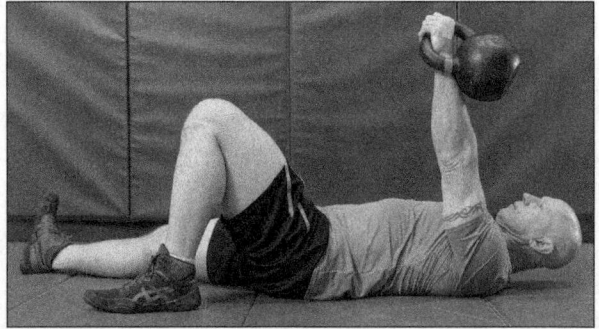

FIGURE 9-10:
Karate-chop the
mat with the
opposite hand.

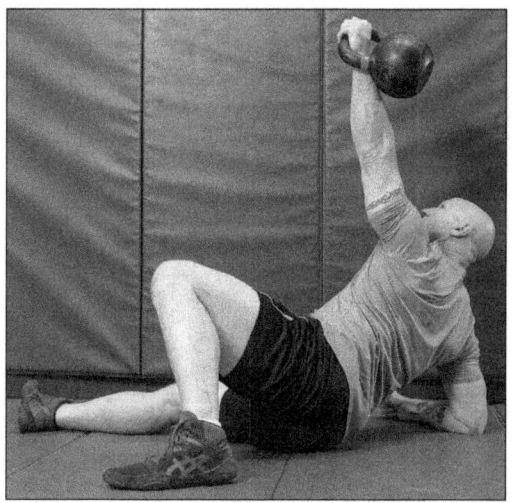

FIGURE 9-11:
Raise your torso
from the mat and
push the bell high
into the air.

60-second abs (B)

Got a minute? Tone those abs! This movement is composed of five positions. Hold each position for 10 seconds.

REMEMBER

Imagine that bolts are driven through your hips, anchoring your hips to the floor. Also, keep in mind that the more muscle tension you put into these positions, the more you get out of them; full-body tension maximizes this movement's return on investment.

Lie flat on your back, and then hold each of the following six positions for 10 seconds each:

> **Position 1:** Flex your abdominal muscles to bring your elbows into contact with the insides of your knees/thighs (see Figure 9-12).
>
> **Position 2:** Hold your elbows about where they are and extend your legs, keeping your feet six inches or less off the ground (see Figure 9-13).
>
> **Position 3:** Extend your arms while keeping your legs extended, as shown in Figure 9-14.
>
> **Position 4:** Bring the right elbow and left knee/thigh together while keeping the opposite limbs fully extended, as shown in Figure 9-15.
>
> **Position 5:** Fully extend your right arm and left leg while bringing your left elbow and right knee/thigh together.
>
> **Position 6:** Flex your abdominal muscles to bring your elbows into contact with the insides of your knees/thighs. (This move is the same as Position 1, bringing the total time to 60 seconds.)

Repeat all six positions at least five times, holding each position for ten seconds.

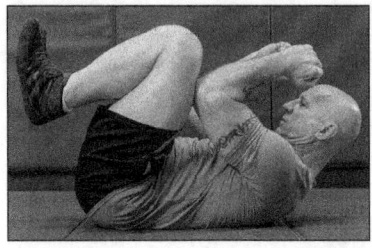

FIGURE 9-12:
Touch your elbows to your knees/thighs.

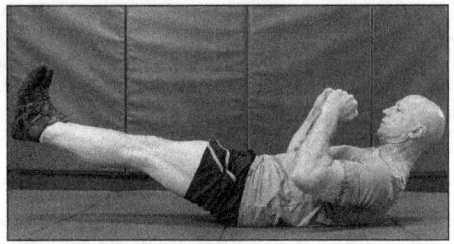

FIGURE 9-13:
Extend your legs, keeping your elbows nearly stationary.

FIGURE 9-14:
Extend your arms.

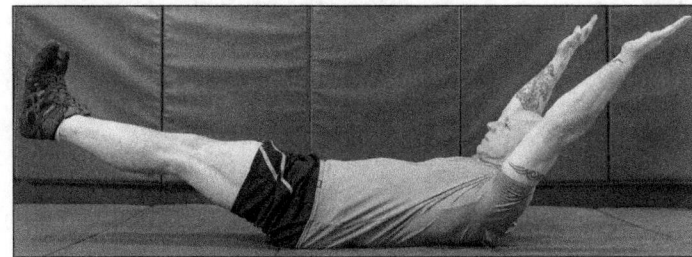

FIGURE 9-15:
Bring your right elbow and left knee/thigh together.

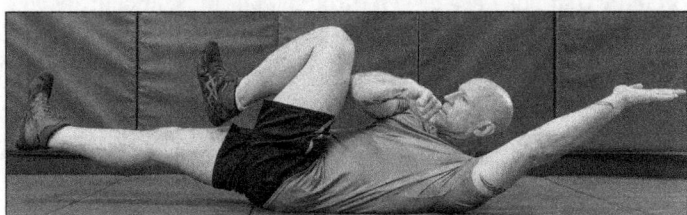

Side crunch (B)

Side crunches are great for developing the obliques (the muscles under those pesky love handles) and improving mobility along the transverse plane (where the upper body meets the hips). Take the following steps to perform a set of side crunches:

1. Lie flat on your back, knees bent, elbows bent, with your hands on either side of your head.

2. Tighten your abs, raising your chest a few inches toward the ceiling, and squeeze your left obliques, bringing your left elbow toward the outside of your left thigh, as shown in Figure 9-16.

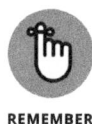

Keep your abs tensed and your chest raised throughout this exercise. Don't twist your torso; move side to side.

3. **Return to the starting position and then squeeze your right obliques, bringing your right elbow toward the outside of your right thigh, as shown in Figure 9-17.** Perform 15–25 repetitions on each side.

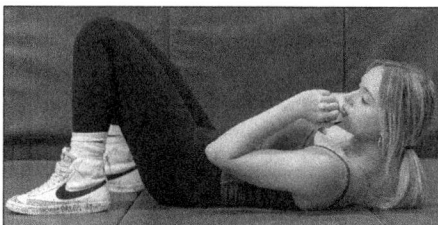

FIGURE 9-16:
Raise your chest and reach your left elbow toward the outside of your left thigh.

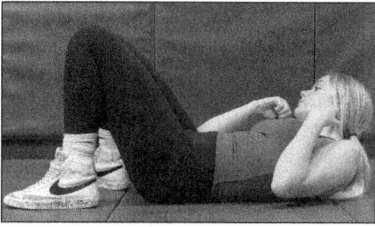

FIGURE 9-17:
Reach your right elbow toward the outside of your right thigh.

Cross crunch (B)

Cross crunches strengthen the core and improve strength and mobility along the transverse plane with its *contralateral movement* (moving one side of the body over to the opposite side). Follow these steps to perform the cross crunch.

1. **Lie flat on your back, knees bent at about a 90-degree angle, hands behind your head, as shown in Figure 9-18.**

Don't apply too much pressure to the back of your head/neck with your hands.

2. **Bring your right elbow to your left knee, as shown in Figure 9-19.**
3. **Slowly lower yourself back to the ground.**
4. **Bring your left elbow to your right knee.**
5. **Slowly lower yourself back to the ground.**
6. **Repeat Steps 2–5 to perform 10–25 repetitions per side.**

Contralateral abdominal training is the *only* type of abdominal training we recommend for women who've had multiple pregnancies and/or cesarean sections. Straightforward abdominal exercise may exacerbate a hernia.

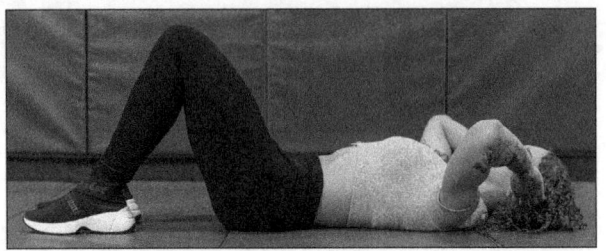

FIGURE 9-18:
Lie flat on your
back, hands
behind
your head.

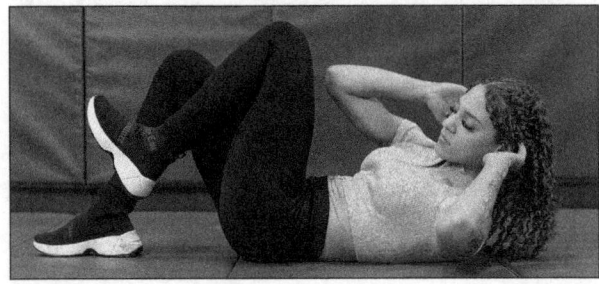

FIGURE 9-19:
Bring your right
elbow to your
left knee.

Dead bug (B)

The dead bug is an excellent isometric tension exercise for maximum abdominal contraction. To do the dead bug, take the following steps:

1. **Lie flat on your back.**

2. **Flex your abdominal muscles to bring your knees up and back and your elbows up and forward until your elbows press against the insides of your knees/thighs, and hold this position for 30 seconds.** (This position is the same as Position 1 of the 60-second abs routine — see Figure 9-12.)

   TIP

   Apply maximum tension throughout the body by forcing the elbows and knees together.

3. **Slowly lower your legs and torso back to the ground.**

4. **Repeat Steps 2 and 3 for ten reps.**

Deadlifts, drags, and swings

Deadlifts, drags, and swings are strength-training exercises that involve moving a loaded barbell or other weight off the ground, along the ground, or through the air. With a deadlift, you lift the weight straight up and then set it straight back down on the ground. With a drag, you slide the weight along the ground. With a swing, you move the weight in an arc through the air. In this section, we present a variety of deadlifts, drags, and swings.

Standard two-hand deadlift (RT)

The deadlift is a staple for developing strength along the posterior chain. Even though it's typified as a lower-body pull, it builds upper-body strength and stability as well. It also lays the groundwork for kettlebell swings.

To perform standard two-hand deadlifts, take the following steps:

1. **Stand erect, feet shoulder-width apart, with the kettlebell directly between them.**

2. **Bend your knees, hip-hinge to maintain a neutral spine position, and grasp the kettlebell's handle firmly with both hands (see Figure 9-20).** Keep your pinkies inside the handle for maximum grip. Your head should be at about the 10 o'clock position and your butt at about the 4 o'clock position.

   Maintain tension throughout your body, bending your knees and hip-hinging just enough to grasp the kettlebell handle.

TIP

3. **Maintaining a neutral spine, pack your shoulders, engage your lats, and squeeze your rhomboids together as you attempt to tear the handle apart, pulling in opposite directions left and right.** (Of course, if you succeed, we will want lessons from you!)

   Maintain full-body tension and keep trying to tear that handle apart for the duration of the exercise.

4. **Stand up, lifting the kettlebell off the ground; tense your kneecaps up into your quads; and tighten your gut and your butt (see Figure 9-21).**

5. **Slowly bend your knees and hip-hinge to bring the bell back down toward the ground without letting it touch the ground.** (If it touches the ground, you're either compromising the integrity of your spine or unpacking your shoulders.)

6. **Repeat Steps 3–5 to complete 10–15 reps.**

Single-arm deadlift (RT)

The single-arm deadlift is nearly identical to the standard two-hand deadlift that we cover in the previous section, with the notable exception that you're lifting the kettlebell with only one arm. This movement pulls unevenly on the side with the kettlebell, engaging your body's stabilizers (shoulder blades, knees, hips) to maintain alignment.

Focus on keeping your hips and shoulders square and not letting that kettlebell touch the ground when you're bringing it down.

REMEMBER

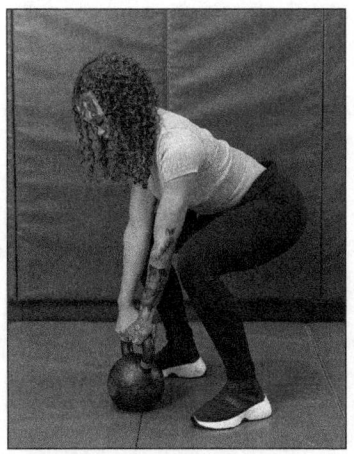

FIGURE 9-20:
Bend your knees, hip hinge, and grasp the kettlebell's handle.

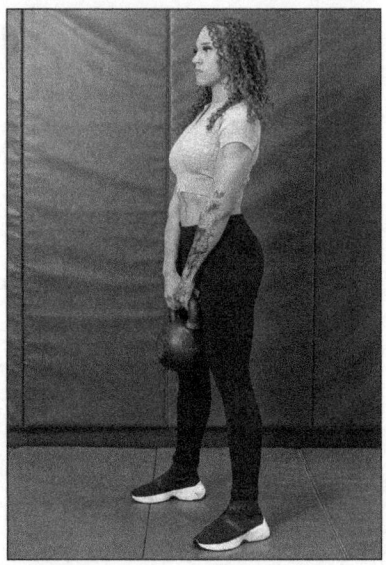

FIGURE 9-21:
Pack your shoulders, engage your lats, and stand straight up.

Deadlift drag (RT)

The deadlift drag reinforces the position of the body used in all deadlifts and swings, as well as the notion of packing the shoulders and engaging the lats. It also serves as a great intermediary movement between deadlifts and swings.

Take the following steps to perform a set of deadlift drags:

1. **Grasp the bell with two hands on the handle so that your arms are outstretched and the bell handle is at about a 45-degree angle, your feet are spaced about shoulder-width apart, your spine is in the neutral position, your head is at about the 9 o'clock position, and your bottom is at about the 3 o'clock position (see Figure 9-22).**

   Position your pinkies inside the handle for a full grip.

REMEMBER

2. **Drag the kettlebell back between your legs, as shown in Figure 9-23.**

3. **Walk or hop backward to return to your starting stance, as in Step 1, and repeat Step 2.** Perform ten repetitions.

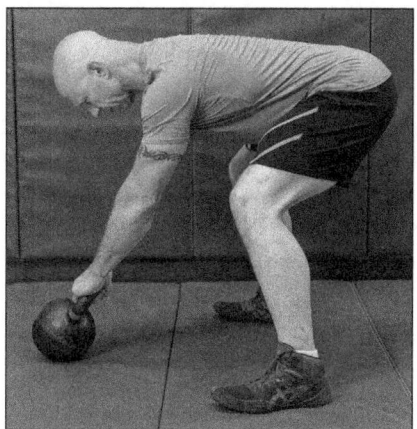

FIGURE 9-22:
Grasp the bell's handle.

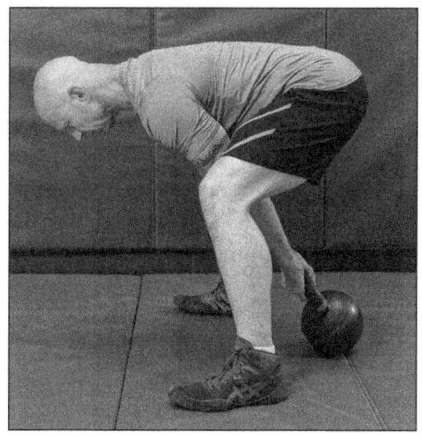

FIGURE 9-23:
Drag the bell back between your legs.

Two-hand swing (RT)

The two-hand swing is the mother of all kettlebell movements and the foundation for all *ballistic* (through the air) kettlebell moves. As kettlebell trainers often say, "If you ain't got the swing, you ain't got a thing!" The two-hand swing requires mastery of multiple fundamental techniques — neutral spine, the hip-pop-and-lock, exhaling hard on the hip-pop, toggling between tension and relaxation, rooting to the floor, tightening the gut and the butt, packing the shoulders, engaging the lats, bringing the ribs down, and firing the bell forward.

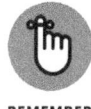

REMEMBER

The *hip-pop* is like a pelvic thrust (yes, that suggestive dance move). You thrust your pelvis forward as you snap your hips back. This motion helps to propel the kettlebell forward while counterbalancing it with a backward motion of your hips.

Here's how you do the two-hand swing:

1. **Grasp the bell with two hands on the handle so that your arms are outstretched and the bell is on its edge, your feet are spaced about shoulder-width apart, your spine is in the neutral position, your head is at about the 10 o'clock position, and your bottom is at about the 4 o'clock position (see Figure 9-24).**

   Position your pinkies inside the handle for a full grip.

REMEMBER

2. **Pack your shoulders (back and down), engage your lats (mid and lower-back muscles), and maintain a neutral spine as you hike the kettlebell back between your legs and swing it far enough so that your elbows reach back between your knees (see Figure 9-25).**

At the bottom of the swing, maintain a big open chest (don't round your shoulders) and gaze at a spot on the floor about six feet out in front of you.

3. **Tighten your gut and butt and keep your ribs down as you fire the bell forward and up and hip-pop to propel the bell forward.** At the lock-out (top of the swing), your arms should be straight out in front of you, as if you were doing a standing plank (see Figure 9-26). Keep your abs tight.

At the peak of the movement, keep your feet firmly planted (rooted to the ground), abs tight, kneecaps tensed up into your quads, and gaze level with the horizon. Use your hips, not your arms, to propel the bell forward. If you're lifting the bell with your arms, you're doing it wrong.

At the top of this swinging-out movement, referred to as the *eccentric* portion of the swing, the bell is essentially weightless for a moment. At this point, you're ready to start the *concentric* portion of the swing to power the bell back between the legs.

4. **Continue to grasp the handle firmly as gravity pulls the kettlebell down, hinging your hips to maintain a neutral spine, packing your shoulders, engaging your lats, and guiding the bell back between your knees.**

5. **Repeat Steps 3 and 4 for 10–20 reps.**

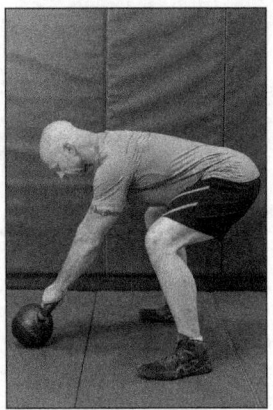

FIGURE 9-24: Grasp the kettlebell's handle and maintain a neutral spine.

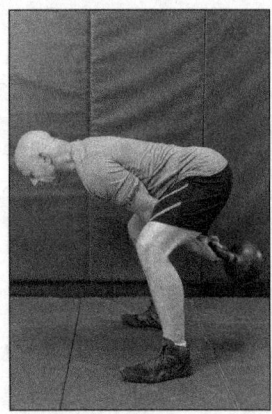

FIGURE 9-25: Hike the bell between your legs.

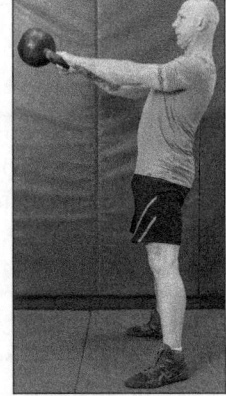

FIGURE 9-26: Swing the bell up and straight out in front of you.

One-arm swing (RT)

The one-arm swing is nearly identical to the two-hand swing except for the obvious difference that you're using only one arm to swing the kettlebell. You use the free arm to maintain balance and keep your shoulders square with your hips.

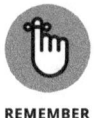

The body tends to twist into the movement, so pack your shoulders, engage your lats, and drive both hips forward at the same rate as you swing the bell up and out from your body. As with all of the other single-side movements, your body recruits the stabilizers (in this case, the shoulders, lats, and obliques) to compensate for the uneven load.

To perform one-arm swings, take the following steps:

1. **Grasp the bell with one hand on the handle so that the arm is out-stretched and the bell is on its edge. Your feet are spaced about shoulder-width apart, your spine is in the neutral position, your head is at about the 10 o'clock position, your bottom is at about the 4 o'clock position, and your opposite arm reaches straight back (see Figure 9-27).**

   Imagine yourself as a professional bull rider — one hand tied to the bull (the kettlebell's handle in this case) and the other hand reaching back for balance.

2. **Pack your shoulders (back and down), engage your lats (mid and lower-back muscles), and maintain a neutral spine as you hike the kettlebell back between your legs and swing it far enough so that your elbow reaches back between your knees (see Figure 9-28).**

   At the bottom of the swing, maintain a big open chest (don't round your shoulders) and gaze at a spot on the floor about six feet out in front of you.

3. **Tighten your gut and butt and keep your ribs down as you fire the bell forward and up, bringing your free hand forward so it touches the bell handle at the top of the movement.** At the lock-out (top of the swing), your arms should be straight out in front of you, as if you were doing a standing plank (see Figure 9-29). Keep your abs tight.

   At the peak of the movement, keep your feet firmly planted (rooted to the ground), abs tight, kneecaps tensed up into your quads, and gaze level with the horizon.

4. **Continue to grasp the handle firmly as gravity pulls the kettlebell down, hinging your hips to maintain a neutral spine, packing your shoulders, engaging your lats, and guiding the bell back between your knees.**

5. **Repeat Steps 3 and 4 for 5–10 reps on each side.**

Romanian deadlift (RT)

The Romanian deadlift (RDL) is a variation of the standard deadlift that targets the hamstrings specifically. It's similar to a standard deadlift but involves more hip-hinge and less knee-bend, strengthening the entire *posterior chain* (the muscles on the backside of the body).

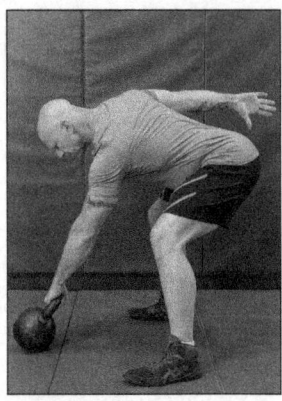

FIGURE 9-27:
Grasp the bell with one hand and reach back with the other hand.

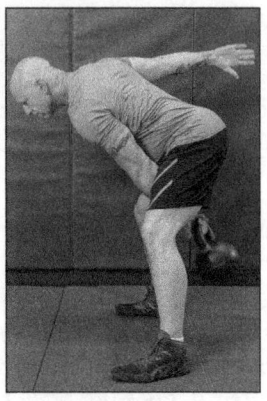

FIGURE 9-28:
Swing the bell back between your legs.

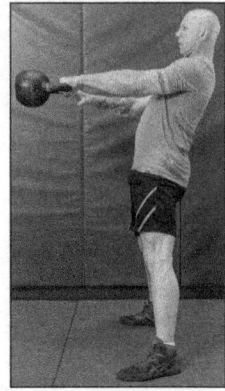

FIGURE 9-29:
Swing the bell forward, out, and up to about chest level.

To perform RDLs, take the following steps:

1. **Perform a standard two-hand deadlift, as explained in the earlier section, "Standard two-hand deadlift."**

2. **Position your feet as close together as is comfortable for you.**

3. **Maintaining a neutral spine, hip-hinge without bending your knees, bringing the kettlebell down toward your feet without allowing it to touch the ground (see Figure 9-30).** Keep the bell close to your body, but not too close; your arms should be nearly perpendicular to the ground.

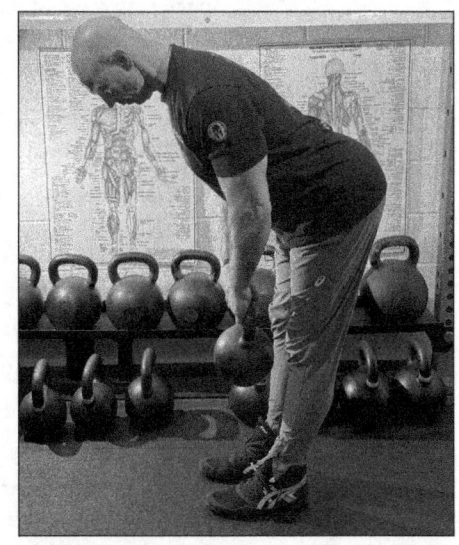

FIGURE 9-30:
Hip-hinge without bending your knees.

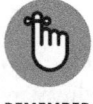

REMEMBER

Keep your shoulders packed, lats engaged, and spine neutral. At the lowest point, your torso should be nearly parallel to the ground, but your thighs should not be parallel to the ground. If they are, you're bending your knees. You should feel tension in your hamstrings.

4. Stand fully erect with the kettlebell in front of you below hip level.

5. Repeat steps 3 and 4 for ten repetitions.

6. When done, hip-hinge and bend the knees as much as necessary to park the kettlebell safely on the floor.

Floor lever (M)

Floor levers are a great substitute for traditional pull-ups, especially for those who are physically unable to do pull-ups or for when a pull-up bar or another suitable apparatus is unavailable. Floor levers engage the lats and strengthen the shoulders and core without the need for any equipment.

To perform floor levers, take the following steps:

1. Kneel down on your mat with the tops of your feet flat against the mat, hips back as far as comfortable, arms extended above your head, palms down against the mat, and fingers spread, as shown in Figure 9-31.

   Apply full body tension to press your hands firmly against the matt. The more muscle tension you put into it, the better the results.

TIP

2. Keep your hands planted firmly into the mat and maintain full body tension as you slowly (over a count of five) raise your body and pivot up and forward until your head is past your hands and your back is fully arched (see Figure 9-32).

3. Maintaining full body tension, slowly (over a count of five) pull your hips back and down to return to your starting position. You should feel more tension in your abdominals as you move back and down.

4. Repeat Steps 2 and 3 for a total of five repetitions.

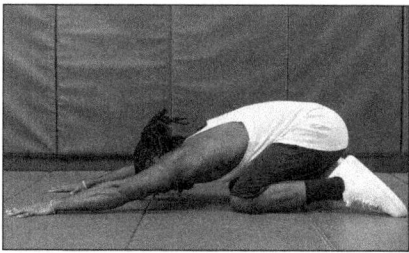

FIGURE 9-31:
Bow down.

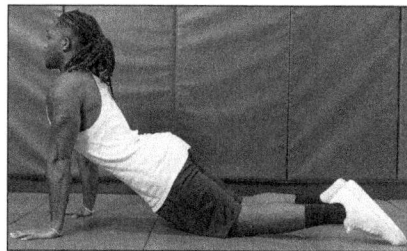

FIGURE 9-32:
Rise up and forward.

Advanced Exercises: "Bullet-Proofing" Your Back

When you're feeling strong enough to take your back-building regimen to the next level, turn to this section for more challenging movements. Don't let words like "advanced" and "challenging" deter you. Assuming that you built a firm foundation by performing the movements in Chapter 8, and you built the first floor of your back-health home by performing the intermediate exercises in the previous section, you're well prepared to move on to the second floor. Embrace the challenge and dedicate yourself to the principle of continual improvement.

REMEMBER

As you move up to the second floor, don't abandon the first floor or the foundation. Continue performing the broomstick movements and joint limbering warmups covered in Chapter 8, along with the beginner and intermediate exercises in Chapter 8 and the previous section, as you add some (or all) of the following exercises to your routine.

Note that bullet-proofing is not intended to eliminate your back pain. Such a result doesn't exist. It is intended to make your daily pain more manageable and to reduce the intensity, duration, and frequency of pain episodes.

WARNING

When it comes to exercise, you need to push yourself. As Michelangelo said, "The greater danger for most of us lies not in setting our aim too high and falling short; but in setting our aim too low and achieving our mark." We've found that most patients fail by playing it too safe. Most exercise manuals come with the disclaimer, "Check with your doctor before taking on these exercises." This warning assumes that your doctor is well-versed in exercise. We've found this not to be the case. If you play it safe, you're less likely to get injured but also less likely to succeed. We recognize that the exercises come with risk. Mitigate this risk through a slow and steady progression, not by going easy on yourself. If you don't take the risk of setbacks, you risk falling short of your goals.

Kettlebell push-ups (B)

To make even the most basic exercise more challenging, all you need to do is add a kettlebell! The kettlebell push-up takes the classic version to a whole new level, reinforcing core stability and strengthening the wrists and triceps. Here's what you do:

1. **Flip a kettlebell over so that the handle is on the floor and is aligned longwise with your body.**

Standing the kettlebell on its handle can make it too unstable for some people to perform this exercise. Feel free to place the kettlebell on its side with the handle facing away from you. As you build balance, you can work up to standing the kettlebell on its handle.

2. **Place your hands on top of the bell and assume the classic push-up pose, elbows bent, as shown in Figure 9-33.** Maintain tension along your entire body (a plank) throughout the exercise.

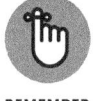

The closer your feet are together, the more challenging this exercise is.

3. **Push up while pulling your chest down toward the kettlebell.** As you reach the top of the movement, contract your chest and shoulder muscles and your triceps and lock your elbows, as shown in Figure 9-34.

4. **Maintain your plank and bend your elbows to lower yourself down to a few inches above the kettlebell (see Figure 9-33).**

5. **Repeat Steps 3 and 4 to complete 10–25 reps.**

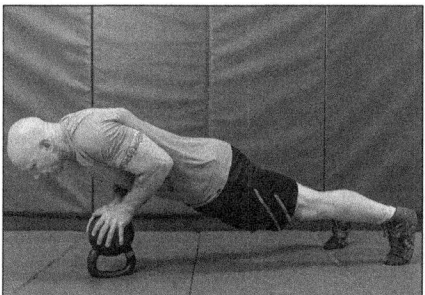

FIGURE 9-33:
Place your hands on top of the kettlebell and do a plank.

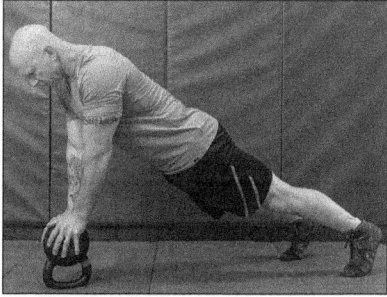

FIGURE 9-34:
Push up to the point at which your elbows lock.

Lateral raises

Lateral raises are strength-training exercises characterized by lifting a pair of weights in an upward arc away from the sides of your body (as if you're flapping your arms like a bird). This movement is great for packing the shoulders and engaging the lats (the low- to mid-back muscles to either side of the spine).

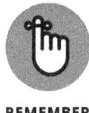

You can use any type of weighted object, such as dumbbells, lump hammers, or sledgehammers. Tension bands also work.

Thor raises (RT)

Thor raises involve lifting a pair of weights in an upward arc from down by your sides to over your head. This movement does an exceptional job of engaging the rhomboids and trapezius muscles.

To perform Thor raises, take the following steps:

1. Stand erect, holding your weights at your sides, palms forward, feet spaced about shoulder-width apart, spine in the neutral position, and a tight gut and butt (see Figure 9-35).

2. Keeping your arms straight, elbows locked, slowly raise the weights out from your sides and up until your arms are fully extended straight above your head and the weights are even with or slightly behind your ears (see Figure 9-36).

3. Keeping your arms straight and elbows locked, slowly lower the weights to your sides.

4. Repeat Steps 2 and 3 to complete 10–15 repetitions.

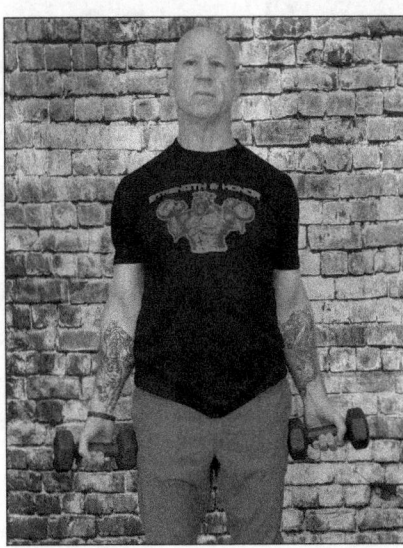

FIGURE 9-35:
Hold the weights at your sides, palms forward.

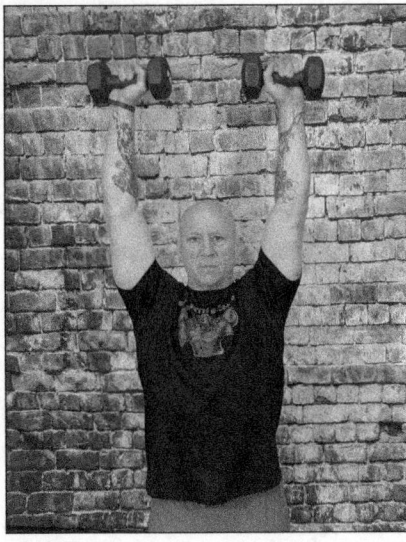

FIGURE 9-36:
Raise the weights in an arc over your head.

Flying monkeys (RT)

Flying monkeys are nearly identical to Thor raises, except that you're hip-hinged forward so that your chest is nearly parallel to the ground. Imagine you're one of the flying monkeys from *The Wizard of Oz* as you take the following steps:

1. Stand erect, holding your weights at your sides, palms forward, spine in the neutral position, and a tight gut and butt.

2. Bend your knees slightly and hip-hinge forward so that your chest is nearly parallel to the ground and your spine is in the neutral position, allowing your arms and dumbbells to dangle down toward the ground without touching it (see Figure 9-37).

3. Keeping your arms straight and elbows locked, slowly raise your arms straight out from your sides, as shown in Figure 9-38.

4. Bring the weights forward so your arms are extended straight out from your shoulders and level with the crown of your head, as shown in Figure 9-39.

5. Slowly bring your arms back so they're straight out from your sides, and then bring them down slowly.

6. Repeat Steps 3–5 to complete ten reps.

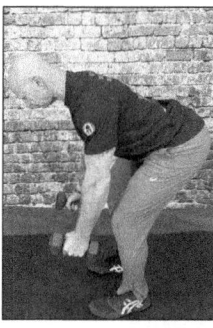 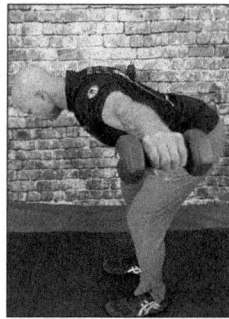 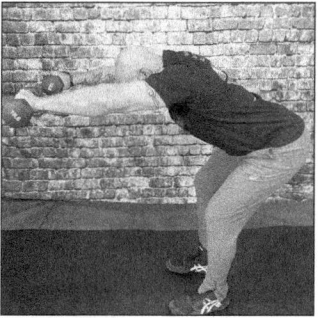

FIGURE 9-37:
Keep your chest nearly parallel to the ground with the weights dangling down.

FIGURE 9-38:
Raise the weights straight out to your sides.

FIGURE 9-39:
Bring the weights forward.

Bridges

Bridges involve arching your body, which strengthens your core muscles and builds mobility and flexibility. They're especially beneficial for conditioning the often-overlooked posterior chain. We present a couple of basic bridge movements in Chapter 8. Here, we present a couple of more advanced techniques.

Thoracic bridge (B, M)

The thoracic bridge may be the most important and most beneficial bridge for counteracting imbalances in the back resulting from modern living. The benefits to the hips, thoracic spine, and shoulders are unmatched by any other unweighted exercise. Do this bridge regularly, and you will be rewarded handsomely:

1. **Start with a tabletop bridge.** See Chapter 8 for instructions on how to perform a tabletop bridge.

2. **Lift your left hand off the ground and bring it toward your right shoulder, as shown in Figure 9-40. Your left elbow should be pointing up at the ceiling, and your left hand should be pointing down toward your right hand, which is planted on the ground.** Look at the hand on the floor. Ideally, your hips are horizontal, and your shoulders are perpendicular to the floor. Hold this position for at least a count of five.

TIP

With your right hand on the floor, focus on firing the right glute to help make the hips parallel to the floor. If your left hand is on the floor, fire your left glute.

3. **Switch sides and repeat this movement for three repetitions on each side.**

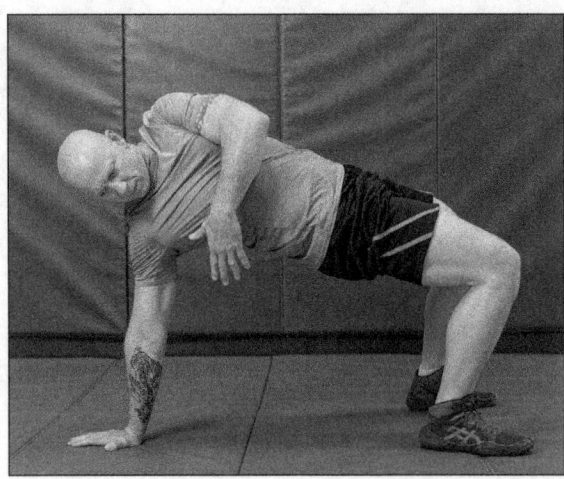

FIGURE 9-40: The thoracic bridge.

Back bridge (B, M)

The back bridge is a classic back movement that can help rid you of back pain caused by sitting hunched over all day long. To perform the back bridge, take the following steps:

1. **Lie on your back, knees bent, feet flat and near your butt, hands to the outsides of your shoulders, palms down, fingers pointing down toward your butt, as shown in Figure 9-41.** Getting your hands in the right position requires some flexibility; do the best you can.

2. **Arch your back, raising your butt and back off the ground and tilting your head back as far as possible to face the ground, as shown in Figure 9-42.**

3. **Exhale at the top of the movement and hold the pose for about five seconds.**

4. **Gradually lower yourself to the ground.**

5. **Repeat Steps 2–4 for a total of 5–10 reps.**

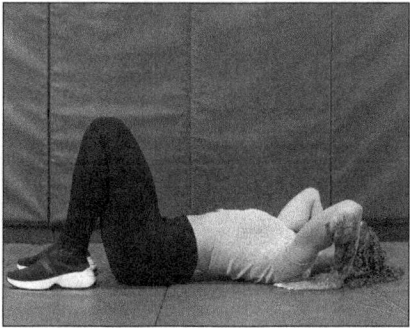

FIGURE 9-41:
Back bridge starting position

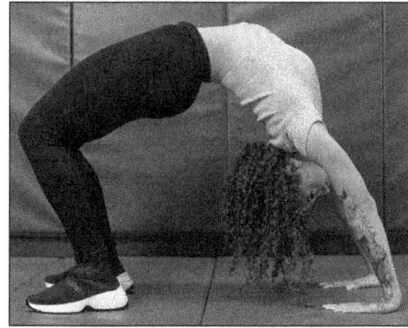

FIGURE 9-42:
Arch your back and tilt your head back as far as possible.

Advanced neck-cercises

We're strong advocates for neck strengthening for two reasons. One is that Phil has a long background in combat sports, where neck strength is essential for self-defense and preventing serious injuries. Another is that neck health is an integral and often overlooked component of back health.

In this section, we present two advanced neck-strengthening exercises.

Neck bridge (B, M)

The neck bridge is a popular exercise among grapplers for strengthening the cervical muscles and improving overall neck health. It involves creating a bridge with your head anchored on one end and your feet on the opposite end. Here's how you do a neck bridge:

1. **Lie flat on your back with your knees bent, your heels close to your butt, and your hands extended just above chest level, as shown in Figure 9-43.**

2. **Drive your hips up, keeping your arms off the ground, and roll back onto your head, as shown in Figure 9-44.** If you need to use your hands to help stabilize your body or relieve some of the weight, that's fine. Hold this position for one or two seconds.

3. **Roll slowly down to bring your back to the mat.**

4. **Repeat Steps 2 and 3 to complete ten repetitions.** Use a one-count hold at the top before bringing them back down to the floor

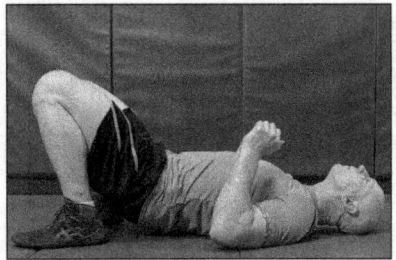

FIGURE 9-43:
Lie flat on your back with your heels near your butt.

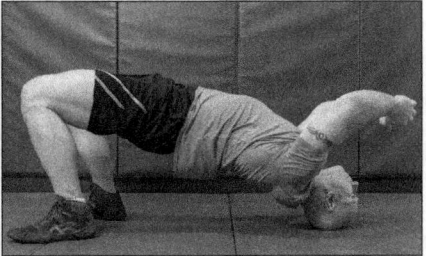

FIGURE 9-44:
Arch upward, rolling back onto your head.

Four-way neck with weight plate (RT)

Chapter 8 introduces you to the four-way neck exercise, which involves using your hands to apply resistance as you lean your head/neck forward, back, left, and right. This plate version of this exercise enables you to use a weight plate to increase the resistance. A *weight plate* (often simply called a "plate") is a disk-shaped metal object that you slip onto a bar to create a dumbbell.

To perform this movement, you need a plate and a towel or other soft material and a workout bench or the equivalent, such as an ottoman. When you're properly equipped, take the following steps:

1. Lie on your left side with the cushioned plate positioned on the right side of your head in a way that's comfortable for your ear, as shown in Figure 9-45.

2. Hold the plate in position with your right hand as you move your head laterally through the full range of motion.

3. Repeat Steps 1 and 2 on the opposite side of your body using your left hand to balance the cushioned plate.

4. Lie stomach down on the bench with your neck and head extending off the end of the bench; place the cushioned plate on the back of your head, and move your head/neck up and down through its full range of motion (see Figure 9-46).

5. Lie flat on your back with your neck and head extending off the end of the bench, place the cushioned plate on your forehead, and move your head up and down through its full range of motion (see Figure 9-47).

6. Repeat Steps 1–5 to complete two sets of 10–15 repetitions in each of the four directions.

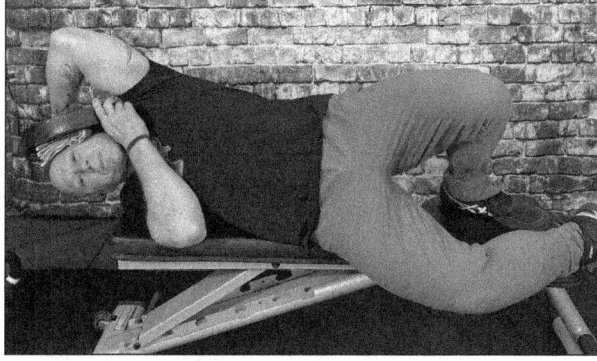

FIGURE 9-45:
Lie on your side and hold cushioned plate to the side of your head.

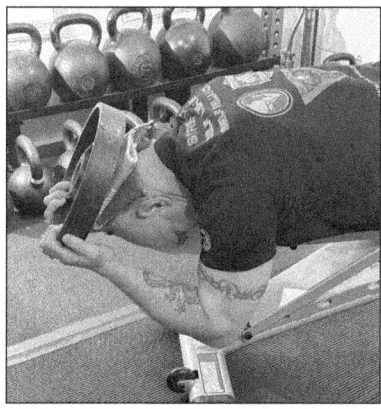

FIGURE 9-46:
Lie on your stomach and hold the cushioned plate to the back of your head.

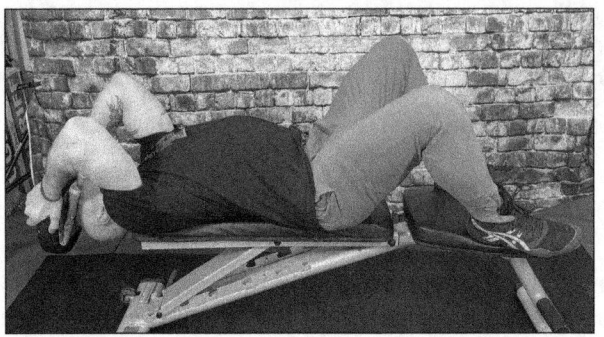

Bite belt lift (RT)

The bite belt lift involves deadlifting a weight with your teeth and (mostly) your neck, although your entire body really gets into the act. It's not an exercise for the faint of heart or, for that matter, anyone who's had extensive dental work. This exercise is great for developing the entire posterior chain, strengthening the jaw muscles, and alleviating stress.

WARNING

If you've had any extensive dental work — bridgework, implants, dentures, braces — you may want to pass on this exercise or at least consult your dentist before attempting it.

To perform the exercise, you need to modify a kettlebell. Take a karate belt or comparable strip of strong fabric (or a rope) about six feet long, hold the two loose ends together, tie them into a knot, and duct-tape the two sides together down from the knot, leaving a loop at the bottom (see Figure 9-48). String the rope through the handle of the kettlebell, thread the knotted end through the loop, and pull tight to cinch the rope to the handle.

REMEMBER

The distance between the knot and the bottom of the kettlebell needs to be just enough for you to squat comfortably and get the knot into your mouth. If it's too long, you'll have trouble getting the bell off the ground. If it's too short, you may have to bend over too far to get it in your mouth.

Take the following steps to perform a set of bite lifts:

1. **Stand over the kettlebell, feet spaced about shoulder length apart, and hold up the knotted end of the belt so that the belt is taut.**

2. **Bend your knees and hip-hinge to reach your mouth down to the knot while maintaining a neutral spine, and bite the knot.** You want the entire knot inside your mouth, as shown in Figure 9-49.

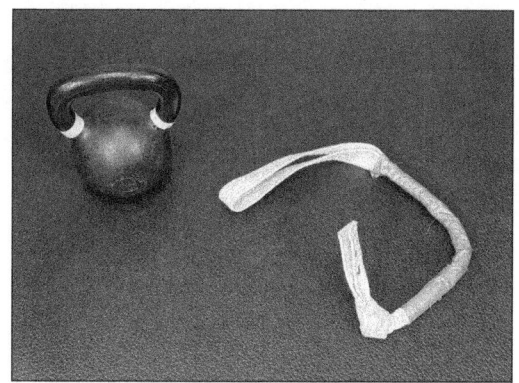

FIGURE 9-48:
Modify your
kettlebell for a
bite belt lift.

3. **Place your hands on your thighs for support (or keep your hands to your sides, shoulders packed, if you don't need the support). Maintain a neutral spine, and raise your upper body just enough to lift the kettlebell off the ground about a foot (see Figure 9-50).**

4. **Bow your head and raise it to move your neck through its full range of motion 10–15 times.**

5. **With your head raised, very slowly turn about 15 degrees to one side, as shown in Figure 9-51, and repeat Step 4.** Turning too fast can make the kettlebell swing into your knee.

6. **Repeat Step 5, turning slowly toward the other side.** You can do left, center, and right multiple times, bowing and raising your head through its full range of motion 10–15 times at each position.

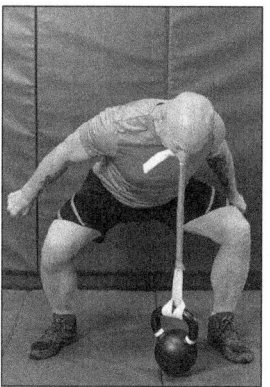

FIGURE 9-49:
Bite the knot.

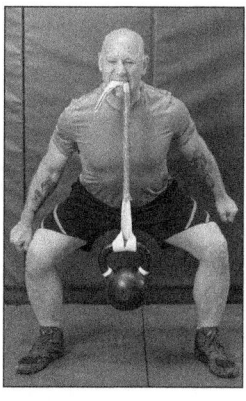

FIGURE 9-50:
Bite-lift the kettlebell
about one foot off
the ground.

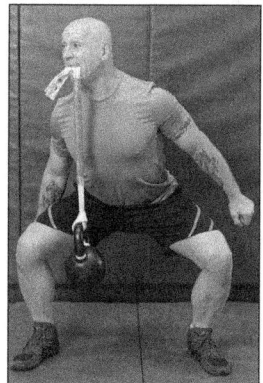

FIGURE 9-51:
Turn slowly to one side.

Pull-ups and chin-ups

Pull-ups and chin-ups are some of the best body-weight-only exercises for developing upper body strength and mobility, improving posture and athletic performance, supporting scapular health and grip strength, and developing mental toughness.

In this section, we present three renditions of this classic body-building exercise — pull-ups, chin-ups, and what we like to call "plank pull-ups."

REMEMBER

To perform any of the following exercises, you need a horizontal bar strong enough to support your body weight as you raise and lower yourself and at least high enough to keep your knees off the ground — preferably high enough to keep your feet from touching the ground when your arms and legs are fully extended.

Pull-ups (B)

No other calisthenic symbolizes upper body strength more than the traditional (overhand) pull-up. Think about it: How many people can do them? If someone can do 20 pull-ups, do you even have to test their ability to do sit-ups? Pull-ups dramatically strengthen the back, shoulders, and arms while helping to tone the core.

WARNING

If you're over age 50 or have shoulder issues, consider doing (underhand) chin-ups, which engage the same muscles but apply less torque (twisting motion) to the shoulder joint.

To do a set of pull-ups, take the following steps:

1. **Grasp the bar firmly, hands spaced about shoulder-width apart, palms facing away from you, arms straight, feet off the ground, as shown in Figure 9-52.**

Pack your shoulders (back and down) and maintain tension in the abs, back, and shoulders throughout the movement.

2. **Slowly pull your body up until your head and neck are above the bar (see Figure 9-53), and then slowly lower your body until your arms are completely straight.**

3. **Perform three sets of 80 percent of the maximum number of pull-ups you can do.** For example, if you can do 10 pull-ups, do three sets of 8.

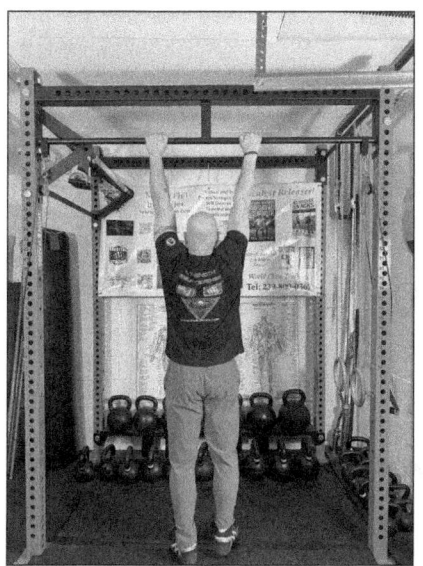

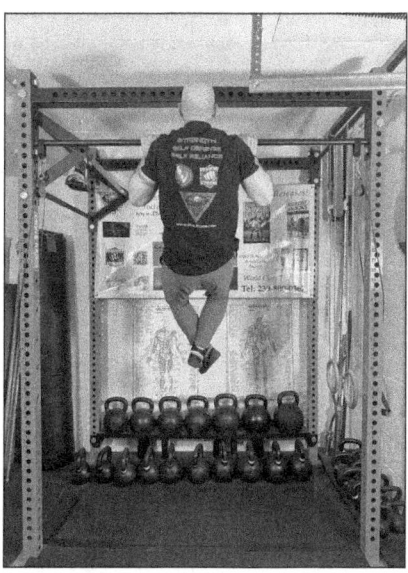

FIGURE 9-52:
Grasp the bar and hang from your arms.

FIGURE 9-53:
Pull yourself up until your head and neck clear the bar.

Chin-ups (B)

Chin-ups (underhand pull-ups) are easier to do and easier on the shoulders than pull-ups, but they're nearly as good for building the back and shoulder muscles, and they deliver the added benefit of engaging the biceps.

Perform chin-ups the same way you do pull-ups (see the previous section) except grasp the bar with palms facing you instead of facing away from you, as shown in Figures 9-54 and 9-55.

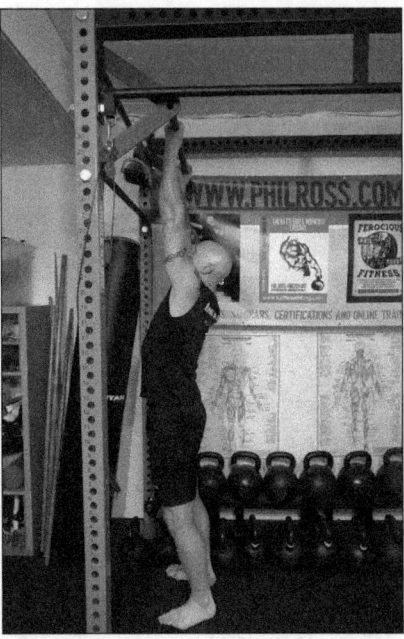

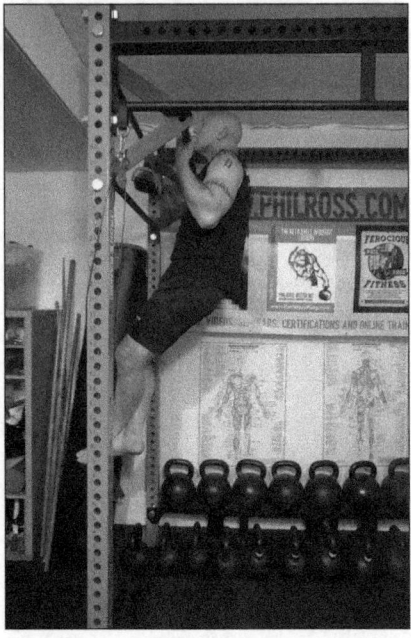

FIGURE 9-54:
Grasp the bar so that your palms are facing you, arms straight.

FIGURE 9-55:
Pull yourself up until your chin is above the bar.

Plank pull-ups (B)

If you can't do a single pull-up or chin-up, don't feel bad — most people can't. Nearly everyone, however, can do a plank pull-up. You can think of it as a gateway pull-up and use it to build upper body strength so that you can transition into doing traditional pull-ups or chin-ups.

To do plank pull-ups, you need gymnastics rings or something comparable to hang from — suspension-training equipment, such as CrossCore or TRX, a rope, or a karate belt — and something to anchor them to — a pull-up bar, a wall or ceiling anchor, or a closed door. Set the length so the part you'll be gripping hangs down from where it'll be anchored to about waist height. (Experiment with the length to find your comfort level and desired resistance later.)

To perform plank pull-ups, take the following steps:

1. **Stand facing the handles/rings about a foot away from them.**

2. **Grasp the handles/rings with an overhand grip, tense your body (plank), lean back on your heels, and extend your arms straight out, as shown in Figure 9-56.**

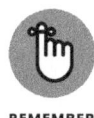
Keep your shoulders square by tensing your shoulder muscles. You don't want rounded shoulders.

3. **Maintain a tight plank and square shoulders while pulling your body up until your chest is nearly even with your hands, as shown in Figure 9-57.** As you pull yourself up, rotate your hands outward so your thumbs are up. When you're all the way up, try to bring your elbows together behind your back to fully engage your rhomboids.

4. **Slowly lower yourself back down to the point at which your arms are straight, shoulders square (don't let them round out), rotating your hands inward so your palms are facing down.**

5. **Perform three sets of 80 percent of the maximum number of plank pull-ups that you can do.** For example, if you can do 10 plank pull-ups, do three sets of 8.

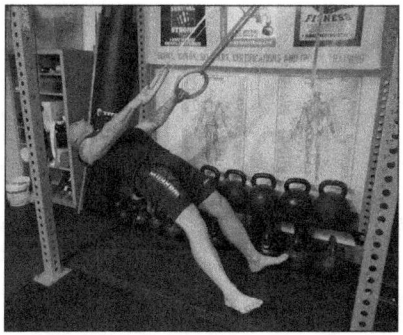

FIGURE 9-56:
Hang loose, heels on the ground.

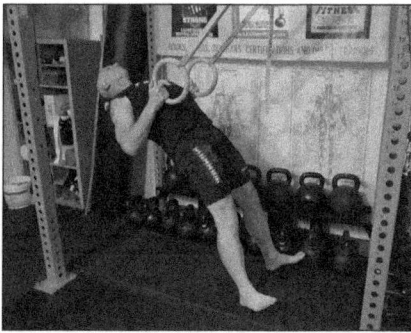

FIGURE 9-57:
Pull yourself up.

Advanced ab work

If you've been doing some of the ab exercises that we cover in Chapter 8 and earlier in this chapter for some time, you should have a well-toned abdomen, maybe even the proverbial "six pack." When you're ready to take your abs to the next level (abs of steel?), try the exercises in this section.

Ab wheel (B)

The ab wheel (aka wheel of death) is a great tool for abdominal and upper body development.

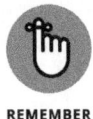
Round your back (as opposed to the normally neutral spine). Imagine arching your back like an angry cat. Many gymnasts refer to this posture as "the hollow" because you're creating an empty space in your midsection.

To use your ab wheel, take the following steps:

1. **Kneel down, press the tops of your feet against the ground, grasp the handles of the wheel, position it directly below your shoulders, and lean down on it (see Figure 9-58).**

2. **Roll the wheel forward slowly (over a count of five) as far as you're able to roll it back, as shown in (see Figure 9-59, keeping your abs tight).** You can use a spot on the floor as your reference point or mark a spot using a pencil or erasable marker.

3. **Roll the wheel back slowly (over the count of five) to the starting position.**

4. **Repeat Steps 2 and 3 to perform five sets of ten reps each.**

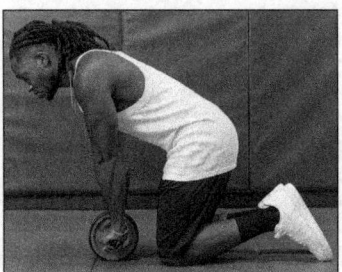 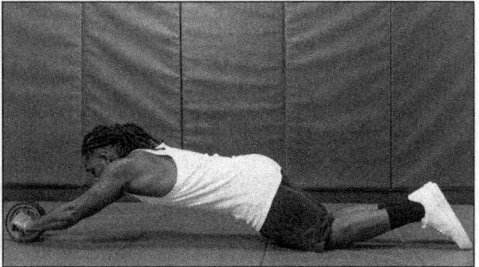

FIGURE 9-58:
Start with the wheel below your shoulders.

FIGURE 9-59:
Roll the wheel out as far as you'll be able to roll it back.

Hanging abs (B)

The hanging ab delivers the "best bang for the buck" among ab toning exercises. The wheel of death comes close, but the hanging ab reigns supreme. In addition to working the abdominal region, the act of hanging is particularly beneficial for overall back health because it helps to decompress the spine. It also strengthens your grip.

To perform hanging abs, you need a pull-up bar that's tall enough to keep your feet off the ground when your arms and legs are fully extended. Follow these steps:

1. **Grasp the pull-up bar with palms facing out (away from you) and elbows and knees locked, as shown in Figure 9-60.** If you have shoulder issues, try grasping the bar with your palms facing you, as you would do for a chin-up.

2. **Raise your knees slowly to your chest (or as close as you can get them), as shown in Figure 9-61.**

For a more challenging hanging ab that's better for developing abdominal strength, keep your legs straight as you raise them.

3. **Slowly lower your legs so they're fully extended down below you (knees locked).**

Avoid swaying or rocking, which can make the movement easier but less beneficial.

4. **Repeat Steps 2 and 3 to perform 5–20 reps.**

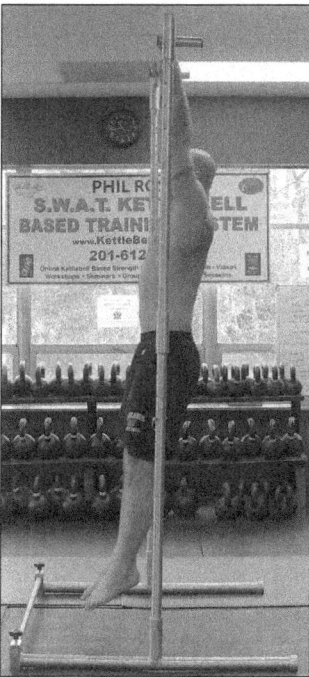

FIGURE 9-60:
Hang straight down from the pull-up bar, palms out.

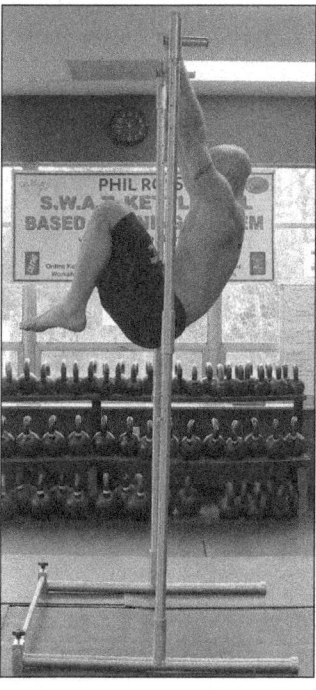

FIGURE 9-61:
Raise your legs (knees to chest or straight legs).

Ab crawls (B)

The ab crawl is a challenging movement but fantastic for core development and abdominal strength. It's also a great deal of fun when you get good at it, giving you the opportunity to channel your inner cha-cha dancer.

To perform ab crawls, take the following steps:

1. **Lie flat on your back, bring your knees up toward your chest, and hold your hands fisted about shoulder level.**

2. **Rotate your knees to one side and reach your arms to the opposite side to do "the twist," as shown in Figure 9-62.**

3. **Repeat Step 2 to alternate sides, moving your body across the floor.** Move the same distance in each direction. If you have a lot of floor space, start by moving 20 feet in each direction, and then add distance or "laps" as you're able.

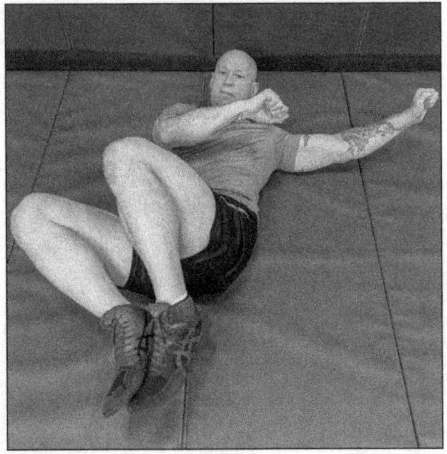

FIGURE 9-62:
Lie flat on your back and do the twist.

Get-ups (RT, M)

The get-up (also known as "Turkish get-up) involves transition from fetal to standing position while hoisting a kettlebell from the floor to over your head with one hand. It's a movement that inspires fear, shock and awe in the hearts and minds of fitness enthusiasts! It's the most difficult kettlebell movement to master and the most beneficial for overall strength and mobility. So even though it takes time and practice to become accomplished at it, we encourage you to stick with it.

To perform get-ups, take the following steps:

1. **Start in the fetal position with the kettlebell on the mat near your right bicep, holding the bell's handle with your right hand, your left hand wrapped over it, and your elbows close to your body, as shown in Figure 9-63.**

2. **Keep your arms flexed tight while rolling onto your back so that the kettlebell follows you, straighten your left leg, and press the bottom of your right foot against the mat (see Figure 9-64).**

3. **Raise both hands toward the ceiling, pushing the bell skyward, as shown in Figure 9-65.**

4. **Deliver a karate chop to the mat with your left hand, creating tension up through your back as you raise the bell straight up with your right arm, locking your wrist and elbow in place (see Figure 9-66).**

5. Roll in the direction of the extended leg and onto your opposite elbow as you "punch" the bell skyward (see Figure 9-67).

6. Plant your left hand on the mat, arm straight, elbow locked, shoulder packed, right foot flat on the mat, left leg extended (see Figure 9-68).

7. Use your left arm and right leg to push up off the mat as you bring your left leg back into a kneeling position (see Figure 9-69), and then raise your torso straight up while remaining in the kneeling position (see Figure 9-70).

   The kettlebell is now above your head, your left knee is on the floor, and the balls of your feet are on the mat, ready to launch you forward and upward.

8. Push off with your left foot and then with your right leg as you stand tall with your feet shoulder-width apart, kettlebell raised in triumph straight above your right shoulder (see Figure 9-71).

9. Repeat the movements slowly in reverse to bring the kettlebell back down to the mat.

WARNING

Keep your elbow (on the arm holding the kettlebell) locked on the way down. It has a tendency to buckle. Don't bend your elbow until you're ready to rest it on the ground. Perform the descent slowly, one count to each movement.

10. Use two hands to slide the bell around your head (not across your chest) to the opposite side.

11. Repeat Steps 1–10. Do a total of five reps per side.

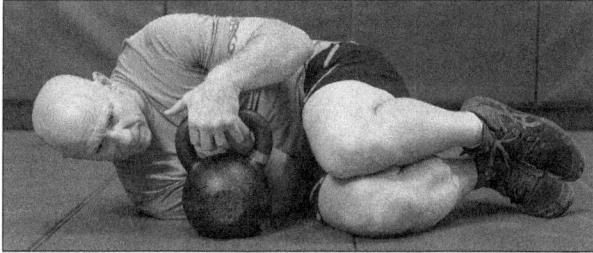

FIGURE 9-63:
Start in the fetal position.

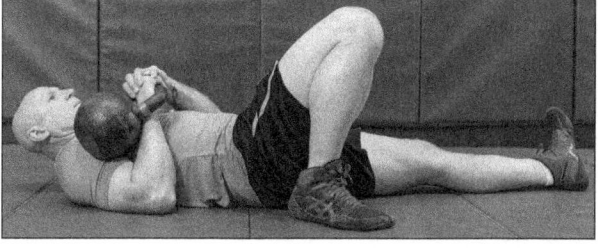

FIGURE 9-64:
Roll onto your back, taking the kettlebell with you.

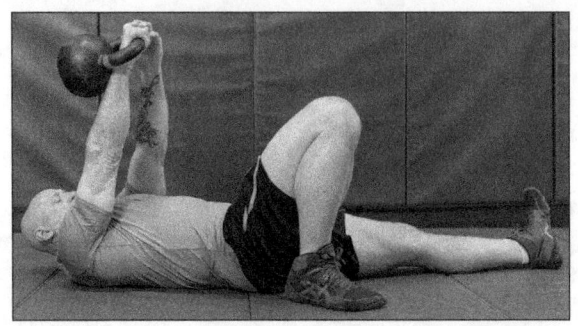

FIGURE 9-65:
Push the kettlebell straight up.

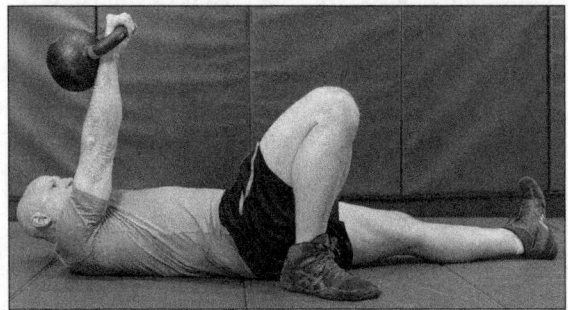

FIGURE 9-66:
Karate-chop the mat with your free hand.

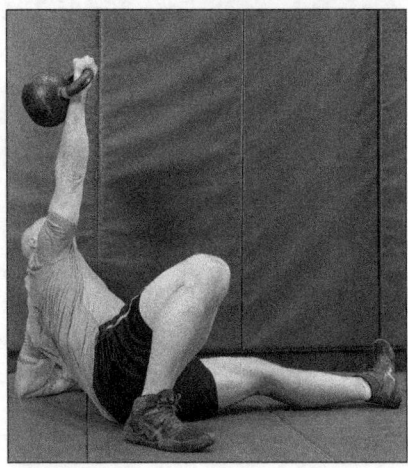

FIGURE 9-67:
Rise up and support your upper body on your left elbow.

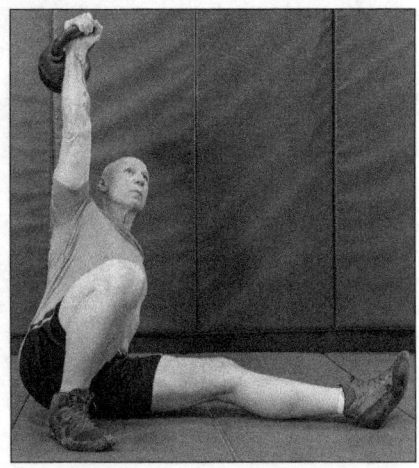

FIGURE 9-68:
Use your left arm and right leg to raise your butt off the mat.

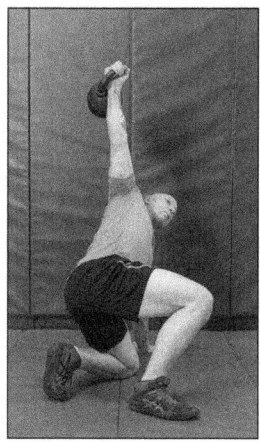

FIGURE 9-69:
Swing your left leg between your left arm and right knee into the kneeling position.

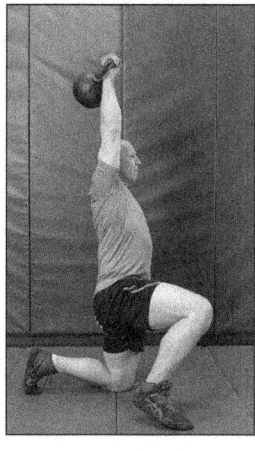

FIGURE 9-70:
Kneel on your left knee and press the balls of your feet into the mat.

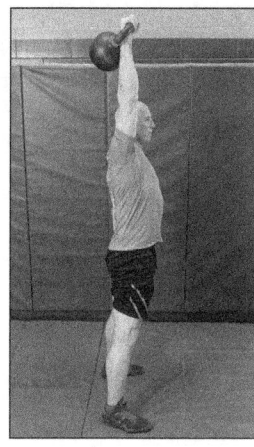

FIGURE 9-71:
Launch forward and up into a standing position.

More kettlebell swings

Kettlebell swings are great for strengthening the posterior chain, increasing mobility, and toning the body's stabilizers. When you're comfortable doing the basic kettlebell movements we present in the earlier section "Deadlifts, drags, and swings," you're ready to move on to the more advanced exercises we cover in this section.

Uneven kettlebell swing (RT)

The uneven kettlebell swing involves swinging two kettlebells of unequal weights, which challenges the core muscles and the body's stabilizers.

To perform uneven kettlebell swings, take the following steps:

1. **Place two different-sized kettlebells on the ground in front of you with the handles at 45-degree angles to the ground and to you; space your feet about shoulder-width apart. Bend your knees slightly and hip-hinge so that your upper body is nearly parallel with the ground, and grasp the kettlebell handles so that the backs of your hands are facing each other, as shown in Figure 9-72.**

   Position your pinkies inside the handle for a full grip.

REMEMBER

2. **Pack your shoulders (back and down), engage your lats (mid and lower-back muscles), and maintain a neutral spine as you hike the kettlebells**

back between your legs and swing them far enough so that your elbows reach back between your knees (see Figure 9-73).

Don't let the kettlebells clang together as you bring them through your legs. Clanging indicates that your shoulders aren't packed. To counter this unpacking, use scapular retraction (try to pull your shoulder blades together).

3. **Tighten your gut and butt, and keep your ribs down as you fire the bells forward and up.** At the lock-out (top of the swing), your arms should be straight out in front of you, as if you were doing a plank, and the kettlebells should be about chest high (see Figure 9-74). Keep your abs tight.

At the peak of the movement, keep your feet firmly planted (rooted to the ground), abs tight, kneecaps tensed up into your quads, and gaze level with the horizon.

At the top of this swinging-out movement, referred to as the "eccentric" portion of the swing, the bells are essentially weightless for a moment. At this point, you're ready to start the concentric portion of the swing to power the bells back between your legs.

4. **Continue to grasp the handles firmly as gravity pulls the kettlebells down; hinge your hips to maintain a neutral spine, pack your shoulders, engage your lats, and guide the bells back between your knees.**

5. **Repeat Steps 3 and 4 for 5–10 reps.**

6. **When you're done with the prescribed repetitions, switch the bells to opposite hands and perform 5–10 more reps.**

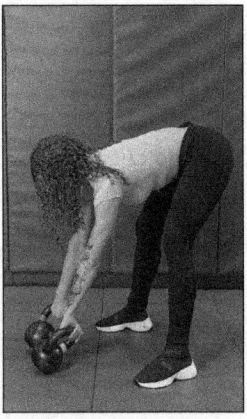 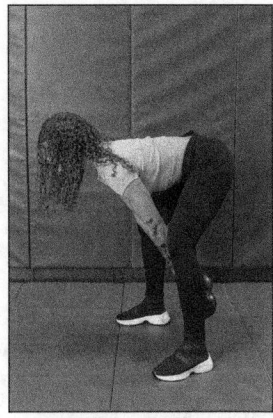 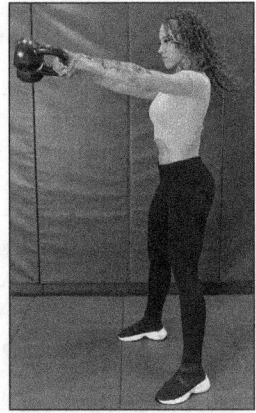

FIGURE 9-72:
Grasp the bells by their handles with the tops of your hands facing each other.

FIGURE 9-73:
Hike the kettlebells between your legs.

FIGURE 9-74:
Swing the kettlebells out and up to about chest level.

Over-speed eccentric swing (RT)

This version of the kettlebell swing accentuates the eccentric (inward) and the concentric (outward) motion of the kettlebell swing while adding a cardiovascular component. You need a partner to perform this movement.

To perform over-speed eccentric swings, take the following steps:

1. **Instruct your partner to stand about a foot to the side of you, a couple of feet in front, and facing you. Your partner should push the kettlebell down when you swing it up to about chest level.**

2. **Grasp the bell with two hands on the handle so that your arms are outstretched and the bell is on its edge, your feet are spaced about shoulder-width apart, and your spine is in the neutral position nearly parallel to the ground (see Figure 9-75).**

   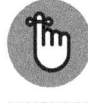
   REMEMBER

   Position your pinkies inside the handle for a full grip.

3. **Pack your shoulders (back and down), engage your lats (mid and lower-back muscles), and maintain a neutral spine as you hike the kettlebell back between your legs and swing it far enough so that your elbows reach back between your knees (see Figure 9-76).**

   TIP

   At the bottom of the swing, maintain a big open chest (don't round your shoulders) and gaze at a spot on the floor about six feet out in front of you.

4. **Tighten your gut and butt, and keep your ribs down as you fire the bell forward and up.** At the lock-out (top of the swing), your arms should be straight out in front of you, as if you were doing a plank (see Figure 9-77). Keep your abs tight.

   TIP

   At the peak of the movement, keep your feet firmly planted (rooted to the ground), abs tight, kneecaps tensed up into your quads, and gaze level with the horizon.

   This is the point at which your partner should push the bell down, propelling it between your legs.

5. **Continue to grasp the handle firmly as the kettlebell launches downward, hinging your hips to maintain a neutral spine, packing your shoulders, engaging your lats, and guiding the bell back between your knees.**

   WARNING

   Be careful not to wrack your groin. As the kettlebell is traveling back between your legs, you may need to hold it back a little to keep it from traveling too far back and up.

6. **Repeat Steps 3 and 4 for 12–15 reps.**

REMEMBER

Employ scapular retraction to keep your shoulders packed (tucked back and down), and prepare to get winded. You have to adapt not only to the additional downward pressure your partner applies to the kettlebell but also to the increased rate at which the "pendulum" is swinging. You're building endurance in addition to strength.

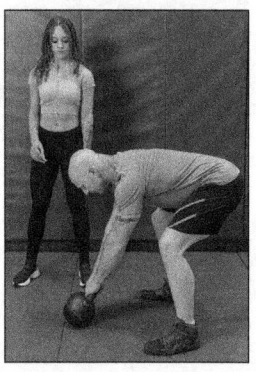

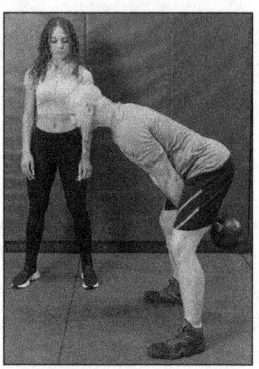

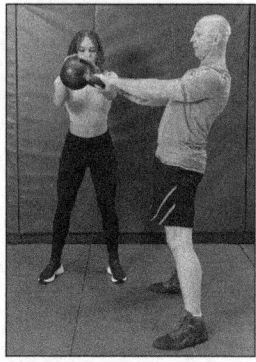

FIGURE 9-75:
Grasp the handle of the kettlebell.

FIGURE 9-76:
Hike the kettlebell back between your legs.

FIGURE 9-77:
Launch the kettlebell forward and up and have your assistant push it back down.

Cleans

A *clean* is a weightlifting movement that involves raising a barbell from the floor up to your shoulders (your *rack*) in one smooth, swift motion. In this section, we present two versions of kettlebell cleans.

Kettlebell clean (RT)

The *kettlebell clean* involves lifting a kettlebell from the ground to the shoulder. It's sort of a cross between a squat and a curl, requiring both lower and upper body strength.

To do a kettlebell clean, perform the following steps:

1. **Grasp the kettlebell handle with one hand so that your arm is outstretched and the bell is on its edge. Your feet should be spaced about shoulder-width apart and your spine in the neutral position nearly parallel to the ground. Reach back with your other arm for balance (see Figure 9-78).**

   Imagine yourself as a professional bull rider — one hand tied to the bull (the kettlebell handle in this case) and the other hand reaching back for balance.

REMEMBER

2. **Stand erect as you bend your arm and rotate your wrist in an outward direction, exhaling as you hip-pop and guide the kettlebell into the rack, as shown in Figure 9-79.** Keep your elbow close to your body as if protecting against someone trying to kick you in your ribs.

3. **Lower the kettlebell to the ground so that you're back in your starting position.**

4. **Repeat Steps 2 and 3 to complete ten reps on each side.**

Your body may tend to twist in the direction of the kettlebell. To prevent it from twisting, drive with both hips simultaneously and square your shoulders with your hips.

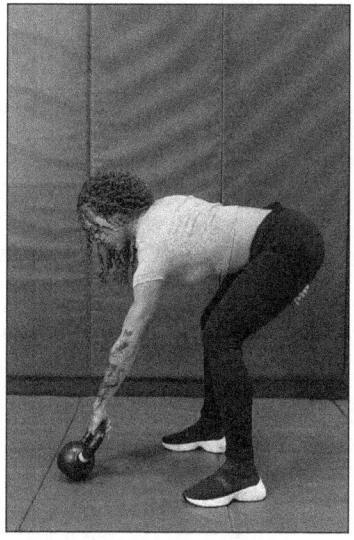

FIGURE 9-78:
Grab hold of the kettlebell's handle and reach back with your other arm.

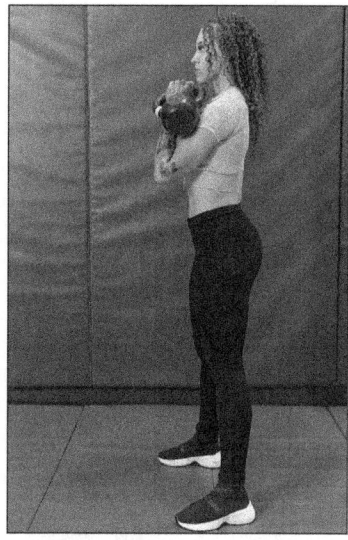

FIGURE 9-79:
Raise the kettlebell into its racked position.

Core clean (RT)

The core clean is an explosive movement that engages the legs, glutes, and lats as it generates movement across the transverse plane like few other movements do.

Here's how you do core cleans:

1. **Position your feet relatively close together, and place the kettlebell close to one foot with the handle parallel to the leg.**

2. **Bend your knees, reach across your body, and grasp the handle of the bell with the thumb toward you, as shown in Figure 9-80.** If the kettlebell is on your left side, grab it with your right hand.

3. **Hoist the kettlebell explosively into the racked position, as shown in Figure 9-81.**

4. **Lower the kettlebell back to the ground slowly, returning it to its original resting position.**

   Be careful not to drop the kettlebell on your foot. That is *not* recommended.

5. **Repeat steps 2–4 for ten reps, and then do ten reps with the kettlebell on your other side.**

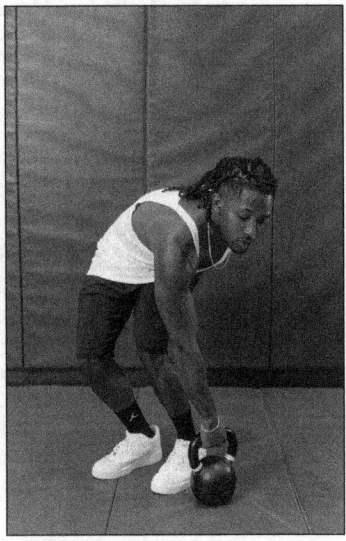

FIGURE 9-80:
Reach across your body to grasp the kettlebell's handle.

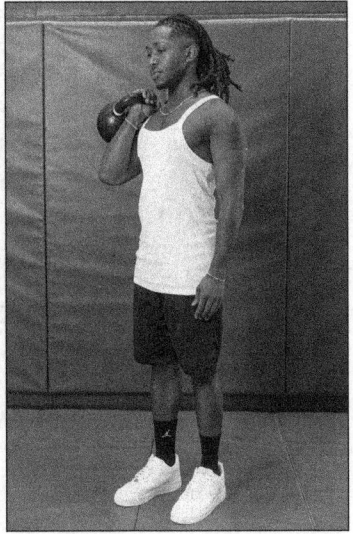

FIGURE 9-81:
Hoist the kettlebell across your body into the racked position.

Rows

A *row* is a weightlifting movement that involves pulling a weight up toward your chest. Rows are great for toning the upper back and biceps. In this section, we present two renditions of rows.

Single kettlebell rows (RT)

The single kettlebell row involves lifting one bell with one arm at a time. We're focusing on it rather than on dual-bell methods because it applies an uneven load, making it better for improving core strength while engaging the core stabilizers.

REMEMBER You don't need a bench for support; you are the bench.

Take the following steps to perform single kettlebell rows:

1. **Adopt a staggered stance (one foot forward, one foot back) and grasp the handle of the kettlebell with the hand that's on the same side as your back foot, palm facing back.** Maintain a neutral spine, with your head at about the 10 o'clock position and your butt at about the 3 o'clock position.

   You can use your other arm to support your upper body by resting your forearm on your thigh or let it hang at your side and rely solely on core strength for support.

2. **Lift the kettlebell straight up toward your chest, keeping your shoulders square with your hips until the handle touches your waist just above the hip (see Figure 9-82).** As you lift the kettlebell, your arm naturally rotates it about 180 degrees so that your palm is facing forward at the top.

3. **Slowly lower the kettlebell toward the ground without letting it touch, keeping your shoulders packed and your lats engaged (see Figure 9-83).**

REMEMBER To prevent the kettlebell from hitting the floor, pack your shoulders and maintain tension throughout the back.

4. **Repeat Steps 2 and 3 for ten reps and then do ten reps on the other side.**

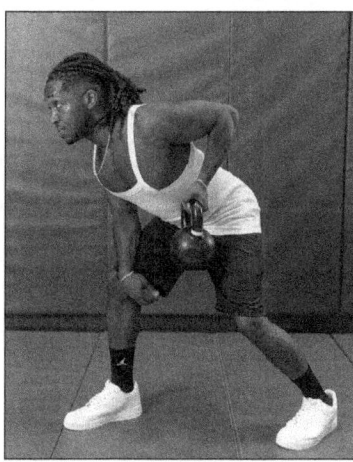

FIGURE 9-82:
Adopt a staggered stance and lift the kettlebell with the arm near your rear leg.

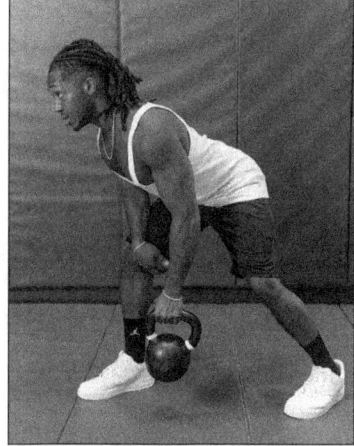

FIGURE 9-83:
Lower the kettlebell toward the ground without letting it touch the ground.

Renegade rows (RT)

Renegade rows require two kettlebells. You assume a push-up position and push down on one while lifting the other with the opposite arm. At first glance, this movement appears to be a pure lat-building exercise, but it's actually incredible at building core strength. As with most kettlebell movements, it's a full-body exercise that strengthens the stabilizers of the core, shoulders, wrists, and support muscles of the spine. Follow these steps:

1. **Place two kettlebells on the ground next to each other, spaced a little less than shoulder-width apart, the handles aligned with your body. Grasp the handles, and assume the push-up position, arms straight, elbows locked, neutral spine, and feet spread about shoulder-width apart, standing on the balls of your feet (see Figure 9-84).**

   If you don't have two kettlebells the same size, you can use two different sizes.

2. **Push down hard on the handle of one kettlebell while lifting the other kettlebell up to your waist (between the hips and the ribs) as you drive the ball of your foot on that same side into the ground for support, keeping your shoulders square with your hips (see Figure 9-85).**

TIP

If you notice that your body is twisting, your core isn't stable enough for this movement. Do one-armed planks and other kettlebell row variations until you've built enough core strength to do renegade rows without twisting.

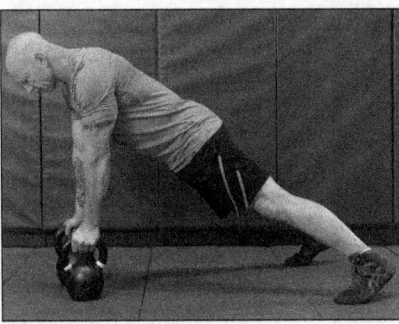

FIGURE 9-84:
Grab the handles and assume a push-up position, arms straight.

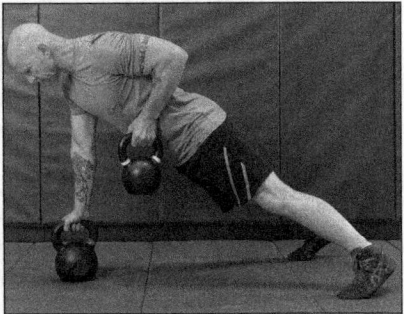

FIGURE 9-85:
Push down on one kettlebell while lifting the other.

Sample Workouts for Bullet-Proofing Your Back

This chapter contains more than 30 intermediate and advanced back-building exercises. We don't expect you to do all the exercises every day. In fact, we don't recommend it. We recommend assembling 3–7 exercises into mini workout routines and rotating them daily. In this section, we provide you with a weekly workout plan consisting of seven daily workout routines, which contain exercises we cover in this chapter (along with a couple from Chapter 8). Feel free to adjust the plan and the daily workouts to suit your needs and tastes, but be sure to engage all your muscle groups over the course of the week and to alternate bodyweight-only (B), resistance training (RT), and mobility (M) exercises.

For optimal results when performing your daily workouts, follow these tips:

>> **Maintain proper form:** Perform the exercises as described and illustrated in this chapter. Proper form is essential for achieving optimal results and preventing injury.

TIP

Work with a qualified instructor or an experienced partner, if possible, at least when you're getting started. An instructor/partner can provide feedback on your form as you're performing the exercises. You can also find instructional videos for some of these exercises on my YouTube channel, @TheMasterPhil.

>> **Adhere to the 80-percent rule:** Do no more than 80 percent of the maximum reps you're capable of performing. You're better off performing more sets of fewer reps than fewer sets of more reps.

WARNING

"No pain, no gain" is a recipe for disaster. It increases your risk of injury and typically results in poor form. Think about it: if the maximum number of pull-ups that you can do is 10, how is your form going to look for reps 9 and 10 compared to your form doing reps 6 and 7? Those last reps are generally not sound in form and are the ones that make you more prone to injury.

>> **Train daily:** You're better off training daily at a lower level than doing an incredibly intense workout that requires two or three days of recovery.

>> **Alternate weighted and unweighted workouts:** Using weights every other day gives your body more time to repair muscles between weighted workouts while also ensuring that you're moving your joints and working your muscles daily.

The goal of these daily workouts is to develop strength and endurance, so gradually increase the weight (for resistance training exercises) or the number of reps (for bodyweight-only and mobility exercises) over time. This approach will stimulate your body's *specific adaptation to imposed demand (SAID)* — physical changes in response to stress — which drives your progression. Here's how to gradually increase the "imposed demand":

>> For resistance training (RT) exercises, start with three sets of 8–12 reps for each exercise unless otherwise specified. When you're able to do 12 reps for all three sets, increase the weight by about five percent.

>> For bodyweight-only (B) and mobility (M) exercises, start with the specified number of reps per set and increase the number of reps if you are able to while also adhering to the 80-percent rule.

REMEMBER

Feel free to do the following workouts as is or add these exercises to your usual exercise routine to augment a more complete training protocol. The purpose of these workouts is to strengthen the core, especially the hidden core, and increase the mobility of the spine and back.

Perform the movements/exercises as a circuit in the prescribed order. If you're unable to do the number of reps and sets we recommend, do as many as you can with the goal of working your way up to the number we recommend. What's important is that you do the exercises daily and gradually improve.

Day 1 workout

Do two sets of each of the following exercises:

1. **Standard scapular push-ups:** ten reps (B)
2. **Full squats:** 15 reps (B)
3. **Glute bridges:** ten reps with a two-second hold (B, M)

Do three sets of 8–12 reps of each of the following exercises:

1. **Standard, two-hand deadlifts** (RT)
2. **Romanian deadlifts (RDLs)** (RT)
3. **Kettlebell cleans** (RT)
4. **Thor raises** (RT)
5. **Dead bugs:** 30-second hold (B)

Day 2

Do three sets of each of the following exercises:

1. **Planks:** 30-second hold (B)
2. **Pull-ups or plank pull-ups:** 80 percent of maximum reps (B)
3. **Thoracic bridges:** three reps, five-second hold (B, M)
4. **Scales:** five reps on each side (B)
5. **60-second abs:** 80 percent of max reps (B)

Day 3

Do two sets of each of the following exercises:

1. **Push-ups (regular push-ups):** ten reps (B)
2. **Full squats:** 15 reps (B)
3. **Cat/cows:** ten reps with a two-second hold (B, M)

Do three sets of each of the following exercises:

1. **Get-up sit-ups:** five reps on each side (RT, M)
2. **Two-hand swings:** 12 reps (RT)
3. **One-arm swings:** six reps on each side (RT)
4. **Kettlebell rows:** 8–12 reps on each side (RT)
5. **Kettlebell push-ups:** 5–10 reps (B)

Day 4

Do three sets of each of the following exercises:

1. **Four-point crawls:** ten forward and back (B)
2. **Lizard crawls:** ten forward and back (B, M)
3. **Floor levers:** five reps, five seconds out and back (B)
4. **60-second abs:** 80 percent of max reps (B)
5. **Single leg bridges:** five reps on each side with a two-second hold (B,M)

Day 5

Do two sets of each of the following exercises:

1. **Standard scapular push-ups:** ten reps (B)
2. **Full squats:** 15 reps (B)
3. **Tabletop bridges:** ten reps with a two-second hold (B, M)

Do three sets of each of the following exercises:

1. **Get-ups:** two reps on each side (RT, M)
2. **Uneven kettlebell swings:** six reps in each direction (RT)
3. **Core cleans:** six reps on each side (RT)
4. **Renegade rows:** six reps on each side (RT)
5. **Hanging abs:** 5–10 reps (B)

Day 6

Do three sets of each of the following exercises:

1. **Pull-ups or chin-ups:** 80 percent of max reps (B)
2. **Push-ups:** 10–25 reps (B)
3. **Ab crawls:** ten reps in each direction (B)
4. **Runner's bridges:** five reps on each side with a two-second hold (B, M)
5. **Neck bridges:** ten reps on each side (B, M)

Day 7

The seventh day is a day of active rest. Go for a hike, bike ride, long walk, swim, or some other type of low-impact activity for at least 30 minutes. Missing a day is okay. Just don't miss too many.

IN THIS CHAPTER

» **Rolling your pain away**

» **Stimulating healing with cupping**

» **Considering red light therapy**

» **Using analgesic ointments**

» **Stretching your spine**

Chapter **10**

Exploring Homespun Therapies

Your back can use some tender, loving care. Unfortunately, chiropractic treatment, massage, and physical therapy can be costly and inconvenient. Besides, with a little knowledge and some inexpensive equipment and supplies, you can get many of the same benefits via self-treatment for a small fraction of the cost without having to leave your home. Two added benefits of self-care options are: 1) the quantity of care is virtually unlimited (it's not constrained to a 15- to 30-minute session once or twice a week) and 2) self-care builds *self-efficacy* — an empowerment mindset, which can improve your health in ways that science is only beginning to understand. (See Chapter 4 for more about self-efficacy.)

In this chapter, we present several self-care alternatives to treatments that otherwise would require a trip to the chiropractor, masseuse, or physical therapist. These self-care techniques can be useful for both alleviating pain and preventing it, and they involve the use of relatively inexpensive equipment and supplies, some of which you may already have.

Massaging Your Back Muscles and Fascia

Your back muscles and *fascia* (the thin, tough connective tissue that encases muscles, organs, and other structures in the body) can develop knots (adhesions and scar tissue) that can lead to muscle stiffness and pain. Applying pressure to these areas helps to break up the knots and make the muscles and fascia more pliable, which can make you more mobile.

In this section, we explain how to use foam rollers, a lacrosse or tennis ball, or a massage gun to give yourself a deep-tissue massage that targets common areas of back pain.

REMEMBER

As we explain in Chapter 2, you can look at pain as having three tiers:

» **Stimulus:** The biological trigger (for example, straining a back muscle)

» **Epiphenomenon:** The biological response to the trigger (for example, inflammation and muscle spasm)

» **Judicial function:** How the brain interprets signals received from the stimulus and epiphenomenon

Massage targets the epiphenomena — sources of the "pain" signals being sent to the brain.

Using foam rollers

Foam rollers are lightweight Tootsie Roll-shaped polyethylene devices that come in various lengths and diameters. Most are smooth; some have a textured surface. The first order of business is to choose a foam roller that's right for you. Here are some guidelines for making a well-informed choice:

» **Hardness/density:** If you're new to foam rolling, have an extremely painful region, or the painful area is bony, consider a softer (lower density) roller. If the painful area is heavily muscled, and you have a high tolerance for pain/discomfort, you may prefer a harder roller. If you can't decide, start with a soft roller and then consider a harder one as you acclimate to using a roller. Check customer reviews for better insight into just how soft or hard a roller is.

» **Length:** For the purpose of addressing back pain, a 12-inch long roller is usually best. At 12 inches, the roller is manageable, suitable for rolling the hip flexors, and easy to take with you and store.

>> **Diameter:** Most foam rollers are 5–6 inches in diameter, which most people are comfortable using. You may want a smaller diameter roller for a more targeted massage or greater stability (closer to the floor).

To use a roller specifically for back pain, take the following steps:

1. **Place the roller on the floor in an area where you'll have plenty of room to roll back and forth.** A hard floor is best because it provides more support.

2. **Sit on the floor with your back end against the roller, hold the roller in place, and lean back to raise your body up onto it.**

3. **Slowly and gently roll forward and then back across the full length of your spine — from the sacrum all the way up to where your neck meets your skull — three times.**

TIP

If you're feeling too much pressure, push off the floor with one or both hands and/or feet so that less of your body weight is on the roller.

4. **Slowly and gently roll back and forth on the specific pain area for at least ten seconds, preferably longer:**

- **Lumbar (low) spine:** Go vertebra by vertebra, feeling each one as the roller slowly moves over the individual bones. You may hear or feel a "pop"; don't worry — popping is a sign that the spine is decompressing.

- **Thoracic (middle) spine:** Follow the same vertebra-by-vertebra approach. In fact, we recommend rolling the lumbar and thoracic spines together in one continuous sweep. The midback is a common area for muscle strain and tightness, primarily due to weak rhomboids and trapezius muscles and poor posture. If you don't strengthen and limber up these muscles, the middle back can become a pain generator, and over time, you could end up looking like Quasimodo.

  For the lumbar and thoracic spine, you can do one side at a time (left then right) or just focus on the more painful side.

WARNING

  Don't roll the cervical spine (neck). It won't benefit that section of the spine, and it could cause injury. It definitely wouldn't feel good.

- **Latissimus dorsi:** These are the large muscles that are located on the sides of the body — the muscles that look like wings on bodybuilders. Start by lying on your side with the roller between the floor and your waist, just below your floating ribs. Slowly roll all the way up to the shoulder joint as you roll over the teres major, teres minor, infraspinatus, and supraspinatus.

When you hit those little muscles, get ready — this may light you up! Be prepared to use your hands and feet to lighten the load on your body by pressing down on the roller. Roll this area for 3–10 seconds at a time.

- **Glutes:** Sitting up tall with your hands on the floor, place the roller under one butt cheek as you roll slowly back and forth, just as you roll your spine. The glutes are large muscles, so expect to feel less pain and discomfort than you feel when rolling your spine. For a deeper massage of the glutes, you need to use a lacrosse ball, as we explain in the next section.

- **Hamstrings:** Sitting up tall with your hands on the floor, place the roller where your glutes and hamstrings meet. Roll slowly down the back of one leg all the way to the knee joint. Repeat this motion at least three times while rolling over the full length of the hamstring and rocking back and forth on pain areas for at least ten seconds. If you need to apply more pressure, place your other leg over the leg that you're rolling. Switch legs and repeat.

- **Hip flexors and quadriceps:** Lie on the floor face down and place the roller between the floor and your hip flexor (where the top of your leg meets your torso). Roll gently back and forth all the way down the quad to the knee and back up.

    Rolling out the quads is essential. If you sit for a large part of each day, you're probably "quad dominant" — your quads are probably tight.

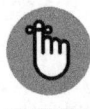

Stay on each target area for at least ten seconds. As a general rule, the longer you roll an area, the more relief you'll experience.

Loosening up with a lacrosse ball

In some areas of the body, a foam roller may not apply enough pressure to penetrate deeply enough into the muscle tissue to deliver the desired therapeutic benefits. Fortunately, we have a solution — the humble lacrosse ball or the softer, gentler tennis ball. We recommend using a lacrosse ball for the following two areas:

>> The muscles of the lower back (thoracolumbar fascia, erector spinae)

>> The muscles of the mid and upper back (rhomboids, trapezius, and elevator scapulae)

When using a ball, don't roll your spine over it. Doing so delivers zero benefits and is unnecessarily painful.

To use a ball for low-back pain, take the following steps:

1. **Lie down on your back.**

2. **Place the ball between the floor and the area of your back where you're feeling pain, discomfort, or tension.**

3. **Gently lower your body weight against the ball.** You don't want to trigger a sudden muscle contraction (spasm).

4. **Roll your back over the ball completely around the area of pain, discomfort, or tension.** Use your body weight to regulate the amount of pressure. Roll the area for about 1–3 minutes up to a maximum of 5 minutes.

TIP

Roll forward and back, side-to-side, and in a circular motion to figure out which of those motions delivers the best results.

For the upper areas of the back, use a wall instead of the floor. Try rolling up and down, side-to-side, and in a circular motion to determine what's most effective. Roll each area where you're feeling pain, discomfort, or tension for 1–3 minutes up to a maximum of 5 minutes. Use your body weight to apply more or less pressure.

Using a massage gun

Another option is to use a massage gun (or similar device), but when you're dealing with back pain, it doesn't exactly qualify as self-treatment; you typically need to lie face down and have someone else use the massage gun on you. You can get massage guns and other devices designed to deliver back massage without the help of another person, but these devices are usually awkward to use and may not provide the same level of benefits.

TIP

If you have a significant other or a friend or family member who's willing to give you a massage, a massage gun can be a very valuable device. A quality massage gun may be a little pricey, but it can pay for itself over the course of a few weeks if you're using it instead of paying a chiropractor, masseuse, or physical therapist.

Use the massage gun to target specific areas of pain. Most of these devices deliver gentle "punches" that can help to break up adhesions and scar tissue. Simply turn on the device and then run it over the painful area.

Stimulating Blood Flow with Cupping

Cupping is an ancient therapy that uses suction to draw blood and other fluids into injured or painful areas of the body to promote healing, alleviate pain, remove toxins, or boost immune function. If you've ever seen athletes at the Olympics or other athletic competitions with big red circles on their skin, you've seen the after-effects of cupping. Cupping methods include the following:

>> **Dry cupping:** Various methods are used to create suction in a cup that's placed over the affected area of the skin.

>> **Running cupping:** Oil is applied to the lip of the cup so that you can slide it around after suctioning it to the skin. This technique is useful for cupping a large area around a sore muscle using a single cup.

>> **Wet/bleeding cupping:** The skin is punctured before placing the cup to extract blood and toxins — not something we recommend unless you've just been bitten by a rattlesnake.

Modern methods involve using manual or battery-powered suction cups, the latter of which provide more consistent suction and stay in place better. Some cups are heated or equipped with red light to further promote healing (skip to the next section for more about red light therapy).

Follow the instructions that come with the device. The process typically involves pressing the rim of a cup against the skin over the painful area and suctioning the air out from the cup. The skin inside the cup rises, pulling blood into the area. You generally leave the cup in place for about 15 minutes.

TIP

If you have any body hair around the area you're treating, consider shaving it to ensure a good seal between your skin and the rim of the cup. Apply oil or body lotion to the area you're treating or to the rim of the cup if you want to slide the cup around during a treatment session.

Shining Red Light on the Problem

Originally developed by the National Aeronautics and Space Administration (NASA) for growing plants in space, red lights have shown promise in space travel for healing wounds that astronauts suffer on missions. Although studies on the benefits of using red light to alleviate muscle soreness and pain are limited, preliminary data suggests that red light delivers notable benefits, including the following:

>> Promotes new cell growth, thereby healing and rejuvenating the skin

>> Stimulates collagen production and reduces inflammation at the cellular level

The clinical evidence for the benefits of red light therapy is impressive. We know many healthcare professionals and patients who've had success alleviating muscle pain and soreness with red light therapy.

Look for a device from a reputable manufacturer that offers the following features:

>> **Combination of wavelengths:** 600–650 nanometers (for red light) and 800–880 nanometers (for near-infrared light) to ensure that the light penetrates deep enough to deliver therapeutic benefits.

>> **Power output:** At least 100 milliwatts per square centimeter (mW/cm²) at the treatment surface. Higher power can deliver quicker results but may be uncomfortable for some people.

>> **Coverage area:** For back pain, you want a device that covers a broader surface area, such as a pad or panel, instead of a small hand-held device that's designed for more targeted applications.

>> **Adjustable treatment time and intensity:** Look for a device that enables you to control the treatment time and intensity. A typical session is 10–20 minutes.

>> **Comfort and usability:** Choose a device that is comfortable and easy to use. You can find cordless therapy belts that wrap around your back and fasten in front.

>> **Safety:** Look for a device that has automatic shutoff or overheating protection for extended sessions.

Bringing the Heat: Heating Pads, Baths, Saunas, and Whirlpools

Heat and hydrotherapy can be very effective for reducing tension, relaxing muscles, improving circulation, relieving pain, and alleviating stress. However, if the pain is due to inflammation or a recent injury, cold therapy may be the better option. Cold tends to reduce inflammation (and slow the healing process), but heat increases inflammation (and may accelerate healing). Here are a few heat and hydrotherapy options to consider:

>> **Warm baths:** Soaking in a warm bath delivers all the aforementioned benefits; plus, thanks to buoyancy, the water reduces stress on the spine. Adding Epsom salt (a source of magnesium) to the bath relaxes the muscles even more.

>> **Heating pad or gel packs:** Lie down with the painful area positioned over the heating pad or gel pack to relax tight muscles and reduce muscle spasms.

WARNING

Be careful when using heat therapy. Follow the instructions that come with the product, and start with the lowest recommended setting/time so you don't burn your skin. Don't place a heating pad or gel pack directly on your skin; wrap it in a towel. And don't fall asleep on a heating pad.

>> **Sauna:** Saunas are great for alleviating stress and relaxing muscles and joints. In addition, they promote sweating, which supports the body's detoxification mechanisms.

WARNING

To sauna safely, drink at least eight fluid ounces of water before you enter the sauna and more water afterward. Avoid drinking alcohol in the hours before or after using the sauna. Remain in the sauna for no longer than 20 minutes at a time.

>> **Whirlpool (hot tub):** A whirlpool combines heat with hydrotherapy and massage and provides buoyancy to reduce pressure on muscles and joints. To use a whirlpool safely, follow the same precautions we provide for using a sauna: drink plenty of fluids, avoid alcohol, and limit your time in the whirlpool to about 20 minutes max per session.

Soothing Your Pain with Arnica and Other Ointments

Numerous ointments and salves have been developed to alleviate pain, including back pain. They include a variety of natural, synthetic, and prescription pharmaceuticals, including Arnica and capsaicin (natural substances), non-steroidal anti-inflammatory drugs (NSAIDs), lidocaine, and a variety of herbs and menthols. Here's our list of top ten salves and ointments for back pain (in no particular order of preference):

>> **Arnica:** Balm, liquid and roll-on

>> **Aspercreme:** Roll-on

>> **Bengay Ultra Strength:** Paste in a tube

>> **Biofreeze:** Cream in a tub

>> **Evil Bone Water:** Base of dit da jow in a spray bottle

>> **Icy Hot:** Roll-on

>> **Tiger Balm:** Low-cost, effective balm

>> **Topricin:** Cream in a tub

>> **Uber Numb:** Cream in a tub (lidocaine)

>> **Voltaren:** Cream in a tube (diclofenac is the generic and is half the price)

Some patients have reported benefits from using topical cannabinoids, such as ointments containing cannabidiol (CBD). CBD is a marijuana extract that's not psychoactive (it doesn't make you high). Tetrahydrocannabinol (THC) is the substance that produces a high. For more about analgesics, including cannabinoids, see Chapter 14.

WARNING

If you're taking pain relievers orally, talk to your doctor about before using topical analgesics. These topical formulations may be absorbed through the skin to some degree.

TIP

For optimal results, apply the salve two or three times daily, preferably after a shower (to aid absorption), and rub it into the area of pain, discomfort, or tension.

Decompressing Your Spinal Column

Allowing your spinal column to decompress improves posture, relieves pressure on nerves and discs, increases circulation, reduces muscle tension, improves mobility, and promotes overall spine health. In this section, we present several techniques and tools for decompressing your spine.

Practicing a simple spinal decompression technique

Here's a simple technique for decompressing the spine that you can do almost anywhere without any special gear:

1. **Lie on your back on the floor or a hard mattress and relax for at least 30 seconds, breathing in and out slowly and deeply.**

2. **Roll to the face-down position and arch your back slightly by supporting yourself on your elbows and forearms. Keep breathing slowly and deeply.** Relax. You may hear or feel your back crack, which is normal and actually a good thing.

3. **Lower your chest back to the floor or mattress, roll onto your back, and slowly "swing" one leg over the other, which remains on the floor/mattress.** Keep your shoulder blades flat on the floor/mattress. Hold this position for 30 seconds.

4. **Return the leg you swung over to its original position and then repeat Step 3 with your other leg.**

Using a yoga/physio ball to stretch your back

You can use a yoga or physio ball to strengthen and stretch your back at the same time. Get a quality ball that's the right size for you. Here are some features to consider:

>> **Size (diameter):** When you sit on the ball, your feet should be flat on the ground with your knees bent at a 90-degree angle. Here's a general size chart:

Your Height	Ball Size
Shorter than four feet, six inches	30 centimeters
Four feet, six inches to five feet	45 centimeters
Five feet to five feet, 5 inches	55 centimeters
Five feet, six inches to six feet, two inches	65 centimeters
Over six feet, two inches	75 centimeters

>> **Material:** High-quality non-toxic PVC that's anti-burst and anti-slip. Whether the surface is smooth or textured is a personal preference.

>> **Weight capacity:** Be sure the ball is rated to support at least the amount that you weigh. Most high-quality balls support over 300 pounds.

>> **Ease of inflation:** Look for a ball that's easy to inflate and deflate. Some come with their own pumps, and the quality of the pump is another consideration.

Yoga/physio balls are versatile, and you can use yours in several ways to build back strength and mobility. Here are a few suggestions:

>> Use your ball as a chair. Make a conscious effort to maintain a neutral spine when sitting on the ball.

>> Place your hands on the floor, palms down, and your knees on the ball as if you're doing a push-up, and roll the ball forward and back and in circles, clockwise and counterclockwise equally.

>> Sit on the ball and do crunches, fingers interlocked behind your head, elbows back.

>> Lie flat on your back, place the ball between your bent legs, squeeze the ball, bring your knees up toward your chest, and guide the ball down and to the right, straight up, and then down and to the left for five repetitions on each side.

TIP

To make this movement more challenging, keep your legs straight, squeeze the ball between your ankles, lift it up as high as possible, and guide the ball down and to the right, straight up, and then down and to the left for five repetitions on each side. Keep your lower back planted firmly on the floor during the entire exercise.

>> Lie with your mid back (thoracic region) on the ball, feet flat on the floor, arms out to the sides, and let your head go back and down. Breathe and relax into the ball. Feel your body "melt" into the ball. Do this for 2–3 minutes or longer.

Hanging around: Inversion tables, traction, and other gear and techniques

Gravity is great for providing the resistance needed to build back strength, but it works against you when you're trying to decompress the spine. Fortunately, you can use gravity to your advantage and use traction to reverse its effects. In this section, we present several options, including inversion tables, dead hangs, countertops, dips, and traction devices to decompress the spine.

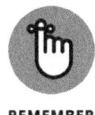

REMEMBER

Whenever and however you're "hanging around" to decompress your spine, relax and focus on your breathing. Breathe deeply and slowly. Most people tend to tense up. Controlled, focused breathing coupled with relaxation enables your vertebrae to "hang loose."

Inversion tables and anti-gravity boots

Inversion tables and anti-gravity boots enable you to hang upside down, like a bat, suspended from your ankles. Inversion tables are usually adjustable for different heights and have different weight capacities and features. Be sure to buy one that's tall enough for you and that can support your weight. Anti-gravity boots typically come with an inversion rack that mounts inside a doorway and boots or braces that wrap around your ankles. Anti-gravity boots are more hard-core; with an inversion table, you have more control over how inverted you are. Do your research and read customer reviews to gain some insight into the perfor-mance and comfort of each device you're looking at.

Another option is to use a sit-up or crunch bench. Instead of using it for an ab workout, you can use it to decompress your spine. You can adjust the angle for your comfort level.

REMEMBER

We recommend that you try an inversion table before you buy one. Inversion isn't for everyone, especially if you've had a knee replacement, hip replacement, or other orthopedic surgery, or you just don't like having a lot of pressure on your ankles or the tops of your feet, or you can't stand the feeling of having blood throbbing in your head. Some people love inversion, some people hate it, and many simply choose to tolerate its discomfort in exchange for the benefits.

TIP

If you're inverting for the first time, ease into it and have a partner on hand to spot you, especially if you're trying boots. Start with small doses of one to two minutes and then come back up. Eventually, you may be able to stay inverted for 10–15 minutes at a time. You may even be able to do crunches or stretches while you're dangling from your ankles. Anti-gravity boots provide a little more free-dom of movement, so you can gently twist from side to side, which can promote spinal decompression.

WARNING

If you have glaucoma, trouble with blood pressure regulation, vertigo, or other health issues that may be exacerbated by inversion, consult your doctor before trying it. If you're using an inversion table, you can start at a slight incline, for example, about 10–15 degrees, and work your way up.

Dead hangs

If you have the grip strength to hang from a pull-up bar, you can do a dead hang. You simply grip the bar (overhand or underhand), lift your feet off the ground, and hang there. For opening up the spine, the dead hang is more effective than an inversion table or anti-gravity boots. Think about it — you have a lot more of your body weight pulling down on your spine when you're hanging from your arms than when you're hanging from your legs. Dead hangs deliver some additional health benefits, including the following:

>> Improve grip strength

>> Stretch the hard-to-stretch lats

>> Lower the risk of cardiovascular and respiratory disease

>> Improve posture

>> Mobilize the entire upper body

>> Relieve shoulder pain (but they can cause shoulder pain, too, so be careful)

Here are a few tips for getting the most benefit from your dead hangs:

>> Before trying dead hangs, work up to doing some pull-ups or chin-ups, as we explain in Chapter 9, to strengthen your shoulder muscles. Strong shoulder muscles can help prevent pulling a muscle when doing dead hangs.

>> If possible, hang from a bar that's high enough to keep your feet off the ground. If it's not high enough for that, bend your knees and let the tops of your feet rest on the ground.

>> Let your body relax and your spine decompress. Breathe slowly and deeply, allowing the tension to leave your body. The grip is the only part of your body that should have tension.

>> Hang for as long as you can retain your grip. If you can hang for only 10 seconds or so at a time at first, that's fine — do 3-6 reps, so that you're getting 30-60 seconds of hang time. Many experts claim that hanging 20 minutes a day is best, which is great, but if you can work up to a total of 5-10 minutes daily, your back will still love you for it!

Countertops and dips

If you don't have a pull-up bar or the grip to do dead hangs (or you just don't like doing them), another option is to do dips. You can buy a dip station or use a countertop or chair — anything that enables you to lift your body upward so that most of your body weight is supported by your arms and shoulders. (Your spine dangles from your shoulders down.)

To do a countertop, stand with your back to the counter, place your hands palms down on the countertop, and push yourself up as far as possible. Hold the position for at least 30 seconds and do a few reps throughout the day. If you're sitting in a chair with strong armrests that are fairly close to your body, you can push yourself up from your armrests and even "bounce" gently up and down a little to promote decompression. Breathe slowly and deeply, allowing your spine to relax.

Chapter **11**

Breathing New Life into Your Back

Human survival is governed by the rule of three: A human can live roughly three weeks without food, three days without water, and only about three minutes without oxygen. Of course, the number three isn't precise, but the message is clear: The need to breathe is far more urgent than the need for food and water.

But you need more than "just enough" oxygen to stay alive. You need enough to stay healthy. Ideally, oxygen content in the blood, measured as *saturation of peripheral oxygen (SpO2)*, should be between 95 and 100 percent consistently. When it drops below 95 percent, you start to experience *hypoxemia* (oxygen deficit), and your health can start to suffer:

» **Mild hypoxemia (90–94 percent SpO2)** may cause increased heart rate, shortness of breath, fatigue, and lightheadedness.

» **Moderate hypoxemia (80–89 percent SpO2)** may result in confusion or disorientation, increased respiratory rate, and *cyanosis* (skin, lips, or nails turn blue).

» **Severe hypoxemia (below 80 percent SpO2)** can cause labored breathing, loss of consciousness, organ damage, and respiratory failure.

With respect to back pain specifically, low oxygen can worsen existing pain and impair the body's repair and recovery processes.

In this chapter, we provide guidance on how to determine whether you're getting a healthy supply of oxygen throughout the day and overnight, and we share several techniques for breathing effectively and efficiently. These techniques help not only to boost your oxygen saturation but also to alleviate stress and reduce muscle tension.

TIP

You can use breathing to support your spine while lifting heavy objects. This technique (called "breathing behind the shield") transforms your torso into a pneumatic pillar of strength, sort of like an air mattress. See Chapter 7 for more about breathing behind the shield.

Monitoring Your Oxygen Saturation Levels

You may be able to tell whether your oxygen saturation level is low based on how you're feeling. If you feel tired all the time, even after a good night's sleep, you feel short of breath or lightheaded, or you're experiencing brain fog (impaired memory or thinking), you may not be getting enough oxygen. You may also be oxygen deprived during sleep, especially if you have a condition called *sleep apnea* — a sleep disorder characterized by repetitive pauses in breathing, periods of shallow breathing, or collapse of the upper airway. Common symptoms of sleep apnea include loud snoring, pauses in breathing, gasping for air, excessive daytime sleepiness, morning headaches, and difficulty concentrating.

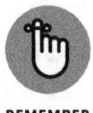

REMEMBER

Proper breathing, particularly during sleep, is a building block of health, along with exercise and diet. Sleep apnea is associated with several medical conditions, including heart disease and dementia, and it may play a role in longevity.

To get a more complete oxygen saturation assessment, use a pulse oximeter. You've probably seen one of these devices in your doctor's office. It clips to the tip of your finger and measures your pulse (heartbeats per minute) and your oxygen saturation. Unfortunately, the reading indicates only what your pulse and oxygen saturation are at that point in time. It doesn't show your oxygen saturation when you're working, exercising, or sleeping. To obtain readings during those times, get your own pulse oximeter.

Pulse oximeters vary widely in price. Inexpensive versions have an LED display that shows your current pulse and oxygen concentration. More expensive versions connect wirelessly to a smartphone app, which can record your pulse and oxygen saturation levels continuously or at intervals. If you can afford it, we recommend buying a more expensive device from a reputable company. If you want a device to help you determine whether you have sleep apnea, make sure it's designed for that purpose — that it provides continuous monitoring and won't fall off if you move in your sleep.

TIP

As an alternative to buying a pulse oximeter to monitor your oxygen saturation while you sleep, consider asking your doctor to order a sleep study. If you have health insurance, check to be sure that your insurance provider will cover the cost. You may also want to check whether your policy covers the cost of a continuous positive airway pressure (CPAP) machine if the sleep study indicates the need for one. If you don't have health insurance, consider ordering an at-home sleep test online. For a one-time fee, the sleep test provider sends you a monitor to wear while you sleep that collects data (including oxygen saturation), typically via an app on your smartphone, and then sends the data to your doctor (or one of their doctors) to interpret the results and offer treatment recommendations.

Brushing Up on Deep-Breathing Fundamentals

Amid the hustle and bustle of day-to-day living, people often forget to breathe, or they forget how to breathe properly. Over time, they may stop using their diaphragm to take deep, full breaths and develop a shallow, chest breathing habit. If you notice that you forget to breathe during the day or that your breathing is shallow, you may need to re-learn how to breathe. In this section, we touch on the fundamentals.

TAKING A LESSON FROM MIDWIVES

Childbirth can be one of the most painful of human experiences. For thousands of years, midwives have been guiding women through that process, helping them manage the pain, relax, and deal with the physical and emotional stress of giving birth. Their techniques often include some form of conscious, controlled breathing.

These same techniques, which promote oxygenation, relax the muscles, and reduce pain, can be very helpful in managing back pain as well. Pregnant women who enroll in Lamaze classes are often taught these techniques, which include breathing through the surges (waves of pain) associated with contractions.

Several times over the course of the day, shift your awareness to how you're breathing at home, at work, while on your computer or phone, when watching TV, and during other activities. Note how deeply you're breathing, whether your breathing is tensed or relaxed, and the rate at which you inhale and exhale. Your observations can help you identify the times of day that you need to work on your breathing technique.

Maintain a posture that facilitates deep breathing

Maintain a neutral spine all the time. This advice, which we drill into you in Chapters 7, 8, and 9, ensures not only that your vertebrae remain in proper alignment but also that your lungs have the room they need to expand fully. If you're slouching, you're compressing your abdominal and chest cavities, leaving your lungs less room to expand.

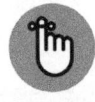

REMEMBER

Stand tall and sit tall — neutral spine, shoulders back, chest out, and head up! No, you're not getting off the bus for your first day of boot camp, and we're not your drill sergeants. We're just reinforcing the fundamentals of good posture, which are essential for deep breathing. Be especially conscious of your posture when sitting; even people who are conscientious about standing tall often slouch or hunch over when they're sitting. Just take a look around when you're sitting on benches in a stadium, and you'll notice that a large majority of the crowd is slouched or hunched over.

Breathe from your diaphragm

The diaphragm is the dome-shaped muscle that separates the chest cavity (containing the heart and lungs) from the abdominal cavity (containing the stomach, intestines, liver, kidneys, and a few other internal organs). It's the muscle that plays (or should play) the biggest role in breathing. It contracts to inhale and relaxes to exhale.

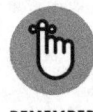

REMEMBER

Breathe with your belly, not your chest. Perform the following exercise to practice belly breathing (also known as diaphragm breathing):

1. **Sit or lie down in a relaxed position and gently close your eyes. If sitting, maintain a neutral spine and relax your shoulders.** If lying down, place one hand on your chest and the other on your belly.

2. **Breathe normally, paying attention to the rise and fall of your chest and belly.**

3. Belly-breathe slowly in through your nose, to a count of about four, so that your belly rises and your chest doesn't move.

4. Exhale slowly through your nose or pursed lips for a count of about six, allowing your abdomen to fall as the air leaves your lungs.

5. Repeat Steps 4 and 5 for several minutes, maintaining a steady rhythm.

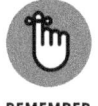

REMEMBER

A strong diaphragm can eliminate or at least significantly calm the symptoms of respiratory ailments, including exercise-induced asthma (EIA), and it can improve athletic performance.

Breathe through your nose

The most natural and efficient way to breathe is through your nose. Your nasal passages filter, humidify, and warm the air before it enters your lungs, and breathing through your nose regulates your breathing, all of which help you absorb oxygen and exhale carbon dioxide more effectively. Breathing through the mouth can dry the airways and stress the lungs, and it encourages shallow breathing.

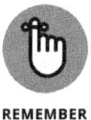

REMEMBER

Breathe through your nose regardless of what you're doing — relaxing, sleeping, working, exercising, you name it. If you can't quite manage to breathe through your nose entirely when exercising, inhale through your nose and exhale through your mouth (pursed lips) as you transition toward breathing through your nose all the time.

Breathe slowly, deeply, and relaxed

Take slow, deep breaths to expand your lungs fully. Rapid, shallow breaths impair the transfer of oxygen to the lungs and can make you exhale too much carbon dioxide (CO_2), which can cause other problems. Work toward establishing a slow, steady breathing pattern, inhaling over the span of about 4–5 seconds and exhaling over the span of about 5–6 seconds.

CO_2 is a waste product produced by cells during metabolism, and it plays an important role in maintaining pH balance in the blood. When you breathe too fast, you may lose too much CO_2, which can cause the blood's pH to become too alkaline. This condition, called *respiratory alkalosis*, can result in lightheadedness, muscle twitching, and tingling in the extremities.

Exploring Deep-Breathing Techniques

Deep breathing is healthy breathing. It takes in more oxygen and expels carbon dioxide more efficiently, synchronizes your breathing with your heartbeat, balances your nervous system, reduces stress, and improves mental clarity. People have developed all sorts of deep breathing techniques. In this section, we share our favorites.

Taking crocodile breaths

Honestly, we don't spend much time watching crocodiles breathe, but apparently, they're experts at diaphragmic breathing. If you search for "crocodile breathing" on YouTube or TikTok, you'll find plenty of videos of people demonstrating how to breathe like crocodiles. Crocs are also good about breathing through their noses, but you would be too if you swam around all day with every part of your body except your nose and eyes submerged.

We don't recommend that you take breathing lessons from a crocodile, but crocodile breathing is an exercise we recommend:

1. **Lie face down on the floor, hands palm down, one over the other, your forehead resting on your stacked hands.**

2. **Breathe in slowly and deeply through your nose so that your stomach rises and your ribs expand out to your sides.** You don't want your chest rising.

3. **Hold your breath for a few seconds and then breathe out slowly through your nose.**

4. **Repeat steps 2 and 3 for at least five minutes.** (Set a timer on your phone so you don't have to keep looking at the time.)

TIP

Crocodile breathing is a great exercise to do before bed or whenever you're feeling stressed or tired. Lying face down encourages you to breathe from your diaphragm and helps you regain your balance and composure.

Practicing meditative breathing

Meditation and breathing go together like peanut butter and jelly. In fact, a certain yoga style called pranayama focuses on developing a variety of breathing techniques. Practitioners of pranayama yoga believe that mastering your breath enables you to master your mind and, hence, master your life. Advanced practitioners can even breathe in through one nostril and out through the other. However, you don't need to be a yogi to practice meditative breathing. You simply need to empty your mind and shift your attention to breathing:

1. **Lie on your back or sit or stand in a comfortable, neutral spine position with your eyes closed.** Consider sitting on a yoga/physio ball, as we recommend in Chapter 10.

2. **Empty your mind of all thoughts and concerns other than your breathing and maintaining a neutral spine.**

3. **Belly-breathe in through your nose over a count of four and out over a count of four.** Repeat for 3–5 minutes, focusing solely on your breathing and posture.

TIP

Before engaging in anything that's potentially stressful or strenuous — such as a challenging exercise session, a presentation you're about to deliver, a test or exam you're about to take, or a discussion about a sensitive issue — take three deep, slow, meditative breaths. Meditative breathing serves several purposes:

>> Oxygenates your body, including your brain

>> Lets your body know it's about to do something important and challenging

>> Clears your mind and enhances your mental focus

Exploring resonant breathing and box breathing

Resonant and box breathing are similar rhythmic breathing techniques. Here, we provide guidance on both of these techniques.

Resonant breathing

Resonant breathing is a deep breathing technique designed to synchronize your breathing with your heartbeat. The theory is that it engages your body's parasympathetic nervous system to trigger the "rest and digest response" (as opposed to the sympathetic nervous system's "fight or flight" response). In the rest-and-digest state, you're more calm, balanced, and focused. Here's a step-by-step guide to resonant breathing:

1. **Lie on your back or sit or stand in a comfortable, neutral spine position.**

2. **Belly breathe in through your nose over a count of four seconds, filling your lungs and allowing your belly to expand fully.**

3. Breathe out through your nose or pursed lips over a count of four seconds, fully emptying your lungs.

4. Repeat Steps 2 and 3 for five to ten cycles.

Box breathing

Box breathing is very similar to resonant breathing, except you're adding a four-second pause after you fully inhale and after you fully exhale. To box-breathe, take the following steps:

1. Lie on your back or sit or stand in a comfortable, neutral spine position.

2. Belly breathe in through your nose over a count of four seconds, filling your lungs and allowing your belly to expand fully.

3. Hold your breath for four seconds.

4. Breathe out through your nose or pursed lips over a count of four seconds, fully emptying your lungs.

5. Wait for four seconds before taking your next breath.

6. Repeat Steps 2–5 for five to ten cycles.

TIP

Another way to enhance oxygenation is to exercise your lungs, which can strengthen your diaphragm and increase your lung capacity. Practicing deep breathing techniques can help. Pranayama yoga is also very effective. You can also purchase devices specifically designed for exercising your lungs.

3

Exploring Professional Back Pain Treatment Options

Chapter **12**

Getting a Diagnosis and Exploring Your Provider Options

At some point in your journey to manage your back pain effectively, you may need professional assistance — a doctor or surgeon, a physical therapist, a chiropractor, or even a psychologist or psychiatrist. And you may need or want a diagnosis to shed some light on what could be causing your back pain and to obtain some professional guidance on what to do about it.

In this chapter, we reveal the potential benefits of getting a medical diagnosis and the limitations of such diagnoses, and we provide guidance on various healthcare providers who can deliver the type of treatments you think would benefit you the most.

Considering the Accuracy and Value of a Diagnosis

When you see a doctor for any health concern, you're looking for clear, accurate answers to questions such as "Why am I sick?" "What's causing my symptoms?" and "What can be done to make me feel better?" In many cases, doctors can answer those questions by asking you a series of questions, performing a physical exam, looking at your medical and family history, and reviewing lab test results. In some cases involving back pain, a doctor can order medical imaging, such as X-rays or magnetic resonance imaging (MRI), and clearly see evidence of a cause. More often than not, however, test results and medical imaging reveal no clear cause of a patient's back pain. And when that happens, the doctor has few options, none of which is very attractive or helpful:

>> Make their best guess about the biological cause of the pain, such as a slipped or herniated disc or a pinched nerve. This is perhaps the worst option because it can give patients false hope and lead them down the wrong path.

>> Admit that they can't find anything physically wrong, the implication being that the pain is all in the patient's head (something no patient wants to hear).

>> Treat the symptoms — the pain and/or inflammation — usually with pain-relief medication or steroid shots, which do nothing to address the root cause(s) of the pain and may cause other health problems.

The fourth option, which is usually the most effective by far, is to help the patient restore their overall physical, mental, and emotional health and well-being, change their focus from eliminating their pain to improving their function, and learn how to manage stress and strengthen and mobilize their back. Unfortunately, most doctors aren't trained or incentivized to provide this type of care, and patients often aren't receptive to it — addressing all the possible causes of back pain can be complicated and requires considerable time and effort.

In some cases, medical diagnosis and treatment are necessary, as explained in Chapter 5. But keep in mind that a diagnosis can be very accurate and valuable, totally useless, or even counterproductive — leading you down a path of treatments that can do more harm than good and cost you considerable time, money, and effort. In the following sections, we present several good reasons to think twice about seeking a back pain diagnosis.

The healthcare system is dysfunctional

Medical diagnoses are often counterproductive due to the nature of today's healthcare system. We believe that doctors and other medical professionals genuinely strive to do what's best for their patients, but they have several factors working against them, including the following:

>> **An industry focus on illness:** Medical professionals are trained to diagnose and treat illnesses primarily with medication, surgery, and other medical interventions. They're not trained so much to encourage and empower patients to become healthier, stronger, and independent.

>> **Expectations for quick fixes:** In the U.S., many patients expect doctors to fix all their health problems. Doctors, pharmaceutical companies, and the media feed this expectation for quick fixes.

>> **Doctors are rewarded for providing treatment, not positive outcomes:** Many providers act independently and are incentivized by a fee-for-service reimbursement system, which can become a source of bias. They have an economic incentive to offer you their own services rather than refer you to a more appropriate provider or enable you to do more self-care.

REMEMBER

Many doctors want to address patient complaints in the quickest possible way — by relieving pain. This may be accomplished through prescriptions and/or surgery — but that may not get to the root source of the issue and may actually mask the true source of the pain.

>> **Doctors are compelled to provide a diagnosis:** To get paid for providing treatment, doctors must first present a diagnosis telling the insurance company what they're treating the patient for. "I don't know what's causing your back pain" doesn't qualify as a diagnosis, even if the doctor knows the steps you can take to manage your pain effectively.

>> **Doctors have limited time to spend with patients:** Profit-driven overbooking of patients gives doctors just enough time to diagnose a condition and write a prescription or make a referral. Little time is provided for the doctor to get to know the patient, educate the patient, or develop a personalized treatment plan complete with recommendations for diet, lifestyle, stress management, sleep optimization, and so on.

REMEMBER

You can counteract these negative effects of a dysfunctional healthcare system by playing a more active role in your healthcare. In addition to taking care of yourself, collaborate closely with your providers and advocate for the treatment you think will be most effective. Let your providers know that you're not looking for a quick fix and that you're willing and eager to play a bigger role in your health and fitness. Don't assume that "doctors know best," and don't be afraid to question them on their knowledge of food choices, fitness, and strength.

Diagnosis isn't necessarily objective

Diagnosis takes many forms, some more grounded in evidence and others more speculative (a doctor's best guess). A diagnosis may be based on a cluster of symptoms characteristic of a certain condition; you may have many of the symptoms and not have the condition associated with them. A diagnosis may also come from one person's interpretation of a medical image, an interpretation that could be skewed by various factors (see Chapter 13 for details). And a back pain diagnosis rarely, if ever, reveals the specific causes of the pain, which may include a composite of musculoskeletal imbalances, weak or tense back muscles, or various medical conditions that can cause inflammation. Thus, the diagnosis is often not helpful in constructing a treatment plan with a predictable outcome.

WARNING

Be cautious of the answer that you receive when you ask your provider what's causing your back pain. Providers love to provide explanations, even when they don't really explain. We like to use the analogy of a parent answering their young child's question, "What is sex?" The parent says, "Sex is your gender; you're either male or female." The parent explained but didn't really answer the child's question. In this case, the child leaves falsely satisfied. Don't make the same mistake with your provider. Chances are good that your provider doesn't really know what's causing your back pain and is just giving you an answer in the hopes that it makes you stop asking difficult questions.

Diagnosis: Friend or foe?

A back pain diagnosis can be a double-edged sword. It can organize symptoms and direct the provider toward treatments with predictable results, but it can also oversimplify and prevent the provider from considering alternative treatments. Not every patient fits neatly into one diagnosis. When you receive a diagnosis, remember that it may not give you the full picture and may be misleading.

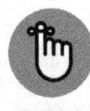

REMEMBER

The diagnosis of "back pain" has never been useful to predictably select treatment. This uncertainty is likely due to the fact that back pain has many different causes. Until the "back pain" diagnosis is divided into more discrete categories, it won't be very helpful in providing patients with effective treatment recommendations. For now, you're responsible for navigating the proposed treatments your providers recommend.

Your diagnosis can change you

Diagnosis is not without a downside; it can change you. Sometimes, patients develop the symptoms of the diagnosis they're given — a phenomenon often referred to as "the chameleon effect." For example, if a patient is told they have the spine of an 80-year-old, they sometimes start to walk and feel like they're 80. In the late 1800s, many people who commuted by train were diagnosed as suffering from a condition called "railway spine." When the theory of that diagnosis was debunked, the incidence of back pain sufferers commuting by train suddenly dropped.

REMEMBER

The power of suggestion can have a tremendous impact on your physical health, and you don't have to be hypnotized to be susceptible to it. Having blind faith in a doctor's opinion can make you very susceptible to accepting as fact whatever that person tells you.

Exploring Your Provider Options

A variety of trained professionals treat various aspects of back pain and have widely differing philosophies and perspectives. In this section, we provide insight into what different doctors and other healthcare professionals offer with respect to back pain diagnosis and treatment so you can make well-informed decisions about the types of providers you may want to add to your treatment team (if any).

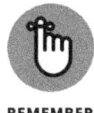

REMEMBER

The training, experience, skills, and treatment philosophy of the medical professionals you choose to consult can have a tremendous impact on the diagnosis and treatment you receive, so choose carefully.

Providers you may want to consider starting with, switching to, or adding to your treatment team include the following (arranged from most to least common starting point):

>> **Primary care physician (or internist):** If you're lucky enough to have a primary care physician who has a sophisticated understanding of back pain and the broad array of treatment options and can spend time getting to know you and working with you, that person can be a tremendous resource. Unfortunately, most are limited to treating acute pain (writing you a prescription) or referring you to a specialist they know. In this case, you won't escape the common trap of receiving treatment based on the provider you start with rather than what's wrong.

>> **Functional/integrative practitioner:** Practitioners of functional and integrative medicine tend to spend more time with their patients and focus on the building blocks of health (an approach we strongly favor) rather than medicines or surgery. They can help you identify and address possible root causes of back pain, such as food sensitivities, nutritional deficiencies, lack of physical activity, emotional stress, poor sleep, improper breathing, and gastrointestinal issues (a common source of inflammation). Unfortunately, they're rarely covered by insurance.

>> **Physical therapist:** We're big fans of physical therapy for back pain because physical therapists are experts in movement and rehabilitation. A skilled physical therapist provides a personalized treatment plan that often includes exercise, deep-tissue massage, postural training, and temporary pain relief, all for the purpose of restoring strength, mobility, and flexibility and empowering you to live fully. Chances are good that your insurance provider will require physical therapy before approving an MRI or escalating your case to treatment by a surgeon or pain management specialist.

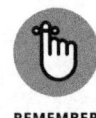

The best physical therapists are not "one trick ponies." Instead, they personalize their treatment for each patient and are willing to change directions if their approach isn't working.

>> **Massage therapist:** Deep-tissue massage can be very helpful in breaking up adhesions and making muscles more pliable, which can improve mobility. If your muscles are stiff, achy, or prone to spasms, massage can help. The primary goal of massage should be to enable you to become more physically active and return to exercise. Professional massage can be costly and is rarely covered by insurance.

>> **Chiropractor:** Chiropractors are often easy to access and effective at providing short-term relief. Their two drawbacks are that they tend to promote dependence (their business model relies on repeat business), and they're usually not part of a larger comprehensive approach to back pain, which we think works best.

Chiropractors, physical therapists, trainers, and other professionals in this list may be certified in Active Release Technique (ART), a hands-on treatment directed at working out the kinks in muscles while they're in a relaxed state. If your back pain is muscle-related, ART can be very beneficial.

>> **Physiatrist:** Physiatry (fizz-*eye*-uh-tree) is a relatively new branch of medicine that focuses on preventing, diagnosing, and treating musculoskeletal and nerve disorders that affect how well patients function in their daily lives. They tend to use nonsurgical treatments, including injections, nerve stimulation, and physical therapy, to improve function and quality of life. They spend more time with patients than is typical, provide more personalized treatment, and often coordinate care with other providers. Not a bad place to start.

- **Surgeon:** Many patients with back pain start with a surgeon. Obviously, surgeons are not exempt from the bias of offering their own limited repertoire of treatment. If you see a surgeon, you risk hearing that surgery is what is needed. I (Dr. Roth) am a surgeon, and I believe strongly that although this bias exists, a surgeon who can overcome it can be a particularly good primary care provider for patients with back pain. Why? Because surgeons are experienced diagnostic clinicians who read their own films (medical imaging), understand pain management, and are familiar with the various therapies. The key to starting with a surgeon is making sure the surgeon can overcome their bias to offer surgery. A surgeon who's part of an integrated group of providers is your best bet.

- **Personal trainer:** Personal training is a seldom used starting point for addressing back pain, but it works quite well. You may worry about the lack of standardized treatment for back pain among trainers, but the same can be said about physical therapy and many other therapies. Ultimately, a little trial and error with your eyes wide open can deliver great results.

- **Psychologist/psychiatrist:** Psychologists and psychiatrists can help patients address the mental aspect of back pain and can play a key role in providing comprehensive treatment.

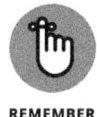

REMEMBER

  Seeing a mental health professional for back pain doesn't mean you're "crazy" or that "it's all in your head." It just provides another avenue for treating the pain. (See Chapter 19 for details on how psychological and psychiatric interventions can help patients manage back pain.)

- **Pain management specialist:** We're very opposed to the idea of simply dialing down pain with either injections or medications. Sometimes, starting with a medication or an injection can help, but it needs to be followed up with treatment that engages both the mind and body to build strength and resilience and make the patient more independent.

- **Acupuncturist:** Acupuncture's efficacy in treating back pain is via the *placebo effect* (the patient's belief that it helps), which doesn't diminish its efficacy. The efficacy of many medical treatments is due, at least in part, to the patient's belief in it. Acupuncture is a reasonable short-term solution to pain but is typically not covered by insurance.

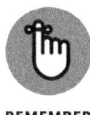

REMEMBER

With the knowledge and understanding you develop through your own experience and by reading this book, you can serve as your own primary care physician, referring yourself to different providers. The only limitation you may face is whether your insurance provider allows you to serve in this role. You may be able to work around any obstacles by calling your insurance provider and requesting pre-approval to consult with a specific provider.

Choosing and Teaming Up with Providers

In Chapter 5, we lead you through a process of conducting a self-assessment and determining whether your back pain is something you may be able to manage on your own or whether it's something requiring professional medical attention. Here, we're assuming you decided the latter, or you tried the do-it-yourself approach and need some professional assistance. Now, you need to know where to start — which provider to consult with first — how to choose a provider, and how to work with providers to achieve the best outcome. In this section, we offer guidance.

Working with your insurance provider

If you want your insurance to pay for your treatment, start with a medical doctor (primary care, physiatry/pain management, or surgeon) or a chiropractor. The doctor you choose will serve as the gatekeeper between you and other providers and services, such as a physical therapist and a radiologist (to obtain an MRI). We recommend starting with a surgeon, a primary care physician/internist, or a function and integrative care provider. If immediate relief is what you seek, a chiropractor may be your best bet.

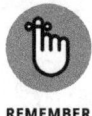

REMEMBER

The insurance company controls the timing of any imaging your doctor deems necessary. Your insurance may require a trial period of physical therapy before approving an MRI or surgery. These barriers are placed ostensibly to fulfill evidence-based protocols but are more likely methods for controlling costs. Insurance companies know that an MRI is not only expensive, but leads to more expensive treatments.

WHAT ABOUT REPUTATION?

Many people try to choose providers based on their reputation, which is something I (Dr. Roth) find amusing. New patients often tell me that they were strongly attracted to me by virtue of "word of mouth." When I probe a little deeper, I often discover that the recommendation came from a single individual. That's not exactly a resounding endorsement.

The scientific community recognizes the limitation of making conclusions based on anecdotes, but in medicine it's very common. As a surgeon, I would prefer that a prospective patient choose me based on observations from a front-seat view in the operating room or on the basis of published outcomes, but these aren't realistic or generally available.

Trust your gut

When searching for a provider, look for a provider who has a good reputation but trust your instincts, particularly regarding the provider's character. Get to know your provider's philosophy of care. Try to understand not only *what* your provider does and *how* but, more importantly, *why*. A provider's *why* always trumps the *what* and the *how*. If your initial consultation with a provider is too brief to sense this, keep looking.

Don't hesitate to seek another opinion

We encourage you to seek a second opinion, especially if a doctor is recommending an invasive medical procedure such as surgery. Another doctor's opinion gives you the benefit of another perspective and perhaps an alternative solution. A second opinion provides you with more information and insight on which to base your treatment decisions.

The only drawback is the possibility that a second opinion will result in paralysis by analysis — you have two conflicting opinions that complicate the decision-making process. However, that could be a good sign that you need a third opinion or you need to think a little more deeply and creatively about your options.

Collaborate closely with your providers

As you meet prospective healthcare providers, be honest and be open-minded and skeptical at the same time. You may have instincts about what's wrong with you and how best to treat yourself, but those instincts can be wrong. Listen carefully to what the provider tells you. Be sure you understand the diagnosis and the proposed plan of care, the benefits and potential risks, and the "natural history" of your diagnosis — what's likely to happen over time without treatment.

At the same time, try to evaluate the provider's character. Your provider should listen to you and demonstrate an understanding of what you're saying, present a reasonable explanation of what's causing your pain, and have the integrity to tell you what *you* need to do to improve your back. If the experience or your sense of the provider's character doesn't feel right to you, don't hesitate to look elsewhere.

WARNING

Beware of the "expert" fallacy. When face-to-face with an expert, people tend to defer to the expert. Don't assume that the expert is always right and has your best interests at heart. Realize that even the most well-intentioned doctor has training, experience, and incentives that could bias their opinion and recommendations. On the other hand, too much suspicion can undermine your capacity to achieve the desired outcome. Strive to achieve the Goldilocks' balance — just enough trust and just enough skepticism.

Chapter **13**

Taking a Peek Inside with Medical Imaging

L ike the comic book hero Superman, modern medicine has X-ray vision. Thanks to the magic of medical imaging, doctors and other medical professionals can see what's inside the body without having to open it up. And the technology has improved immensely in recent decades, progressing from plain old X-rays to three-dimensional reconstructed X-rays (CT scans) to MRIs to functional MRIs (employing glucose utilization to identify functional anatomy) to the single photon emission computed tomography (SPECT) scans, which uses the energy of radioactive tracers to create three-dimensional images showing areas of inflammation.

More recently, artificial intelligence (AI) has entered the field, greatly enhancing the ability to interpret these images. Powerful computers are now being trained, using massive amounts of data, including medical images and reports of clinical outcomes, to produce readings that are often more comprehensive and accurate than a human can generate. And, as more data becomes available, the better those readings become.

When you're experiencing chronic back pain, these advances in medical technology work to your advantage, helping to ensure that you receive the most comprehensive and accurate information and insight possible. In this chapter, we focus on the different types of medical imaging commonly used to evaluate the back and spine so you can communicate more effectively with your healthcare providers when discussing which types of medical imaging solutions would likely be best for evaluating the pain you're feeling.

Checking Out Your Bones with Plain Ol' X-Rays

X-rays have been around for more than a century, and they're generally best for assessing bones. They work by sending an invisible beam of radiation through the body, which is *attenuated* (weakened) by different bodily tissues to a different extent. A detector on the opposite side of the body captures the beams that pass through. The beam easily passes through soft tissues, such as skin and muscle, and not so easily through bone, producing an image that's sort of like a shadow of the bone. In the world of back pain, X-rays are a valuable way of evaluating bones for the following conditions:

>> Vertebral alignment, spinal shape, and posture

>> Deformities, such as scoliosis

>> Degenerative conditions, such as osteoarthritis and spondylosis

>> Fractures

>> Laxity (the looseness or flexibility between vertebral bodies — the weight-bearing portion of each vertebra)

X-rays are less helpful for diagnosing conditions related to soft tissues, such as herniated discs, nerve compression, and damage to muscles or ligaments.

To evaluate for laxity, the radiologist performs X-rays of the spine with the patient assuming different postures, for example, flexion and extension of different parts of the spine (typically the cervical spine and lumbar spine, which are the mobile parts of the spine). *Flexion* refers to a forward movement that decreases the angle between body parts, and *extension* refers to a backward movement that increases the angle. Laxity is very helpful for analyzing the etiology (origin) of back pain. If laxity is an issue, exercise, injections, and surgery (when a clear anatomical pain generator has been confirmed) are all predictable ways of reducing the pain.

WARNING

Flexion and extension X-rays are contraindicated for anyone who's suspected of having a potentially dangerous spinal instability.

TIP

When having your spine X-rayed to evaluate for laxity, push yourself to perform a full flexion and extension and bend the whole cervical and lumbar spine when flexing. The major drawback of flexion and extension X-rays is a lack of consistency with respect to the posture the patient assumes when the X-ray is taken. This inconsistency is primarily due to two factors: lack of standardization in terms of instruction to the patient (for example, how hard the patient should push the flexion and extension of the spine) and the fact that bending the neck and lower back isn't simple. For example, when bending the neck, you want to distribute the bend throughout the cervical spine, not just by hinging your skull down from your spine. Likewise, when bending the lumbar spine forward, you want to distribute the bend throughout your lumbar spine; you don't want to hip-hinge so that the rest of your back remains straight.

WARNING

X-rays have a downside — the radiation is toxic in large doses, and exposure is cumulative over the course of your life. X-rays are often obtained during emergency room visits because they're cheap, quick, available, and usually don't require insurance approval. Some insurance companies bundle the charge in an emergency room visit. This incentivizes the ER to not order more expensive imaging modalities out of fear of not being paid. Far too many X-rays are done in emergency rooms — they're often unnecessary. Unfortunately, many insurance companies insist on a plain X-ray evaluation before approving an MRI.

Upgrading to 3-D with a CT Scan

A *computed tomography (CT) scan* is a medical imaging technology that uses X-rays and a computer to generate detailed cross-sectional images of the body showing bones, organs, and soft tissues. Rather than measuring attenuation from a single beam of electromagnetic radiation, spinning the beam around the patient produces a three-dimensional image. Like plain X-rays, CT scans are particularly helpful for looking at the anatomy of bones — they show everything you can see in a plain X-ray and then some. They're more expensive and generally less accessible than plain X-rays, but they offer the following advantages:

>> Greater detail (although less than an MRI, which we discuss in the next section)

>> Clearer images of soft tissues

>> Ability to detect issues often missed on X-rays, such as small fractures, herniated discs, spinal tumors, infections, and nerve compression

The choice between an X-ray and a CT scan or MRI depends on the specifics of the patient's symptoms, clinical history, and the need for detailed information. In many cases, X-rays are used first, followed by a CT scan or MRI if more detailed imaging is required.

WARNING

CT scans expose patients to higher levels of radiation than plain X-rays, but they serve as a good alternative to an MRI when that option isn't available or affordable.

Cranking Up the Detail with an MRI

Magnetic resonance imaging is a medical imaging technology that uses magnets to disrupt molecules in the body and then measures their energy as they return to their resting state. This technology produces spectacular windows into an individual's anatomy, revealing muscles, nerves, discs, and other soft tissues in exquisite detail.

REMEMBER

MRIs are best for imaging soft tissues such as spinal discs, nerve roots, ligaments, and the spinal cord. They show cysts, areas of inflammation, infections, narrowing of the corridors through which nerves traverse, and much more. They are not as helpful as CT scans for assessing bone health and structure, spine shape, and posture.

MRIs have three limitations with respect to their use in back pain diagnosis:

>> Although MRIs show soft tissue anatomy beautifully, they don't identify what's causing the pain. Your doctor may be able to infer the location of the pain source from the anatomical picture created, but the MRI rarely points to a specific origin of the pain.

>> MRIs can show too much detail. Aging can result in normal changes that may appear as abnormalities on an MRI, but these changes don't necessarily represent the origin of the pain. Having a single provider (or a group working closely together) perform the physical exam, review the patient's medical history, and read the MRI can help mitigate this limitation. Interpreting the MRI in the context of the patient's medical history and physical exam can help to determine whether the MRI finding is relevant or is merely incidental to the patient's complaint.

>> Interpretation of medical images isn't a precise science. Three radiologists looking at the same MRI may present three very different reports. Differences may be due to one or more factors, such as the following:

- **Cognitive bias:** Bias is any tendency to favor a certain idea or perspective. Bias compromises a person's ability to remain objective. For example, the radiologist may notice a bulging disc early in their MRI review and focus on it to the point of overlooking a more significant issue, such as a spinal tumor or nerve compression.

- **Lack of standardization in language:** For example, one radiologist may describe a certain anomaly in a disc as a "bulge," whereas another describes it as a "herniation."

- **Radiologist's mood or mindset:** A radiologist's interpretation of an MRI may be influenced by how tired, hungry, or emotionally upset the radiologist is or by other factors that impair rational thought.

- **Noise:** Noise encompasses everything from image quality to disruptions and distractions that may impact the radiologist's ability to perform an objective review.

WARNING

To some extent, the MRI report has been weaponized. Because abnormalities are so easy to see on an MRI, doctors often use the report as a definite diagnosis, and lawyers use the MRI findings as evidence in a trial. Keep in mind that although an MRI provides a detailed picture of what's inside the body, it rarely offers unequivocal proof of what's causing the pain. The value of any medical imaging technique depends on the detail shown in the image and the skill of the person interpreting that image. The art of caring for back pain is the provider's ability to correlate the radiographic studies with the patient's history and physical exam to identify the pain generator when possible.

Evaluating Inflammation with a SPECT Scan

The *single photon emission computed tomography (SPECT) scan* uses radioactive tracers (such as iodine, xenon, gallium, and technetium) injected intravenously and a special camera to take detailed three-dimensional images of the bones, tissues, and organs inside the body. The tracers emit energy that the camera detects.

One of the tracers, technetium, which is absorbed into areas of *bone remodeling* (creation and absorption of bone), serves as a *surrogate marker* for inflammation; that is, it's a measurement that correlates with inflammation but isn't a definitive indication of it. Someone reading the SPECT scan may infer that areas absorbing the technetium are pain generators.

Although the CT scan and the MRI provide exquisite anatomic detail, the SPECT scan offers the following benefits:

>> Better answers to questions such as "Why does my back hurt?" and "Where is the pain coming from?"

>> Help in diagnosing *pseudarthrosis* (failure to fuse after a fusion operation)

>> Help in diagnosing pain arising from the sacroiliac joint and pain in other skeletal bones and bones and joints outside of the spine

>> Insight into bone metabolism, which may shed light on conditions such as spondylitis, spondylosis, and facet joint arthritis

>> Guidance for making treatment decisions, such as whether a specific area may benefit most from physical therapy, injections, or surgical intervention

Overall, the SPECT scan is typically used when other imaging methods (X-ray, MRI, or CT scan) don't provide sufficient information or when doctors (typically a surgeon or spine specialist) are looking for a more detailed understanding of bone and joint conditions related to back pain.

Discography

Discography is a diagnostic procedure for identifying whether an intervertebral disc is the source of a patient's back pain. It involves injecting a contrast dye into a disc and then taking an X-ray or performing a CT scan to check the disc for bulging, herniation, tears, or degeneration (as indicated by abnormal disc height or structure). In addition to providing a clear image of a disc (a *discogram*), the procedure may also provoke a pain response that can be helpful in the diagnosis. The procedure is done with the patient awake. The patient is asked to describe the induced pain as the disc is injected. The more similar the pain is to the patient's presenting pain complaints, the more likely that the disc is the pain generator.

Discography has several drawbacks, including the following:

>> Variations in technique produce variations in the diagnostic value of the results.

>> Subjectivity (bias) in the interpretation of the discogram and in how patients express their pain can impact the diagnostic value of the results.

>> The procedure can be very painful.

>> Injections carry a slight risk of infection.

>> Some studies suggest that the trauma of a needle inserted into an intact disc as a control level in discography may contribute to deterioration in that disc.

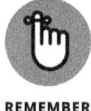

REMEMBER

For identifying a painful disc, we prefer the SPECT scan over discography because SPECT scans are less subjective. Many spine specialists no longer consider discography a viable or predictable way to determine a patient's origin of pain.

Chapter **14**

Launching a Three-Pronged Approach

I n theory, making back pain go away should be a simple two-step process:

1. Identify what's causing the pain.

2. Fix what's causing it.

Unfortunately, it's never that simple. Half the time, the doctor can't identify a definitive biological/anatomical cause. In nearly all other cases, even when the doctor identifies a clear biological/anatomical cause — a herniated disc, infection, or some other problem — and fixes it, the pain doesn't fully resolve, or it moves to some other area of the back.

So, what's the solution? In this chapter, we present a three-pronged approach we have found most effective. This approach targets three key components of back pain — the pain generator, the pain, and the patient.

Finding the Pain Generator or Abandoning the Search for It

The first prong in our three-pronged approach to managing back pain is to perform an all-out search for what's causing the pain and then stop looking if that search doesn't reveal a clear origin of the pain.

REMEMBER

We believe that when patients present with pain over a long period of time — particularly when the pain is significantly affecting their quality of life — the best approach is as follows:

1. **Conduct a deep dive to identify the pain generator.** Perform a comprehensive physical evaluation, examine the patient's medical and family history, order targeted lab tests, and order medical imaging, including an MRI, plain X-rays done in flexion and extension, and a SPECT scan. (See Chapter 13 for more about medical imaging.) Occasionally, imaging of the abdomen, shoulder, hip, and other areas is added to look for non-spinal origins of the pain.

2. **If the deep dive reveals a definitive pain generator, provide treatments that target it.** Treatments should be limited to those that are predictably helpful, such as treatment for an isolated spondylolisthesis, spinal instability, a large herniated disc, or an infection.

3. **If the deep dive fails to reveal a definitive pain generator, abandon the search and shift gears to treat the pain and the patient.** Note that effective treatment for back pain is still possible, even in the absence of a clear pain generator. Doctors can still treat the pain and help restore patient health and fitness, which can do wonders for alleviating back pain, as we discuss in the next two sections.

This approach gets a lot of pushback from insurance companies who believe that the search for a pain generator is costly and doesn't amount to better results. We disagree. The reason the search for the pain generator has traditionally been expensive is that providers often misuse whatever they find on a patient's MRI to justify unnecessary, expensive, and ineffective treatments. However, if the search for the pain generator is used instead to either identify the pain generator or rule it out, subsequent treatment can be both more affordable and more effective.

REMEMBER

MRIs often reveal incidental findings — not necessarily related to the pain. For example, suppose you have back pain, you get an MRI of your lumbar spine, and your doctor says you have back pain because of a herniated disc shown on the MRI. The problem is that MRIs on people *without* back pain routinely show those same herniated discs. In other words, having a herniated disc doesn't mean it's the cause of your back pain.

Most insurance companies now require conservative treatment (physical therapy and medicine) prior to authorizing an MRI or invasive targeted treatment such as surgery. This approach is based on it being cost-effective. Because conservative treatment and time will heal a percentage of pain, the insurance company avoids paying for the more invasive treatment, even if that treatment is necessary. We believe that adherence to this strict protocol often leaves patients in pain for longer. A more effective and affordable approach is to identify the pain generator, if one is clearly present, and offer patients a predictable targeted treatment, and then follow up with therapy for mind and body. If no pain generator is clearly present, skip to treating the pain and the patient with therapy for mind and body.

SEARCHING FOR THE HOLY GRAIL

Patients with back pain are often disappointed to discover that in a large percentage of cases, modern medicine, with its advanced technology, is unable to determine unequivocally what's causing the pain — the pain generator. In many cases of chronic back pain, no clear cause shows up on any lab tests or medical imaging. At this point, the patient and doctor need to decide whether to keep looking for the pain generator or try to reduce the pain without knowing specifically what's causing it and work on restoring function.

To continue searching for the pain generator after comprehensive lab tests and medical imaging fail to identify it is like searching for the Holy Grail. It can be exhausting, time-consuming, expensive, and, in the end, all for naught.

Part of our job as healthcare providers is to help our patients decide whether to keep looking or change gears and begin treatment without knowing the specific cause. In our experience, if the pain generator isn't plainly obvious on an MRI (magnetic resonance imaging), the odds of identifying it, even through extensive testing, are low, and to continue the search is a waste of time, effort, and money. In addition, it sends the patient a message that successful treatment requires first identifying the cause, and that's not always the case.

Treating the Pain — or Not

The second prong in our three-pronged approach to managing back pain is to decide whether to treat the pain itself. This decision depends on the severity of the pain and the patient's preference.

Treating the pain covers everything from taking pain relieving medication to applying a topical analgesic to seeing a chiropractor for an adjustment. It can be a very effective short-term solution that improves your mobility and enables you to exercise and strengthen your back. For example, suppose you're experiencing a muscle spasm that's causing excruciating pain. You start taking ibuprofen, which alleviates the pain and relaxes the muscles, and the next day, you head to the gym to do the movements and exercises that we recommend in Chapter 8. Three days later, you continue the exercises and stop taking the ibuprofen because you no longer need it. That's a good approach to treating the pain.

Treating the pain is bad if that's all you do. For example, you've been in excruciating pain for months. Your primary care physician refers you to a pain management clinic, where the doctor prescribes an opioid and/or shots to alleviate the pain. You feel better, so no need to hit the gym, right? Eventually, you stop feeling better, so you return to the clinic for a prescription refill and more shots. That's bad. You're not doing anything to be healthier, strengthen your back, or increase mobility, so you're not getting any better. All you're doing is becoming more dependent on medication.

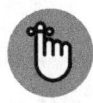

REMEMBER

Treating the pain alone, especially with medication, has two main drawbacks:

>> It can make you dependent on medications, which have many negative side effects, some of which can be fatal.

>> It doesn't improve your condition. Your back remains in the same state, or it becomes weaker and possibly suffers more damage. Likewise, your state of mind fails to improve or worsens; you're not building self-efficacy, as we discuss in Chapter 4.

REMEMBER

Sometimes, the intensity of the pain demands pharmaceutical medications and/or shots, but even in these cases, treating the patient with therapy for mind and body is essential. Even if the pain generator is identified and treated, or the pain medications reduce the pain, the patient should be treated. Pain is never as simple as signals from a pain generator, and treatment of pain is never as simple as merely reducing the pain.

Patients have high expectations for modern medicine. After all, NASA landed a man on the moon more than 50 years ago. Given all the advances in medicine and science, certainly, today's doctors must have the tools to diagnose and fix the cause of the pain or at least make the pain go away, right? Well, modern medicine *does* have powerful tools to treat pain. The question is whether making the pain go away without making the patient any healthier (in mind and body) is the *best* that the medical community can offer.

In the mid-1990s, the American Pain Society pushed the concept of pain as the fifth vital sign. The idea was that patients were entitled to be relieved of pain and that doctors should simply "dial down" the pain just as they dial down blood pressure, heart rate, and respiration. This concept, coupled with aggressive marketing from narcotics producers, helped to create the current opioid epidemic in the U.S., which has resulted in hundreds of thousands of deaths and tremendous costs in healthcare, human suffering, and productivity.

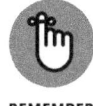

REMEMBER

Doctors prescribe pain medication with the best of intentions. They don't like to see their patients suffer. Unfortunately, these medications have several downsides, including the following:

>> **Risk of dependency or addiction:** Narcotics, in particular, can lead to dependency.

>> **Reduced pain tolerance:** As you build up a tolerance for pain medication, your body's natural ability to control pain is impaired. Over time, pain medication can make your pain worse. (See the nearby sidebar "How Narcotics Work.")

>> **Impaired cognitive and physical function:** Narcotics can impair mental clarity, coordination, and motor skills, which may impact your ability to perform everyday tasks such as working, driving, and spending quality time with loved ones.

>> **Other health issues:** Long-term use of narcotics can cause liver damage, kidney issues, and hormonal imbalances, along with mental health problems, such as mood swings, depression, and anxiety.

HOW NARCOTICS WORK

Your body has a built-in pain reduction system consisting of pain receptors and opioids that your body produces naturally. These opioids bind to the receptors, triggering several processes, one of which results in pain reduction. As part of your body's ability to self-regulate, it maintains just the right number of pain receptors and opioids for proper function.

If you ingest opioids, over time, they disrupt this balance, and your body responds by producing fewer opioids or reducing the number of opioid receptors. Either way, you reach a point at which you need to take more opioids just to feel normal. Eventually, you may reach a point at which the amount you need to take to feel normal is very close to the amount that will kill you.

As people struggling with chronic pain become aware of the risks of narcotics, they are beginning to search for new and better drugs to dial down the pain. Cannabis seems to be the substance of choice. Although the side effects are different from those of opioids, cannabinoids (various chemicals present in marijuana) come with their own host of undesirable side effects. (See Chapter 15 for more about using medications and other substances to manage back pain.)

Treating the Patient — Always

The third and final prong in our three-pronged approach to managing back pain is to treat the patient. It's also the only one of the three approaches that we consider essential in all cases. Regardless of whether your back pain is new or something you've been struggling with for a long time, whether you've gotten surgery to repair damage due to an injury, or whether you need medication to alleviate the pain or relax the muscles, your back pain will get better by improving your overall health, strengthening your core, and developing the right mindset.

In Chapter 2, we divide pain into three tiers: stimulus, epiphenomenon, and judicial function. Almost regardless of what's causing your back pain, the most effective treatment targets all three tiers:

>> **Stimulus:** The pain generator, if it can be identified.

>> **Epiphenomenon:** The secondary physical adaptations of the body, such as muscle spasms, weakness, or musculoskeletal imbalances. Epiphenomena responds to movements and exercises such as those we present in Chapters 8 and 9.

>> **Judicial function:** The cognitive and evaluative role the brain plays in interpreting pain and determining the appropriate response. You can improve judicial function by educating yourself about back pain (such as by reading this book) and by taking advantage of therapies that target thoughts and mental function, such as those we describe in Chapter 19.

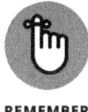

REMEMBER

As long as you live, your mind and body are inseparable. Your thoughts, moods, and emotions affect your body, and how you feel physically has a tremendous impact on your thoughts, moods, and emotions. (See Chapter 4 for more about the mind-body connection.)

Treating the patient also involves other factors that can contribute to back pain, including hydration, diet/nutrition, sleep, stress, smoking, alcohol consumption, posture, weight, and so on. See Chapter 6 for details. Your overall physical health is not a minor concern. Any of these factors, alone or in combination, can be a significant source of back pain — and they don't show up on X-rays or MRIs.

Chapter **15**

Targeting the Pain

How doctors and patients approach back pain depends largely on which of those two words they choose to focus on — "back" or "pain." The approach we recommend focuses more on the back and less on the pain. Our approach is based on the belief that if we can help the patient improve their back, the pain will largely resolve on its own. However, when you're in extreme pain and you don't know what to do about it, dialing down the pain may become your primary objective. This is true for both doctors and patients.

We're not against using medication to alleviate pain, so long as it's used as the means to transition to more robust and sustainable mind-body treatments that improve the patient's condition. Pain relief should never be the only treatment for back pain. If it gets you back on your feet and is followed up with education, exercise, and other whole-health and back-strengthening therapies, pain relief can be very valuable.

In this chapter, we provide information and guidance on using medication, targeted injections, and *ablation* (intentionally damaging nerve tissue) to relieve back pain and on weighing the potential benefits and drawbacks of using these tools as part of your back pain management protocol.

Relieving Pain with Medication

Nearly everybody has used pain medication at some point in their lives to treat everything from headaches and minor aches and pains to more severe pain. In this section, we provide general guidance on which pain medications are most effective for treating back pain and those that have questionable benefits, and we touch on the potential downsides of these pain relievers.

REMEMBER

Many medications have a *rebound effect* — the symptoms the medication is used to treat tend to worsen after the medication is stopped or its effects wear off. The rebound effect can extend to medication side effects as well. For example, if a medication causes constipation, when you stop it, you may experience diarrhea.

WARNING

Be careful with pain medication. Many classes of medications are abused. Narcotics are the worst of the groups, but you can get into trouble with muscle relaxers and even over-the-counter pain medications, such as acetaminophen and ibuprofen, if you take too much or use them for too long. Try to use as little medication as possible for as short a duration as possible — just enough to get mobile and start exercising to achieve more substantive and sustained relief.

Anti-inflammatory medications

Anti-inflammatory medications, which include steroids and non-steroidal anti-inflammatory drugs (NSAIDs), reduce pain, inflammation, and fever. In most cases, if medication is to be used to treat back pain, these are the medications that should be used.

NSAIDs

NSAIDs are aspirin and variants of aspirin, including ibuprofen (Advil) and naproxen (Aleve). Many NSAIDs have different effects at different doses. At lower doses, they function more like analgesics — they reduce pain. At higher doses, they become true anti-inflammatories — they reduce both pain and inflammation. Most are available over the counter, but some require a prescription. You may also need a prescription for high-dose versions of NSAIDs that are otherwise available over the counter.

REMEMBER

Acetaminophen (Tylenol) isn't an NSAID. It works primarily as a pain reliever and fever reducer. It doesn't have significant anti-inflammatory properties.

NSAID side effects include platelet inhibition, which increases the risk of bleeding. NSAIDs can also cause gastrointestinal tract irritation and kidney toxicity.

Steroids

Steroidal anti-inflammatories (corticosteroids) require a prescription. They're stronger than NSAIDs and very effective for quickly reducing inflammation and swelling. They're also effective for modulating overactive immune responses characteristic of autoimmune diseases.

Unfortunately, although corticosteroids are very effective, they come with potentially harmful side effects, especially when used for extended periods, including the following:

>> Weight gain

>> Elevated blood sugar, which can lead to or worsen diabetes

>> Osteoporosis (weakened bones)

>> High blood pressure

>> Suppressed immune function (increased susceptibility to infections)

>> Mood changes (for example, irritability, anxiety)

>> Stomach irritation (ulcers or gastritis)

>> Cushing's syndrome (characterized by symptoms such as a round face, thinning skin, and fat redistribution)

WARNING

If you've been taking corticosteroids for several weeks, don't stop them abruptly. Taper off your usage slowly and gradually under a doctor's supervision.

Narcotics

Narcotics (opioids) are primarily used to relieve pain. They bind to opioid receptors in the brain and spine, blocking pain signals and altering the way the brain perceives pain. Common narcotics used to control back pain include morphine, oxycodone (OxyContin, Percocet), hydrocodone (Vicodin, Norco), codeine, fentanyl, and tramadol.

Narcotics are controlled substances because of their propensity for abuse. They're addictive and tend to lose their effectiveness over time, so the patient must take more and more to achieve the same desired effect. The way our medical system has over-prescribed narcotics is both an embarrassment and a tragedy. (See Chapter 14 for a more in-depth discussion on this topic.)

Narcotics reduce pain and can play a very useful role in helping patients manage back pain, especially acute and severe pain, so doctors should be careful not to throw the baby out with the bathwater. If prescribed, narcotics should be used as part of a personalized whole-health plan of care designed to make the patient less dependent on them. Prescribers should track their use and find ways to educate patients who request repeated prescription refills. One of the difficulties controlling the use of narcotics is that the educational piece requires time and energy.

Muscle relaxers

Muscle relaxers (also called muscle relaxants) are intended to relax tight muscles and alleviate muscle spasms. This class of medications includes cyclobenzaprine (Flexeril), methocarbamol (Robaxin), tizanidine (Zanaflex), and diazepam (Valium). Unfortunately, muscle relaxers don't really relax muscles. They mostly reduce anxiety and cause fatigue, they can be very addictive, and they can be dangerous when mixed with other central nervous system (CNS) depressants, including alcohol.

In our experience, like with many of the medications mentioned in this chapter, other than anti-inflammatories and narcotics, the efficacy of muscle relaxers is hard to predict, so doctors generally prescribe them using trial and error. When they work, their effect on pain may be due to their effectiveness at removing the angst often associated with pain.

Topical analgesics

An analgesic is any medication or substance used to relieve pain, including NSAIDs, acetaminophen, and narcotics. Topical analgesics are those applied to the skin in the form of ointments, sprays, or patches. See Chapter 10 for a list of topical analgesics that have some evidence of helping people manage their back pain.

Topical analgesics may provide pain relief that's only skin deep. How deeply they penetrate the skin to reach muscles, nerves, and other tissues is unclear, but plenty of anecdotal evidence supports their use in treating muscle pain.

Antidepressants

The fact that certain antidepressants have been shown to be effective to some degree in pain management supports the notion of a mind-body connection. Antidepressants, which may be helpful for improving mood, may also be helpful for reducing the perception of pain. They've been used to treat pain for more than half a century and can be especially helpful for managing chronic pain when it has a nerve-related or psychological component or when traditional pain relievers aren't effective.

Three classes of antidepressants are used to support back pain management:

>> Tricyclic antidepressants (TCAs) such as amitriptyline (Elavil), nortriptyline (Pamelor), and doxepin (Sinequan) increase the levels of certain neurotransmitters in the brain, which can help reduce pain signals.

>> Serotonin-norepinephrine reuptake inhibitors (SNRIs) such as duloxetine (Cymbalta) and venlafaxine (Effexor) increase levels of serotonin and norepinephrine in the brain, which may reduce the perception of pain.

>> Selective serotonin reuptake inhibitors (SSRIs) such as fluoxetine (Prozac), sertraline (Zoloft), and paroxetine (Paxil) increase levels of serotonin in the brain, which may play a role in modulating the perception of pain.

WARNING

Antidepressants can cause a wide range of negative side effects, including metabolic disorders, insomnia, sexual dysfunction, headaches, anxiety, and increased heart rate and blood pressure. They may also trigger a shift to bipolar mania or cause psychosis, and have demonstrated links to suicidal and homicidal ideation. Discuss potential side effects with your doctor. Don't stop taking an antidepressant abruptly; withdrawal can have serious side effects as well.

Anti-seizure medications

Anti-seizure medications are used primarily for treating patients with epilepsy, but they're being used more and more by pain management doctors. Their increased use is likely a response to the opioid epidemic, as fear of prescribing opioids has made anti-seizure meds the "go-to" drug after anti-inflammatories. Their efficacy is quite limited despite their being widely prescribed.

The first of these drugs to hit the market, gabapentin (Neurontin), was originally designed for epilepsy, but when it was found to be less effective than some of the other medications for epilepsy, the producer, Pfizer, looked for other potential uses for the medication given the enormous cost of bringing it to market. Initially, some evidence showed it useful for treating neuropathy, but its use has morphed into many other pain syndromes and made it one of the most prescribed medications in the world.

WARNING

If you're taking an anti-seizure medication and you want to stop, wean off it gradually under your prescribing doctor's supervision. Sudden withdrawal can cause seizures, which can be serious and even fatal.

Cannabinoids

Cannabinoids are chemicals found in hemp and marijuana plants that have some medicinal purposes. Hemp has more cannabidiol (CBD), the pain reliever, and marijuana has more tetrahydrocannabinol (THC), the mind intoxicator. CBD is the main chemical used for pain, but THC may enhance CBD's pain-relieving trait.

Cannabinoid use has increased significantly over the past decade for both medical and recreational use. Plenty of anecdotal evidence supports its efficacy for the treatment of back pain, but for various reasons, scientific evidence to support its efficacy and safety is lacking.

Although we can't predict whether cannabinoids will ultimately prove safe and effective for managing back pain, we have some concerns that they will mimic the use of opioids.

REMEMBER

No drug is perfect. If it's powerful enough to relieve pain, it's powerful enough to cause harmful side effects, and cannabinoids aren't an exception. Prolonged use has been linked to malaise, sexual dysfunction, psychosis, and schizophrenia, to name a few. For more about cannabinoids, including their potential health benefits and risks, check out *Cannabis For Dummies*, by Kim Ronkin Casey and Joe Kraynak (Wiley, 2019).

Alleviating Pain with Targeted Injections or Ablations

If your doctor can identify the pain generator, and nothing can be done to repair it, a targeted injection or *ablation* (destruction of nerve tissue) may help prevent pain signals from reaching the brain. In the following sections, we explain what these two different procedures involve and highlight the four areas of the spine that are generally more amenable to these treatments.

Understanding your options

Injections and ablations have the same general objective — to prevent pain signals from reaching the brain. In this section, we cover the pros and cons of each option so that you're better equipped to discuss these procedures with your doctor and make well-informed treatment decisions.

Injection

Injection involves delivering medication (steroids, local anesthetics, or nerve blocks) directly into spinal joints, discs, or nerve roots to reduce inflammation, dull the pain, or decrease swelling. Injections typically provide relief lasting a few weeks to a few months. They don't treat the underlying cause of the back pain.

Injections are minimally invasive and relatively low risk. Risks include infection, nerve damage, and side effects of steroids (if that's one of the medications used). Injections may be limited to 3–4 times a year to reduce the risks of side effects (see the earlier section "Steroids" for more about their potential side effects).

TIP

Injections can also be helpful for confirming the identification of a pain generator before proceeding with a more invasive procedure such as ablation.

Ablation

Ablation involves using heat (radiofrequency) or cold (cryoablation) to destroy nerve tissue responsible for transmitting pain signals. It offers longer-term pain relief than an injection, with relief lasting from several months to several years; however, nerves can regenerate over time, so the pain may return.

Ablation is considered minimally invasive, but it's more complex than injection. In some cases, it can also be more painful. Potential side effects include nerve damage and infection.

Targeting the four main spinal pain generators

Injection and ablation target the four main spinal pain generators — the space around a disc, the facet joint, the spinal canal, and the muscle and fascia (see Chapter 3 for more about the anatomy of the back). In the following sections, we take a closer look at why each of these areas is important.

The disc space

Back pain that arises from the disc space can be the result of a herniated disc. In this case, the back pain arises from distortion or irritation of the *annulus,* the ligament that forms the outer portion of the disc and surrounds its gel-filled nucleus. The annulus has pain fibers and is a source of pain in the back and extremities (arms, hands, legs, feet). It can be targeted by an *epidural injection* (an injection into the spinal space outside of where the nerves traverse). Although injection into the disc space is primarily used to treat extremity pain, it may help with back pain as well, particularly acute back pain.

The disc space may also be subject to inflammation (discitis), which may result from infection or non-infectious causes.

A relatively new basivertebral nerve ablation procedure involves entering the disc space s (through a needle stick in the skin) and using radiofrequency energy to injure the *basivertebral nerve* (a nerve that runs through each vertebra). This procedure has two limitations:

>> Identifying the painful disc may be difficult.

>> The person performing the procedure can't see the nerve, so they need to position it as close as possible to where the nerve typically resides. The efficacy of the procedure depends on spreading sufficient heat to damage the nerve.

The facet joint

The facet joint is another source of back and leg pain. Facet joints are relatively easy to access for injection or radiofrequency ablation. Insurance companies typically require evidence that the facet joint is the pain generator before authorizing the ablation. Evidence consists of a positive result from one or two facet injections, also called medial branch blocks — the *medial branch* is the small nerve that innervates the capsule of the facet joint (see Chapter 3 for details).

The spinal canal

Spinal stenosis (narrowing of the spaces within the spine, which puts pressure on the spinal cord and nerve roots) is a source of both back and leg pain. An epidural injection has a positive effect on back pain about 70 percent of the time and a higher percentage on leg pain. (See Chapter 3 for details about spinal stenosis.)

Fascia and muscle

Trigger point injections are a medical treatment used to relieve muscle pain and muscle spasms that arise from *trigger points* — tight, knotted areas within the muscle fibers and fascia that can cause localized pain and referred pain in other areas of the body. These trigger points are typically in injured muscles.

Trigger point injections into the fascia and/or muscle can alleviate back pain. Effects are less predictable and less localized compared with the injections in the previously mentioned locations. The use of ultrasound to enter particular fascial planes may optimize the chance of success.

Weighing the Pros and Cons of Pain Relief

Pain management is a growing field focused on using medications and injections to treat pain. It offers patients three attractive benefits:

» **Accessibility/convenience:** Pain management clinics are within driving distance of most patients, making it easier for patients to get an appointment to see someone for help in managing their pain. Most are covered by insurance.

» **Quick pain relief:** Medication, injections, and ablations provide quick pain relief.

» **Low risk:** Most pain management treatments are non-invasive or minimally invasive. The biggest risk is that of developing a dependence. All medications also carry risks of producing certain side effects. Compared to major surgery, however, the risks are relatively low.

Pain management also has several potential drawbacks, including the following:

» Relief is generally short-term.

» Pain relief alone doesn't improve the patient's health or fitness.

» Other treatment options may be neglected.

» Patients face an increased risk of dependency/addiction.

» Pain clinics aren't immune to fee-for-service bias that plagues other health-care providers; they have an incentive to prescribe the treatments they offer.

» Some pain clinics give patients little or no autonomy in their care. They may even require you to sign a contract agreeing to whatever treatment they recommend and allowing them to drop you as a patient if you refuse a specific treatment. You could end up being prescribed a variety of powerful pain medications and then having to wean yourself off those medications when you decline an expensive treatment that's not covered by your insurance.

WARNING

Approach any form of pain relief carefully. Medications, injections, and ablations all have risks, and none of them will improve the condition of your back. We strongly recommend that if you use any of these treatments to help manage your back pain, you combine them with education and whole-health treatments for improving back strength and mobility.

IN THIS CHAPTER

» **Deciding whether you need a physical therapist**

» **Exploring and comparing different physical therapies**

» **Knowing what to look for in a physical therapist**

» **Teaming up with your therapist for optimal results**

» **Knowing when to stick with a therapist and when to try something else**

Chapter **16**

Restoring Mobility with Physical Therapy

M ost people, in most situations, can manage their back pain on their own by following the guidance we provide in Part 2 of this book. They don't need a physical therapist, and many people just prefer to do it on their own. You may need or prefer to work with a professional, especially in situations such as the following:

» Your doctor recommended physical therapy or referred you to a physical therapist, and you think it's a good idea.

» Your doctor recommended surgery, and you'd like a second opinion from someone likely to have a different perspective.

» You've consulted with one or more doctors who haven't helped you to the degree you expected or haven't provided a clear enough explanation of why you're feeling this pain.

>> You feel that you're unable to do even the basic movements that we recommend in Chapter 8, or you've tried the do-it-yourself approach and you're not getting the results you expected or hoped for.

>> You feel that you would benefit from assistance in setting goals, structuring sessions, creating a schedule, and holding yourself accountable.

>> Insurance requires that you try physical therapy before it will approve coverage for a specialist or even medical imaging. Increasingly, insurance companies are demanding a trial of conservative treatment prior to any invasive treatments and, on occasion, before allowing imaging of the spine to be done.

Whatever your reason, you're considering the option of consulting a physical therapist. In this chapter, we help you make that decision, explore different types of physical therapy and massage, and provide guidance on how to collaborate closely with your physical therapist to achieve the best possible outcome.

TIP

Even if you choose to forego physical therapy, you may be able to accelerate your recovery by adding massage sessions to your recovery routine, as explained in the later section, "Adding Massage to Your Physical Therapy Regimen: Don't Get Rubbed the Wrong Way!"

Recognizing What a Physical Therapist Brings to the Table

Whenever you're considering a healthcare option, you need to look at its potential value — what you stand to get out of it. A highly skilled and knowledgeable physical therapist offers the following benefits:

>> **Expertise:** A therapist who has a long track record of successfully helping patients manage their back pain can provide valuable insight into the *etiology* (origin) of the pain and how to address it. Experts have a better idea of what works, what doesn't, and what's likely to worsen the condition. They know how much to stress your body to improve mobility and strength without causing injury.

>> **Personalization:** A physical therapist can help you tailor your treatment to your specific condition and goals. Your treatment plan may combine exercise with rest, massage, pain relief (heat, ice, electrical stimulation), strategies for improving posture, and other treatments and guidance.

>> **Structure:** A physical therapist can help you develop a progressive recovery plan, complete with an overall goal and benchmarks or milestones for achieving that goal. Progression should be challenging yet attainable.

DEVELOPING EXPERTISE: IT'S NOT EASY

Expertise in healthcare is harder to develop than you may think because medicine is such a wicked learning environment — medical professionals often lack the feedback they need to improve. Patients who aren't progressing as quickly as they would like will seek out different providers without giving a reason why. Others may tell their provider that they're getting better just because they're afraid of offending the provider. Practicing medicine in such an environment is like trying to fly an airplane without any gauges, sensors, or GPS.

As a consequence, the learning curve for providers is often not as steep as it could be, and expertise develops slower than it should. In addition, medicine lacks well-developed databases to track outcomes. This lack of feedback results in a lack of knowledge and insight that negatively impacts the efficacy of treatment. Even a very experienced provider can lack the expertise necessary to provide quality care.

>> **Education:** A good therapist engages both your body and mind. Knowing why you're doing a certain set of movements, what sensations you should be feeling, how to engage the pertinent muscle groups, and what benchmarks you should be meeting all help in the healing process. See Chapter 19 for more about therapy for the mind.

>> **Motivation/accountability:** If you struggle to stick with your own do-it-yourself recovery program, having a physical therapist can help you stay on track by encouraging you, motivating you, and holding you accountable. Sometimes, having someone to answer to, such as a therapist or a workout partner, can keep you from getting lazy.

Knowing What Physical Therapy Typically Entails

Physical therapy typically involves several different treatment modalities (methods), including the following:

>> Heat or cold to relieve pain and reduce inflammation.

>> Transcutaneous electrical stimulation (TENS) — applying weak electrical impulses to help muscles and nerves recover.

>> Spinal manipulation to relieve pain and improve mobility.

- » Exercises to strengthen the core and musculoskeletal balance — prioritizing posterior (backside) strength over anterior (frontside) strength.

- » Low-impact aerobic exercises (stationary bike, treadmill, rowing, bicycling) to increase endurance.

- » Education on proper body posture for sitting, standing, and lifting to reduce back strain and injury.

- » Stretching to improve range of motion and mobility. (Be sure to prioritize strength and mobility over flexibility, as explained in Chapter 8.)

- » Information on movements and exercises to perform at home.

REMEMBER

Your physical therapist should provide a personal treatment plan that specifically addresses the back pain you're feeling and the suspected origin of that pain.

Adding Massage to Your Physical Therapy Regimen: Don't Get Rubbed the Wrong Way!

Massage can be a very helpful part of physical therapy. It relaxes muscles and alleviates muscle spasms, increases blood flow to promote healing to injured tissues, facilitates lymphatic drainage to remove toxins and reduce inflammation, and stimulates the body's parasympathetic nervous system to promote the release of *endorphins* (the body's natural pain relievers), breaks up muscle *adhesions* (scar tissues that form in the muscles, often as a result of injury or repetitive strain), and reduces stress and anxiety.

Many different types of massage are available, including deep tissue, Swedish, reflexology, hot stone, sports, Shiatsu, prenatal, aromatherapy, myofascial release, Thai, chair, trigger point, craniosacral therapy, manual lymphatic drainage, medical, Reiki, neuromuscular, and cupping. We've found the following massage types to be the most effective for managing back pain:

- » **Deep tissue massage** involves applying firm pressure, slow and steady, to reach the deep layers of muscle and connective tissue. It's effective at relieving chronic aches and pain as well as stiffness of the back, neck, arms, and shoulders.

REMEMBER

One of the benefits of deep tissue massage is that it helps break up adhesions. Adhesions occur when collagen fibers stick to adjacent tissues, leading to stiffness and discomfort.

- **Sports massage** targets one or more areas that have been injured or affected by a particular activity. This type of massage is used to augment training, facilitate rehabilitation, and aid in recovery. It can be especially useful for athletes who have sustained a back or neck injury during competition or training.

- **Myofascial release** is gentler than deep tissue and sports massage. It involves manipulation of the fascia, or connective tissue, as opposed to the skeletal muscles. The focus is on the release of tension in the fascia.

- **Thai massage** employs a combination of passive stretching and acupressure as the therapist moves your body into positions that enhance your range of motion. The therapist applies pressure with their hands and feet to stimulate the nerves and massage the muscles. Instead of lying on a massage table, you're on a mat with your massage therapist.

- **Trigger point massage** targets specific areas of muscle pain (*myofascial trigger points*, which are like tiny cramps, often referred to as "knots"). There are three types of trigger points, most commonly in the neck, shoulders, back, and hips:

  - **Active:** Always painful when touched and can cause pain in other areas of the body

  - **Passive:** Not always painful when touched but may cause pain in other areas of the body

  - **Satellite:** Similar to active trigger points but not as painful

- **Medical massage** targets a specific area based on a medical assessment with the goal of achieving a predetermined outcome. The therapist may use other techniques described in this list, such as deep tissue massage, myofascial release, or trigger point massage to target specific muscle groups, sections of the spine, or related areas such as the hips.

- **Neuromuscular massage therapy** applies firm, sustained, and controlled pressure to painful trigger points to relieve muscle tension and increase blood flow to affected areas to facilitate healing.

- **Cupping therapy** is an ancient healing method that involves placing glass, plastic, or silicone cups against the skin near painful areas and suctioning the air out of the cups to lift this skin and promote healing by increasing blood flow and drainage of the lymphatic fluids. Draining lymphatic fluids encourages the removal of toxins and can help reduce inflammation.

REMEMBER

Other massage therapies, including the most popular, Swedish massage, may also be useful for promoting relaxation, but the massage techniques in this list provide therapeutic benefits beyond relaxation. Therapeutic benefits include breaking up adhesions, improving circulation, restoring health and function to nerves and muscles, and increasing range of motion. You may experience some discomfort with these forms of massage, but we encourage you to become "comfortable with being uncomfortable" — some degree of pain or discomfort is often a sign that the therapy is working. Pain also triggers the body's healing mechanisms.

Choosing a Physical Therapist Who's Right for You

Choosing a physical therapist can be a challenge. You have no objective data to distinguish one therapist from another. Most therapists don't track or publish their outcomes. As a patient, you're left to either trust an individual recommendation or rely on reputation, and reputation is usually attached to a practice rather than an individual. You can choose a great practice and be assigned to a therapist who doesn't meet your needs. Often, choosing a physical therapist becomes a process of trial and error, and for that process to work, you need to know how to evaluate the physical therapist and the therapy you're receiving.

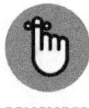

REMEMBER

Don't hesitate to leave a therapist who is not delivering the results you desire, but don't leave for the wrong reasons. Therapy often takes time to work, and abandoning a treatment just because it's difficult or painful early on can undermine your ultimate success. Three or four sessions should be enough to determine whether the therapy is producing the desired results. You may struggle to decide whether to stay or leave, but making difficult decisions is better than relinquishing your autonomy and simply following what your doctor or insurance company tells you to do. Taking responsibility is a big part of successfully managing back pain. Taking charge reflects *self-efficacy* (the belief that you can accomplish what you set out to do), which plays a crucial role in managing back pain, as explained in Chapter 4.

Evaluating the therapist

Although we can offer no objective metrics for distinguishing one therapist from another, here are some traits to look for in a therapist:

>> **Willingness to listen and collaborate:** Your therapist may have training and expertise in physical therapy, but you're the expert when it comes to your body. Avoid any therapist who has an arrogant "my way or the highway" attitude. If your therapist asks questions, listens carefully to your answers, and responds thoughtfully to your questions and concerns before presenting you with a treatment plan, those are all good signs. If the therapist seems to ignore you and treat you like a generic patient instead of a unique individual, that's a warning sign.

>> **Structured:** Your therapist should discuss your goal (desired outcome) and work with you to develop a reasonable plan for achieving that goal within a certain time frame. The fee-for-service model creates an incentive for the therapist to make you dependent. "Stick with me, and I will make you better." Look for a therapist who transcends this bias and promotes your independence. This type of therapist will promote self-efficacy as well as restore function and reduce pain.

>> **Flexible:** A good therapist doesn't have a generic treatment plan for all patients with back pain. You should receive a personalized treatment plan, and your therapist should be willing to adjust that plan over the course of your treatment. Look for a therapist who's willing to do a little trial and error. The source of the pain or the best corrective movements for your affliction may not be immediately apparent. Your body has a natural tendency to heal with exercise and respond to many different therapies; you and your therapist need to find the ones that work best for you.

>> **Aggressive:** Therapists have a bias to avoid hurting you. The problem is that, at times, success requires you to be pushed. If the therapist adapts the mindset of "first, do no harm," treatment may fall short. Pick a therapist who's willing to set you back. Success often requires this risk.

We subscribe to the advice of Michelangelo: "The greatest danger for most of us lies not in setting our aim too high and falling short; but in setting our aim too low and achieving our mark." If you are not "pushing the envelope," so to speak, you may never know how far you can go. Additionally, if scar tissue is involved, you need to experience some measure of pain to achieve the desired level of mobility and performance.

>> **Hands-on:** Therapists may select treatments based on what's easiest for them. Although we believe that therapy should be educational and aim to make you self-sufficient, you cannot do certain things yourself, such as deep tissue work. A good therapist does the hard work of tissue work (deep tissue massage or other forms of massage, as explained in the earlier section, "Adding Massage to Your Physical Therapy Regimen: Don't Get Rubbed the Wrong Way!").

Part of back pain is always the *epiphenomenon* (how the body changes in response to physical sensations such as pain); for example, pain can make muscles tense. But epiphenomenon works both ways; your tissues can change in positive ways when physically manipulated. Heating and manipulating the tissues through massage triggers the body's healing mechanisms.

>> **Positive:** Good therapists have a positive attitude and appreciate the value that a positive mindset has on the body. Your therapist should be encouraging, motivating, and supportive. If your therapist tries to manage (lower) your expectations so you'll be satisfied with an outcome that falls short of what you want, start looking for another therapist.

You may also want to include as part of your therapist's evaluation their treatment priorities and philosophy. We presented our treatment priorities for back pain in Chapters 7 and 8:

>> Posterior (backside) strength over anterior (frontside) strength — back and shoulder muscles over abdominals and pecs

>> Strength over flexibility

>> Endurance over power

>> Mobility and neuromuscular enhancement

As for our philosophy, it can best be summed up in the words of German philosopher Fredrich Nietzsche: "That which doesn't kill me makes me stronger." Your physical therapist should seek to stress your body in a way that provokes positive adaptations — adaptations that improve mobility, strength, and flexibility. A good therapist can help you find the sweet spot — what we like to call the Goldilocks, "just right," amount of stress — *eustress* (good stress).

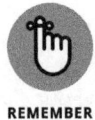

REMEMBER

When the body experiences stress, it adapts to the stress and becomes more resilient. The body is designed to "heal itself." When you train and workout, your muscles break down and then are healed, making them stronger and more resilient. Too little stress causes the body to weaken and muscles to atrophy; too much stress can lead to injury.

Evaluating the therapy

Evaluating the therapy you receive can be even more difficult than evaluating a therapist because no therapy has been proven to be best for back pain. Too many variables come into play, including the origin of the pain, the patient's attitude toward the therapist and the therapy, what the patient does outside therapy, and many other factors. The most objective way to gauge the effectiveness of therapy is to compare your goal and outcome and look at the progress you've made (or the lack thereof). Are you better off now than when you started therapy? Have you made reasonable progress toward achieving your treatment goal? If you haven't, you need to change what you're doing. You may need to take a different approach or change therapists. Also, be honest; if you're the reason the therapy hasn't worked (because you didn't follow the therapist's recommendations), admit it and commit to doing better.

Evaluations such as these can be subjective and may be influenced by how you contextualize your back pain, which can change over the course of your therapy sessions. Ideally, you'd fill out an assessment prior to therapy and a few months later that includes more objective criteria, such as the following:

>> Pain scale

>> Disability index

However, even these criteria can also be subjective. Future assessments may include more objective criteria, such as measures of strength, agility, coordination, and balance, as well as changes in medical imagery and laboratory results, but the medical field has not yet reached that point.

Here are some additional factors you can use to evaluate the effectiveness and value of the physical therapy you're receiving:

>> Whether you have a clearer understanding of your condition now than when you started therapy.

>> Whether you have a clearer understanding of the anatomy and physiology of your condition now than when you started therapy.

>> Whether you feel better prepared to take ownership of your continued treatment.

>> Whether you've been given the information and resources necessary to treat yourself going forward. (Some physical therapists will continue to treat for billing purposes even when you're ready to go it alone or the therapy isn't working.)

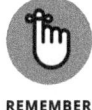

REMEMBER

As the Chinese philosopher Lao Tzu said, "Give a man a fish, and you feed him for a day. Teach a man how to fish, and you feed him for a lifetime." Therapy should be helpful, educational, empowering, and sustainable. It should also be humble. Remember the words of wisdom of Voltaire, the French philosopher, "The art of medicine consists in amusing the patient while nature cures the disease." Granted, physical therapy involves much more than merely amusing the patient, but the best therapists are humble; they know that their role is not to heal their patients but to empower their patients to heal themselves.

Teaming Up with Your Physical Therapist

Physical therapy is a team sport. To optimize the outcome, team up with your therapist by doing the following:

>> Set clear goals and expectations and discuss those goals and expectations with your therapist. Be sure to include milestones. (See Chapter 4 for guidance on setting goals.)

>> Share your philosophy of health and fitness with your therapist. Let your therapist know that you understand how the mind and body work together and how the body responds to stress. Also, communicate your understanding that physical therapy may be difficult and painful and your willingness to endure some degree of pain for long-term improvements. (You're essentially telling your therapist not to "baby" you and permitting them to be more aggressive in their approach.)

>> Demand a personalized treatment plan from the get-go, review the plan, and offer your input if you think the plan would benefit from some adjustments. If you think the plan is too aggressive or not aggressive enough, for example, discuss your concerns with your therapist.

>> Ask questions until you have a clear understanding of what your therapist has determined to be the origin of your pain and how the treatment plan recommendations specifically address that origin of pain. If the therapist expresses some uncertainty, that's okay. Finding the origin of pain can be a learning process.

>> Follow the plan and keep your appointments. You can't fault the therapist if you fail to follow the therapist's recommendations when you leave the clinic.

>> Let your therapist know what's working and what's not and whether you feel you're progressing. Don't expect your therapist to be a mind reader. Report any relevant improvements, setbacks, new symptoms, or other changes. If you're not making progress, do your best to navigate the space between giving it more time and changing direction (or changing therapists).

REMEMBER

By reading this book, you're better equipped to team up with your therapist. Don't be passive. Let your therapist know how you want to be treated, and make it a topic for ongoing discussion. Be prepared to grow in your knowledge and to influence your therapist. Listen to your body and pay attention to how it responds to the different therapeutic applications. As you get to know your therapist, you will begin to grasp their understanding of what's going on with you and their approach to facilitating your recovery. Tension will always exist between what feels right to you and what your therapist believes is right. This tension is often magnified when treatment initially doesn't seem to be working or is even making things worse. Deciding whether to trust your instincts or your therapist can be quite a challenge at times, and only you can make that decision.

Chapter **17**

Considering a Chiropractor

*C*hiropractic medicine focuses on diagnosing, correcting, and preventing mechanical disorders of the musculoskeletal system, particularly the spine, to relieve pain and optimize the health, fitness, and function of the entire body. The idea behind the practice is that proper alignment of the spine is necessary for healthy nerve function, which is essential for the proper function of all other systems of the body, including circulatory, respiratory, digestive, muscular, and lymphatic (immune) systems. Simply put, a healthy nervous system is a healthy body. However, most doctors of chiropractic (DCs) also offer guidance on diet, exercise, and lifestyle and promote a mind-body approach built on the notion that a healthy body can heal itself.

In this chapter, we explore the pros and cons of chiropractic care in the context of back pain management and explain the valuable role it can play. We also caution against becoming dependent on it exclusively for long-term relief.

REMEMBER

Bottom line: Chiropractic adjustments, like medication and shots, can be great for alleviating acute, short-term pain, but they shouldn't be treated as an end in themselves. Chiropractic care should be combined with self-care, as we recommend in Chapter 7, and exercises, such as those we present in Chapters 8 and 9.

Is the Crack a Quack?

Chiropractic medicine and DCs generally don't get the respect they deserve from the rest of the medical community. Chiropractic is often treated as a second- or third-rate approach to treating patients when everything else has failed. Some people consider it a form of alternative or complementary medicine.

When practiced by licensed professionals, chiropractic is a legitimate form of healthcare that focuses on diagnosing, treating, and preventing musculoskeletal disorders, particularly those involving the spine. Plenty of clinical evidence supports its effectiveness in treating acute back pain, neck pain, headaches, and joint issues. In addition, DCs are highly trained and educated. DC certification requires a bachelor's degree along with three to five years of training at a chiropractic college, followed by an internship. So, the answer to the question of whether the crack (chiropractor) is a quack (fraud) is no. DCs have helped many patients manage their aches and pains and are usually covered by insurance.

What many people in the medical community have issues with is that chiropractic practitioners often claim that realigning the spine is effective for treating illnesses that are unrelated to musculoskeletal issues, such as asthma and digestive problems, and such claims are *not* unequivocally supported by medical research. We believe that chiropractic can serve a very valuable role in managing back pain, but that it's not a cure-all, and it's not a long-term solution in and of itself.

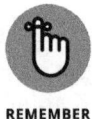

REMEMBER

The two key benefits of chiropractic care are that chiropractors are typically more accessible (and often more affordable) than conventional medical doctors, and that they provide quick relief for acute pain.

ALLOPATHIC, OSTEOPATHIC, CHIROPRACTIC

Chiropractic is a discipline that has evolved in parallel with allopathic and osteopathic medicine:

- **Allopathic:** The conventional approach to medicine. Healthcare providers are medical doctors (MDs) who focus on diagnosing and treating illnesses using drugs, surgery, and other interventions.

- **Osteopathic:** A more comprehensive approach to medicine that considers diet, lifestyle, and other factors to restore health and prevent illness. It's similar to allopathic medicine in that it uses medications and surgery to treat illness, and it's similar to chiropractic care in that doctors of osteopathic (DOs) are trained to perform hands-on manipulation of the spine and other areas of the body to restore alignment and proper nerve function.

- **Chiropractic:** Chiropractic care focuses on diagnosing and treating musculoskeletal disorders, particularly those related to the spine, with the goal of alleviating pain and restoring healthy function to the body.

As you can see, our philosophy and approach to managing back pain align most closely with the osteopathic and chiropractic disciplines. Their approach is generally more holistic and hands-on; it embraces the concept of the human body's ability to heal itself, and it depends less on medications and invasive medical procedures, such as surgery.

As the three disciplines evolved, competition took place, and politics intervened. The chiropractors ended up suffering the most in that power struggle. Many chiropractors are thriving today, however. We believe that their success is partially due to the fact that they provide quick and easy access to care, they treat both mind and body, and they're often effective at relieving acute pain.

Recognizing the Aliments Chiropractic Helps Best

The bread and butter of any chiropractic clinic is the manual manipulation of the spine (adjustments) to address subtle misalignments referred to as *subluxations*, some of which may be so subtle that they aren't visible on X-rays or via other medical imaging. The purpose of adjustments is to realign the spine to restore alignment and relieve pressure on support structures. Chiropractic manipulation is most effective at treating the following conditions:

>> Acute low back pain

>> Acute neck pain

>> Headaches

>> Sciatica (low back pain that radiates down a leg)

>> Whiplash (neck trauma common in car accidents and falls)

>> Joint pain (shoulders, hips, and knees)

>> Postural issues

>> Sports injuries (sprained ankle or wrists, pulled muscles, dislocations)

>> Pinched nerves

>> Carpal tunnel syndrome (pressure on nerves around the wrist due to repetitive stress)

REMEMBER

Acute back pain usually doesn't resolve fully and often returns, so even if you see a chiropractor who successfully treats your acute back pain, be sure to follow up with the self-care advice we provide in Part 2. Building back strength and mobility prevents future flare-ups.

Gauging Treatment Frequency

We believe that the goal of any treatment should be the elimination or significant reduction in the need for treatment, and chiropractic is no exception. The treatment goal should be your independence from your chiropractor.

Initially, if you're experiencing intense pain, you can expect to see your chiropractor at least two to three times a week. The goal at this stage is to reduce pain, inflammation, and muscle spasms and restore mobility. Sometime during that first week, with your provider's approval, you should be re-engaging in physical activities and exercise.

As your pain improves, your chiropractor may schedule you for visits once a week or every other week and recommend an increase in physical activity and exercise.

When you're feeling almost back to normal, you may schedule visits on an as-needed basis. In addition, you should be armed with a home-based program and prepared to take ownership of that program.

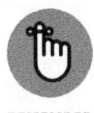

REMEMBER

Regardless of how good those repeated visits to your chiropractor make you feel, try weaning yourself off them and taking on more of the responsibility for your back strength and mobility. If you continue to build strength, mobility, and resilience, you shouldn't need to continue seeing a chiropractor. Independence from chiropractors, therapists, and medication is an independent determinant of health.

Exploring Chiropractic Techniques

DCs use a variety of techniques to restore proper alignment to the spine and manipulate the soft tissues — muscles, fascia, tendons, and ligaments. Common chiropractic techniques include the following:

>> **Spinal manipulation (chiropractic adjustment)** is mostly hands-on adjustments of the spine and other joints to improve mobility and relieve pain caused by *subluxations* (subtle skeletal misalignments).

>> **Flexion-distraction technique (Cox Technique)** is often used for patients with herniated discs or spinal stenosis. The DC positions the patient on a special table that gently flexes and decompresses the spine to reduce pressure on the spinal discs and nerves, improve circulation, and alleviate pain.

>> **Activator method** is a gentler form of spinal manipulation that's commonly used with patients with weaker bones, such as those with osteopenia or osteoporosis, or patients who tend to tense up in response to more traditional hands-on adjustments. The DC uses a small, spring-loaded instrument called an *activator* to deliver quick, targeted impulses to specific joints.

>> **Drop-table (Thompson) technique** is used to treat misalignments, especially in the lower back and pelvis and the sacroiliac joint. The patient lies face down on a special table that's raised slightly at the hips. The DC applies a gentle thrust downward, and the table drops to apply an additional gentle force targeting the pelvic area. It's loud and sounds dramatic, but it's actually a gentle adjustment.

>> **Active Release Technique (ART)** is effective for treating soft-tissue injuries, such as muscle strains and knots, sprained ligaments, and tension in the back. This deep-tissue massage releases tight muscles and breaks up adhesions and scar tissue. It's especially useful for addressing muscle-related back pain and restoring mobility to the affected area. Although ART is primarily in the realm of massage, many chiropractic clinics offer it.

>> **Myofascial release** is another deep-tissue massage technique that targets specific pain and *myofascial trigger points* (tight areas in muscle and fascia that cause pain). The DC applies sustained pressure to the trigger points to release tension, break up adhesions and scar tissue, and promote relaxation.

>> **Graston technique** Is another deep-tissue massage technique for breaking up adhesions and scar tissue. The DC uses a special tool, sort of like a thick butter knife, with a scraping motion to smooth out any bumps or ridges in the soft tissue beneath the skin. This technique is often used for sore calf, thigh, and hamstring muscles, but it may also be useful for treating tight neck and back muscles.

Chiropractic isn't strictly standardized. Different DCs may employ different styles, techniques, and treatments and may use heat, vibration, ultrasound, transcutaneous electrical nerve stimulation (TENS), acupuncture, and other tools and methods in addition to adjustments to alleviate pain and improve mobility.

TIP

If you're interested in adding chiropractic care to your back pain management protocol, shop around to find a DC who recommends exercise and self-care in addition to the in-office treatments. Don't approach chiropractic care as the entire solution to your back pain. Long-term results require strengthening the back, not merely correcting subluxations and tight muscles.

IN THIS CHAPTER

» **Asking the right questions**

» **Exploring surgical options for discs**

» **Understanding the basics of decompressive and fusion surgeries**

» **Mending compression fractures**

» **Looking at surgical options that target pain**

Chapter **18**

Evaluating Surgical Options

S pinal surgery is typically viewed as a last resort, or worse, as a four-letter word. Many people, even those with debilitating back pain, won't even consider it. Some are convinced that it won't do any good, or they're afraid that if something goes wrong, they'll suffer even more — maybe even end up paralyzed.

We ask you to let go of any preconceived notions you may have about spinal surgery. Surgery can play a very useful role in getting patients back on their feet and on the path to strengthening and mobilizing their spine. However, surgical options should be pursued only after carefully considering the predictability of success and formulating a plan for what happens after surgery — what you're going to do to build on the benefits of surgery.

In this chapter, we discuss several surgical procedures that can help correct spinal issues that may be functioning as pain generators and provide guidance on how to decide whether the potential benefits outweigh the risks.

Making an Informed Decision

If your surgeon or another provider tells you that you "need" surgery, view that as a red flag. Surgery is *needed* in very few situations. It's usually more a choice than a necessity. To decide whether it's an option you'd like to pursue, consider its potential advantages and disadvantages, along with your condition's *natural history* (what's likely to happen if you don't have the surgery). Part of your surgeon's job is to educate you and help you weigh the pros and cons of your options. The decision is ultimately yours. If you ask the surgeon, what they would do, they can and should provide a frank and honest answer.

In the following sections, we provide additional guidance about factors to consider when deciding whether to proceed with a proposed surgical procedure.

Weighing the predictability of success

One factor to consider when deciding whether to proceed with a recommended surgical procedure is its predictability of success in relation to its risk. If you have a condition that has a 100 percent chance of being alleviated with zero risk, surgery would be a no-brainer (assuming the cost isn't prohibitive). Unfortunately, that situation doesn't exist. Every surgery has less than a 100 percent success rate and more than zero risk.

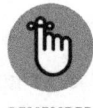

REMEMBER

Spinal surgery tends to be much more predictably successful when aimed at improving extremity (arm or leg) pain than back pain, so if your main complaint is back pain, be more wary of surgery. Here are some numbers to consider:

>> Decompression of the canal in cases of spinal stenosis has about a 70 percent chance of improving back pain compared with a 95 percent predictability of helping the extremity pain.

>> Microdiscectomy in younger patients also has a 70 percent chance of improving back pain.

Of course, these numbers don't really tell you much. Presumably, 70 percent means that seven out of ten patients report an improvement, but how much of an improvement? The claim that surgery has been shown to "improve back pain" says nothing about how much improvement a patient can expect to experience. It could be an improvement ranging from 1–100 percent. Would you be willing to go under the knife for a 70 percent chance of only a 10 percent improvement?

We recommend spending some time in self-reflection to figure out what successful surgery would mean to you and discuss what success looks like from your surgeon's perspective. Does surgery mean your pain will be reduced from eight to two on a scale of ten? Does it mean that you'll be able to return to doing the activities you enjoy but with some degree of pain? And when can you expect to feel better and experience the full benefit of the surgery (days, weeks, months, years)?

TIP

Avoid the temptation to define success as a complete resolution of your back pain because an outcome like that is unrealistic. Instead, think of it in terms of whether you'd be glad you had the surgery a month, a year, or five years after having it.

Considering safety and post-operative pain

Every surgical procedure carries some risk, and recovery can be painful, but modern techniques and technologies have made spinal surgery safer and less invasive and have accelerated recovery and reduced the pain associated with it. In spinal surgery, the use of an operating microscope provides ideal magnification and illumination, and new fast-speed drills enable the surgeon to more safely and precisely contour bone removal to decompress the nerves.

One risk that often comes up is the possibility of developing scar tissue. Although scar tissue is an inevitable consequence of surgery, it's rarely the cause of post-operative pain. Its presence is more often used as a distraction — a way to explain away post-operative pain. The surgeon may try to explain the reason for the pain by saying something like, "It's the way you scarred." The truth is more likely that the surgeon doesn't know the reason for the pain.

Bottom line: Yes, spinal surgery carries some risk, and recovery can be painful. Discuss the risks and what to expect during recovery with your surgeon.

PAIN TOLERANCE

Pain tolerance refers to the maximum level of pain a person can endure before it becomes unbearable or overwhelming. It varies from one person to another based on differences in genetics, psychological state, cultural background, and previous experiences with pain, and it can vary from one situation to another. For example, in the heat of battle, a soldier may not even feel the pain of being shot.

Many patients tell their providers that they have a "high pain tolerance." They want their provider to understand that when they say they are in pain, it's real. The truth is objective measures of pain tolerance reveal that it's about the same for most people.

REMEMBER

Surgeons often use the term "minimally invasive" to alleviate the fear of surgery, but we prefer the term "minimal access," which is more accurate. In gaining entrance to the surgical site, we try to disturb as little of the surrounding and supporting tissues as possible, which results in less pain and faster recovery. However, at the surgical site, being invasive is sometimes a necessary part of the surgery.

Clarifying your understanding

To ensure that you fully understand what to expect from surgery, ask your surgeon the following questions:

>> Where is my pain coming from, and how will this procedure address it?

>> What can I expect if I decide not to have the surgery you're recommending? (What's the natural history of my condition?)

>> What are the consequences of surgery over the next ten years?

>> What is the predictability of success for this procedure?

>> What does a successful outcome look like? Ask more specific follow-up questions, such as "When will I be able to [fill in your favorite activity]?"

>> (If you're feeling pain in your back and in one or more arms/legs): Is success different for my back and my arm or leg pain?

>> What are the risks, and how likely and potentially serious are they?

Evaluating your surgeon

Surgery success depends a great deal on the skills and experience of the surgeon. Your surgeon should be board-certified in neurosurgery or orthopedic surgery and specialize in spinal surgery. Find out how long the surgeon has been in practice and the number of times the surgeon has performed the recommended procedure. Ask about the surgeon's success rate, metrics for determining success, and complication rates. Check for patient reviews online on platforms such as Health grades.com, and check with people you know in your area to find out whether they've had any experience with this surgeon.

Short of being able to observe the surgeon at work from a front-row seat in the operating room, you have to rely on the surgeon's reputation and on your own instincts when deciding whether you trust that person to perform the procedure. Ask the surgeon to share their philosophy on the recommended surgical procedure. (A surgeon's *philosophy* refers to their thinking about whether, when, and how to perform a procedure.) A discussion of the surgeon's philosophy regarding a specific procedure enables you to gauge your level of trust more accurately than relying solely on reputation.

Approaching surgery as a preparation for therapy

We encourage you to think of surgery as merely a preparation for therapy. It's a first step on the road to recovery. This sets the stage for you to learn the anatomy and physiology of the spine, to understand the proposed surgery fully, to think of surgery as part of a "long game," and to take ownership of the therapy that follows surgery.

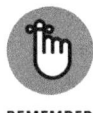

REMEMBER

Surgery takes a pain generator out of the equation or makes it less of a factor, but it rarely eliminates the pain entirely, and it does nothing to strengthen your back. It enables you to do what's necessary to improve your back strength and mobility, which will make you stronger, healthier, and more resilient and help to reduce your pain in the process.

REMEMBER

After surgery, spend some time with your surgeon (not a substitute) to follow up on the outcome of the surgery and your recovery progress. Follow-up discussions are a very important part of surgery, especially if the results have been disappointing. Whatever the short-term outcome, your surgeon can help you contextualize the situation and provide a plan for moving forward.

Considering Disc Surgery

Disc surgery is commonly called *microdiscectomy* (micro refers to magnification and illumination, allowing the surgery to be done through a small incision). This procedure primarily involves removing the portion of the disc that's irritating the nerve while largely sparing the adjacent structures.

Candidates for microdiscectomy typically complain of arm or leg pain that's worse when sitting and better when standing. The ideal candidate for a microdiscectomy has a distinct and recognizable pattern of back pain radiating from a disc herniation in the spine into an extremity (arm or leg) and an MRI showing a herniated disc pushing on the nerve corresponding to the pain, with the rest of the spine looking normal. As we explain in Chapter 3, your doctor can trace the pain back from where it terminates in the arm or leg to the disc where the pain originates.

Among "ideal" candidates, microdiscectomy is approximately 95 percent successful in significantly relieving the pain in the extremity and possibly some of the back pain as well, with a slightly lower chance of maintaining the benefits long-term. Post-operative back pain and recurrent disc herniation account for the lower rate of maintaining the benefit. The predictability of success is lower among patients who are not ideal candidates for the procedure.

REMEMBER

If your surgeon recommends microdiscectomy, ask about their philosophy of removing the disc herniation. Details should include the size of the incision, the amount of bone that will be removed, if any (*laminotomy*), the amount of disc removed (just the fragment that's herniated or some of the disc between the vertebrae that has not herniated), and any post-operative activities to expect (such as physical therapy).

WARNING

You and your doctor should try conservative treatments before considering surgery. If your surgeon recommends surgery without attempting conservative options first, strongly consider seeking a second opinion. Avoid making the decision when you're experiencing severe pain. In such a condition, you may be so distraught that you'll choose surgery before even considering non-surgical solutions.

Relieving Pressure with Decompressive Surgery

Decompressive surgery is performed on patients with *spinal stenosis* — narrowing of the spinal canal through which the spinal cord or spinal nerve roots pass (see Chapter 3 for details). This surgery involves removing some of the bone of one or more vertebrae to provide more space for the spinal cord and/or nerve roots, which branch off from the spinal cord.

Candidates for decompressive surgery typically complain of back pain that radiates to an arm or leg, with the pain being worse when standing and better when sitting. Ideally, the MRI shows an isolated picture of a nerve, or nerves, that corresponds to the distribution of pain that is being compressed by bone and ligament as it traverses through the spinal canal.

Among ideal candidates, decompressive surgery is approximately 95 percent successful in significantly relieving extremity pain. In some cases, fusion is recommended in addition to decompression (see the next section for more about fusion surgery).

If your surgeon recommends decompression surgery, ask about their philosophy of the procedure. What's the natural history of your condition without surgery? How many levels (vertebrae) should be decompressed? Is a fusion recommended in addition to the decompression?

Stabilizing the Spine with Fusion Surgery

Fusion surgery involves permanently joining two or more vertebrae together. Patients tend to think of fusion as the placement of metallic screws, but fusion is the biological process that occurs after surgery. The body attempts to create a bridge of bone with its own blood supply between two parts of the spine that were designed to move relative to each other. Screws create stability while the biological process of the fusion occurs. Originally, screws were designed to be removed after the fusion occurred, but modern screws are lightweight and biologically compatible, so they're typically left in the body.

Fusion is the real four-letter word in spine surgery. It has developed a reputation for being dangerous and painful. Patients fear they will lose significant mobility. Fusion has earned this terrible reputation not so much because of the danger, pain, and loss of mobility patients fear but because too much surgery is done in this country indiscriminately. Pain and loss of mobility are certainly possible and should be part of the discussion, but fusion can be very beneficial when properly indicated (meaning that the surgeon has good reasons for performing the procedure). The following are well-established indications for fusion:

>> Demonstrable instability (laxity) between two vertebrae, as seen on dynamic X-ray evaluation

>> *Foraminal stenosis* (narrowing of the canal that the root traverses through while exiting the spinal canal) that won't respond to simple decompression

>> Recurrent disc herniation

>> Infection of a disc space

>> Correction of a spinal deformity, such as *scoliosis* (excessive side-to-side curvature of the spine) or *kyphosis* (excessive convex curvature of the spine)

Note that mild scoliosis is usually benign. Surgery is generally indicated only when the abnormal curvature is severe or progressive.

>> Decompression of a segment adjacent to a fused segment of the spinal column

More nebulous indications include

>> Pain coming from a degenerative disc

>> Pain coming from an arthritic facet joint

>> Non-specific low back pain

The predictability of success for fusion surgery is difficult to estimate. Success varies according to several factors, including the following:

>> The outcome depends on both the surgeon's technique and on the patient's biology, health, participation, and commitment. Physical therapy is essential for regaining strength, mobility, and function after surgery. Not following rehabilitation guidelines can decrease the likelihood of success.

>> Fusion puts adjacent vertebrae at risk for accelerated degenerative changes over the ensuing years, so it increases the potential for future surgical interventions.

>> The fusion process occurs over several months following surgery, and fusion doesn't always occur; even when the surgeon does everything right, the bones may not fuse as intended. A fusion operation can be successful even if the bones don't fuse, but it's more likely to be successful if fusion occurs.

Understanding the surgeon's philosophy prior to deciding on a fusion or choosing a surgeon to perform the procedure is essential. Recovery is never as simple as having the operation. The patient's participation and commitment are key to success. You and your surgeon need to carefully manage your expectations going into surgery and throughout recovery, which can be a long process.

Exploring Surgery for Compression Fractures

With age, the spine becomes more susceptible to osteoporosis and compression fractures, which can be very painful. For years, doctors treated them with rest and bracing, but *kyphoplasty* has emerged as an alternative treatment. The procedure involves inserting a balloon into the fractured vertebra and then injecting medical-grade cement to stabilize the bone, thus reducing the pain.

Successful kyphoplasty requires identifying the fracture as *acute* (occurred recently) or *subacute* (occurred weeks to months ago and has started to heal). An MRI or single-photon emission computed tomography (SPECT) scan is best for determining whether the fracture is acute or subacute. If the compression fractures are neither acute or subacute, they're chronic, in which case, kyphoplasty would be useless.

If you have osteoporosis, your doctor needs to determine how likely it is that the fracture is the pain generator; many people with osteoporosis have incidental compression fractures, which aren't producing any pain. The other issue with kyphoplasty is that it seems to place adjacent vertebrae at increased risk for compression fractures. Even with these limitations, kyphoplasty is a reasonable option if you have an acute compression fracture that's causing extreme pain.

TIP

Try to give the fracture 6–12 weeks to heal. Patients often start feeling better within 4–6 weeks of this injury. One can consider kyphoplasty sooner if the pain is quite severe or the bone is collapsing to the point at which the window of opportunity will be missed.

Implanting Pain-Relief Devices

Although your surgeon may not be able to identify the source of your pain based on your symptoms and medical imaging, a couple of options are available for targeting the pain.

One of these options, called *modulation surgery,* involves implanting a battery-powered device, such as a dorsal column stimulator, into the body to deliver electrical stimulation to the spinal cord or an individual nerve root. This approach is based on the gait theory of pain; it takes advantage of the brain's capacity to block painful stimuli. As pain signals ascend the spinal cord, they must pass through nerve synapses called gaits. This natural system is hijacked by supplying an electric force to the spinal cord or nerve root. Flooding the brain with sensation from the electrical stimulation causes it to reflexively exert its capacity to block the ascending pain. The process is similar to the instinct to rub your head when you experience "brain freeze" from eating a large bite of ice cream.

Many pain experts are quick to use dorsal column stimulators, but others don't even consider them. One of the barriers to their use is that many patients don't want a battery-powered device implanted in their body. One thing to consider is that unlike a fusion, which can't be reversed, a dorsal column stimulator can be removed if you don't like it or it doesn't work well enough.

Another commonly used implant is an *intrathecal pump* — a device that automatically pumps a narcotic or muscle relaxer into the spinal fluid that surrounds the spinal column and nerve roots. An intrathecal pump provides a continuous, targeted delivery of medication, which can provide the same pain relief with less medication and a lower risk of medication side effects. But again, some patients don't like the idea of having a battery-powered device implanted in their body, and for some patients, the pump doesn't deliver the desired relief.

IN THIS CHAPTER

» **Recognizing the signs that you may need professional help**

» **Shifting your thinking to mitigate the pain**

» **Considering repressed emotions as a possible pain generator**

» **Treating the brain to reduce the pain with psychiatric medications**

» **Finding a therapist who's a good fit**

Chapter **19**

Getting Your Head in the Game with Psychological Interventions

As we explain in Chapter 4, your mind and body are one; your thoughts and emotions affect your physical health, and your physical health affects your thoughts and emotions. People have been known to literally "worry them-selves sick." We're not suggesting that your pain is all in your head or diminishing the role that biology plays in generating pain. We're only pointing out that the mind can also play a significant role.

The good news is that the same power that the mind has to inflict pain can be used to alleviate it. Managing stress more effectively can relax your muscles and improve circulation to promote healing, building confidence can improve your posture, and developing *self-efficacy* (a belief in your ability to overcome chal-lenges) can compel you to engage in physical activities that alleviate the pain. We provide several do-it-yourself techniques in Chapter 4 to improve your mindset, including using the power of suggestion to your advantage. However, if these self-help strategies haven't delivered the desired results, you may benefit from professional help. In this chapter, we cover a few psychotherapies along with psychiatric medications that have helped some people manage their back pain more effectively.

WARNING

Don't relinquish your autonomy and leave it up to the provider to make all the treatment decisions. Assuming a passive role in your treatment is a mistake. Like physical treatments (physical therapy, chiropractic, and surgery), mind therapies (psychology and psychiatry) are subject to the same bias we refer to as the *Maslov principle* — when all you have is a hammer, everything looks like a nail. Mind therapies may be even more difficult to navigate than body therapies. Options are more limited, they're often not covered by insurance plans, and they're even more lacking in an underlying predictive science. To some extent, you're at the mercy of the abilities and philosophy of your provider. Therefore, we recommend that you be even more circumspect and autonomous when adding mind therapies to your treatment plan.

SHIFTING THE PARADIGM

In the current medical system — at least in the U.S. — the treatment you receive for back pain depends more on where you start (the provider you see) than on what's wrong with you. This unfortunate reality makes your original choice of where to look for help all the more critical. Providers are human and are opportunistic to some extent. They lean toward recommending the treatments that they're trained to provide. You need knowledge, confidence, and a willingness to be an active participant in order to obtain the treatment that's likely to be most effective for you.

We hope that the back pain care model changes in the future. We imagine the patient presenting to a large, integrated, and coordinated group of providers. Once you've arrived, they use state-of-the-art techniques to determine what's going on with you and evidence-based medicine to refer you to the optimal provider(s) for the optimal treatment. For example, if your medical history reveals that you're dealing with stressful situations in your life, and your magnetic resonance imaging (MRI) shows no physical issues with your back, you may be prescribed mental therapy to manage your stress, physical therapy to improve mobility, and targeted exercise to strengthen your core.

The current approach to diagnosing and treating back pain (and many other medical conditions) is expensive, self-serving, disconnected, and often ineffective. Doing almost anything other than the current status quo is likely to be an improvement, so we encourage you to gather the confidence to fully and actively participate in your own journey.

Evaluating Psychosocial Factors That May Be Contributing to Your Back Pain

Back pain, like health in general, is physical, psychological, emotional, and social. Although you may interpret the pain as physical, the source of that pain may be a combination of factors, including how happy you are at work, whether you're dealing with relationship conflicts, and your overall attitude — whether you're generally optimistic or pessimistic.

In this section, we help you identify factors beyond the physical that may be causing or contributing to your back pain. Collectively described as psychosocial factors, these are a combination of psychological states (such as being afraid or confident) and social factors (such as having an overbearing or supportive supervisor). Here, we introduce you to a flagging system that can help you identify various psychosocial factors potentially related to back pain and provide guidance on how to move from flag to action.

Flagging psychosocial issues

Occupational health (OH) practitioners commonly use psychosocial flags to help identify mental, emotional, and social factors that may be getting in the way of a person returning to work after an absence due to illness or disability. The flags help to identify different classes of obstacles to recovery so that the OH provider and employee can figure out what additional support the employee may need to return to work. You can use this same flag system to identify potential psychological and social factors that may be causing or contributing to your back pain.

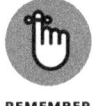

REMEMBER

Don't confuse these flags with the red flags we present in Chapter 5. Those flags are used to help determine whether you need a doctor to evaluate for physical damage or anomalies. The flags we discuss in this section are for evaluating psychosocial factors that may be hindering recovery.

Yellow flags

Yellow flags are counterproductive beliefs, feelings, and behaviors about your pain or your situation, such as the following:

» Believing that your pain is from an injury rather than an ordinary "part of life" when it hasn't been caused by an injury

» Being preoccupied with the pain to the exclusion of thinking about anything that could get your mind off it

>> Believing that treatment is only going to aggravate your pain

>> Worrying about how the pain is negatively impacting your life

>> Looking at your glass as half empty rather than half full

>> Avoiding activities out of fear of producing or worsening the pain

>> Expecting other people or interventions to resolve the pain (being passive in the process)

Yellow flags often indicate a need for psychotherapy, such as cognitive behavioral therapy or mindfulness — therapies developed to change thought processes, attitudes, and mood.

Orange flags

Orange flags are clinically defined psychiatric conditions, including the following:

>> Major depressive disorder (MDD)

>> Anxiety disorders

>> Post-traumatic stress disorder (PTSD)

>> Drug or alcohol use disorders

>> Major personality disorders

These are mental conditions that typically require professional psychological or psychiatric help.

Blue flags

Blue flags are counterproductive thoughts specific to work, such as the following beliefs:

>> You believe that the nature of your job inherently produces back pain.

>> You think your coworkers or supervisors are not as supportive as they should be.

>> You feel that your job is stressful.

>> You don't like your job.

>> You have unreasonable expectations for accommodations that enable you to return to work.

>> You feel as if you're being singled out.

Although blue flags are specific to work, you can apply them to your personal life as well. Any situation that results in frustration and dissatisfaction, such as a toxic relationship, can be a source of blue flags.

Addressing blue flags can be complex. It's not always a simple matter of changing your attitude or thought patterns. Creative problem-solving may be necessary. For example, in the workplace, you may need to consult with someone from your human resources department for support, or you may need to resolve conflicts with coworkers. You may even need to look for work that you find more rewarding.

Black flags

Black flags are concerned with factors that may be outside your immediate control or the control of others who are trying to help you. Here are a few examples of black flags:

>> Your health insurance company doesn't cover a treatment you think would help alleviate your back pain.

>> The claim you filed for worker's compensation has been denied.

>> Your requests for workplace accommodations are being ignored or have been denied.

Black flags are generally outside your control, providing you with limited options, such as appealing to a higher authority, consulting an attorney, or resigning from your current position.

Pink flags

In 2005, physiotherapist Louis Gifford suggested adding pink flags to the model, reflecting his concern that medicine focuses too much on what makes people unhealthy and not enough on what makes them well. Pink flags are positive thoughts and emotions that improve a person's outcome, such as the following:

>> Enjoying what you're doing

>> Having supportive friends, family members, and coworkers

>> Finding physical activities that make you feel better

>> Looking for opportunities to improve the world around you and the lives of others

>> Playing a more active role in managing your pain

Moving from flag to action

One of the biggest mistakes people make in life is to remain in a situation that's causing them distress and either suffer in silence or complain about it without doing anything about it. You basically have three productive options for dealing with anything distressing:

>> Accept it (or ignore it)

>> Fix it

>> End it (or leave it)

Being angry, upset, or frustrated with a person, organization, or situation isn't going to help you, and you have little to no control over what other people think, feel, say, or do. All you have control over is what *you* think, decide, and do.

To determine your course of action, answer the following questions:

>> **What are my flags?** List your yellow, orange, blue, black, and pink flags. Use your flags to determine the type of help you need, if any. For example, yellow flags indicate that mind therapies may help, whereas blue flags indicate external conditions that may need to be changed.

>> **What's the problem?** Define the problem so that you know what you're dealing with. Is the problem a perception/mindset issue (yellow flag), a psychiatric condition (orange flag), a situational or coworker issue (blue flag), or a bureaucratic issue (black flag)?

>> **What can *you* do about it (if anything)?** Think about actions you can take to improve your situation or your thoughts and feelings about it. List your options.

>> **Who (people) or what (resources) would you need to resolve the issue?** List the people and resources (money, insurance, sick days, vacation days, equipment, supplies, and so on) that can empower you to overcome the challenge you're facing.

>> **What's your desired outcome?** Imagine what your situation would be and how you would feel if the issue were resolved. Sometimes, starting with a goal, as we explain in Chapter 4, can help you brainstorm solutions and identify people and other resources that can help you achieve it.

>> **What modifications can you make on your own?** Think about ways you can modify your workspace, posture, and the way you do your work that can alleviate your back pain. You may not need to wait for your organization or your supervisor to take action.

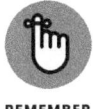

REMEMBER

Effective pain management involves changes to both body and mind. In the long run, this approach is more effective and efficient than trying to identify and treat a specific *etiology* (cause) or reducing the pain with a quick fix such as medication or surgery. Here's the overall approach we recommend:

1. Try your best to identify the etiology of the pain, but don't assume that you'll ever get a definitive answer. In many cases, despite what your doctors may tell you, they may have little to no idea what's causing your back pain.

2. Do as much as possible to manage your back pain on your own by following our guidance in this book, especially in Part 2. Look for pockets of help when you're not successful on your own or when you notice one of the warning flags we describe in this section.

3. Adopt an empowerment mentality; that is, view your body and mind as adaptable, not vulnerable, and remain actively involved even when seeking professional help.

Reprogramming Your Thought Process with Cognitive Behavioral Therapy

Cognitive behavioral therapy (CBT) is a psychotherapy that helps people change their perceptions, thoughts, emotions, and behaviors so they think and act more rationally and productively. For example, if you're avoiding physical activity because you're thinking, "Everything I do makes it worse," your therapist may lead you through a process of challenging the accuracy of that statement. The process can look something like this:

1. **Identify the faulty logic.** In this case, the thought is an overgeneralization. Words like "everything," "nothing," "everyone," "nobody," "always," and "never" are characteristic of overgeneralization, which is rarely reflective of reality.

2. **Challenge the thought.** The therapist may ask, "It sounds like you're assuming that any physical movement at all will make your pain worse, but can you think of any movement you do that doesn't make it worse or makes you feel better?" The therapist may also challenge the assumption that pain is always bad by asking something like, "Is pain always a negative? Can you think of instances in which pain can be necessary for healing or improving mobility?"

3. **Explore the evidence.** The therapist may ask whether you can engage in any activities that don't make the pain worse or whether you've tried anything to manage the pain when doing certain activities.

4. **Reframe the thought.** The therapist may help you formulate a more rational thought by saying something like, "Although your back pain is real and is challenging, you can do something to improve it. Maybe instead of thinking you can't do anything without making the pain worse, we can explore trying more manageable activities that don't hurt as much or actually alleviate the pain with the understanding that some degree of pain may be healthy."

5. **Encourage action.** The therapist may encourage the patient to test the new belief by engaging in activities that feel safe, such as taking short walks during the day or starting with some gentle movements like the ones we recommend in Chapter 8.

CBT employs a variety of techniques that can help manage back pain, including the following:

>> **Cognitive restructuring:** People often frame their pain according to their upbringing and culture. For example, they may think pain is debilitating. Cognitive restructuring challenges negative beliefs about pain to help patients view it as less distressing and more manageable.

>> **Stress management:** Chronic pain often leads to stress and anxiety, which can make the pain worse. CBT helps patients develop relaxation techniques such as deep breathing, progressive muscle relaxation (tensing and then relaxing muscles), and guided imagery (envisioning peaceful settings) to reduce anxiety and stress, helping to alleviate some of the pain.

>> **Coping skills:** CBT helps individuals develop coping skills, such as problem-solving, goal-setting, and communication, to deal more constructively with challenges and with potentially stressful situations and relationships.

REMEMBER

Relaxation techniques and coping skills empower you to respond to situations more calmly and assertively so that you can have your needs met without having to feel anger or angst, both of which can exacerbate back pain.

>> **Exposure therapy:** Individuals with back pain often experience *kinesiophobia* (fear of movement). Exposure therapy helps patients overcome this fear by gradually increasing their activity levels.

>> **Redirection:** Pain is an important component of the fight-or-flight response, which has been key to human survival. However, paying too much attention to pain can cause the expectation of it, which can result in chronic muscle tension. Redirection helps the patient shift attention from the pain to more productive and pleasant thoughts, interests, and activities. Think of redirection as a distraction. When you're focused on other things, you think less about the pain.

ACCEPTANCE AND COMMITMENT THERAPY

A relatively new outshoot of CBT is acceptance and commitment therapy (ACT). It encourages you to *accept* pain and *commit* to living a fruitful and meaningful life despite of it. In the process, you shift your focus from the pain to whatever you value in life, such as spending quality time with family members and friends, gardening, cooking, working, hiking, playing pickleball, or whatever you find enjoyable and rewarding.

When you're fully engaged in whatever you're doing, your mind remains in the present moment, preventing it from drifting into "What if?" scenarios, "Why me?" cognitions, and thoughts about how miserable you feel. Think about the last time you injured yourself doing something you love, like playing your favorite sport or engaging in a hobby. You may not even have felt it until you saw the blood or the bruise. ACT works by encouraging you to re-engage with what you enjoy.

>> **Sleep enhancement:** Pain can interfere with sleep, and poor sleep can exacerbate pain. CBT often includes techniques to improve sleep hygiene, such as setting a regular sleep schedule and creating a relaxing bedtime routine, which can help improve sleep and reduce the intensity of pain. For more about the benefits of sleep and suggestions for improving sleep, turn to Chapter 6.

For more about CBT, including techniques you can do on your own, check out *Cognitive Behavioural Therapy For Dummies* by Rob Wilson and Rhena Branch (Wiley).

Addressing Subconscious Stressors with Psychodynamic Therapy

Psychodynamic therapy helps patients identify and address subconscious conflicts, past traumas, and repressed emotions that may be causing or contributing to their pain. The idea behind psychodynamic therapy is that repressed emotions find physical expression. In many cases, just knowing that the cause of one's back pain is related to an emotionally traumatic event in the past or an unresolved conflict you're trying not to think about is enough to disrupt its physical expression. In other cases, the "cure" is more complex. For example, if you've been raised in a culture that discourages emotional expression, that upbringing could negatively impact your ability to communicate your needs and expectations at work, leading to frustration and anxiety. This can increase muscle tension and reduce circulation to certain parts of your body, including your back. Therapy would begin by identifying the thoughts and behaviors instilled during your childhood, but it would also involve developing emotional intelligence and communication skills and techniques that you hadn't learned over the course of your childhood and young adulthood.

REMEMBER

Psychodynamic therapy is most effective with people who are looking for insight into why they think and behave in certain ways. For example, if you're wondering, "Why don't I stick up for myself?" or "Why do I feel like I'm my own worst enemy?" psychodynamic therapy can help you answer those and similar questions. If you're not interested in developing this deeper understanding, you'll probably find that CBT is better suited for your needs.

During your psychodynamic therapy sessions, your therapist will encourage you to speak about whatever's on your mind, including problems you're having at home or work; your biggest fears and regrets; your hopes and dreams; your relationships with parents, teachers, and coworkers; what your life was like growing up; and other personal topics. Your therapist may also engage you in free association, prompting you with a picture or a word and asking you to respond with whatever thoughts or images pop into your mind. Free association can help uncover issues you may not consciously think are important to mention.

If psychodynamic therapy sounds like Freud's psychoanalysis to you, you're on the right track. The only difference is that psychodynamic therapy is more focused on problem-solving than on uncovering the origin of a patient's psychosis (characterized by hallucinations or delusions) or neurosis (characterized by excessive mental anguish).

Altering Your Brain Chemistry and Function with Psych Meds

If one of your doctors suspects that your back pain is related to a neurological or psychiatric condition, such as anxiety, major depressive disorder (MDD), attention deficit hyperactivity disorder (ADHD), bipolar disorder, schizophrenia, or post-traumatic stress disorder (PTSD), they may prescribe a medication to help with both the psychiatric condition and the chronic pain. Medications may include one or more of the following:

>> **Antidepressants:** Certain antidepressants, especially serotonin-norepinephrine reuptake inhibitors (SNRIs), such as duloxetine (Cymbalta), and older tricyclic antidepressants (TCAs), such as amitriptyline and nortriptyline, may help to reduce back pain. To a lesser extent, selective serotonin reuptake inhibitors

(SSRIs) may be prescribed to help treat pain thought to be associated with conditions such as depression or fibromyalgia.

>> **Anticonvulsants:** Medications such as gabapentin (Neurontin) and pregabalin (Lyrica), used primarily to treat seizures, may be effective for treating nerve-related pain, such as sciatica, by stabilizing nerve function and reducing abnormal nerve firing.

>> **Anxiolytics (anti-anxiety medications):** Benzodiazepines, such as alprazolam (Xanax), lorazepam (Ativan), and diazepam (Valium), are used primarily to treat anxiety and panic disorders but may also relax the muscles, alleviating muscle tension. Buspirone (Buspar) is another anti-anxiety medication, but unlike benzodiazepines, it doesn't cause significant sedation and isn't addictive.

WARNING

Be careful about using benzodiazepines in combination with muscle relaxants such as tizanidine or substances like alcohol that depress the central nervous system. Such combinations can be fatal.

>> **Antipsychotics:** Medications such as quetiapine (Seroquel) and olanzapine (Zyprexa) are prescribed primarily to treat schizophrenia and bipolar disorder, but they may be used off-label to treat chronic pain that's not responding to other treatments. (*Off-label* means that the medication hasn't been approved specifically to treat the condition it's being prescribed for.)

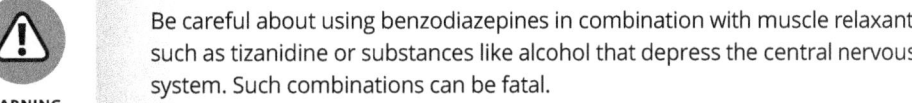
WARNING

Psychiatric medications may be necessary for treating severe mental illnesses, but we believe that they are grossly overprescribed in the U.S. These medications are powerful, and they influence brain function, meaning that they can affect your thoughts and behaviors in both positive and negative ways. Some also impair nerve function, which can negatively impact coordination, muscle strength, and your ability to exercise. We recommend using medication only when necessary and in the lowest doses needed to manage a medical condition. And don't let your doctor dictate what's necessary for you; be an active participant in that conversation.

OVERMEDICATED

People in the U.S. consume more prescription medications than any other population, and antidepressants are some of the most frequently prescribed therapeutic medications in the United States today. Approximately 20 percent of women over the age of 18 and 25 percent of women over the age of 60 are taking antidepressants. Even more alarming is that a growing number of children and teenagers, whose brains are still developing, are on antidepressants.

(continued)

(continued)

Much of the literature supporting antidepressants and other psychiatric medications is flawed and self-serving (the studies are often funded by the pharmaceutical companies that stand to benefit from the results). And certain classes of these pharmaceuticals have many adverse side effects. SNRI side effects include anxiety, diarrhea, constipation, dizziness, poor sleep, fatigue, and low libido. Anxiolytics can cause slurred speech, low heart rate and blood pressure, irregular breathing, sleep problems, fatigue, and a host of other negative side effects. SSRIs carry a black box warning for suicide ideation, and antipsychotics are notorious for causing metabolic disorders, leading to significant weight gain in some patients.

You have many of the chemicals you need for mood and pain management in your own body. You simply need to provide the stimulus to release your "feel-good" hormones — dopamine, serotonin, oxytocin, and endorphin. By "stimulus," we're referring to loving relationships, exercise, hobbies, interests, and other things in life you find worthwhile and enjoyable. Recent studies have demonstrated that exercise is as effective in treating anxiety and depression as medication.

We're not advising against taking an antidepressant. We're only advising caution. For some individuals, antidepressant medication may be a lifesaver and improve their quality of life. Also, if you're currently taking an antidepressant, don't stop taking it suddenly. Consult your doctor to discuss other options, and if you decide to stop taking a medication, work with your doctor to withdraw the medication gradually.

Choosing a Provider

If you think that you may benefit from psychotherapy, you'll need to find a provider who has the right combination of philosophy, training, and experience. Look for a therapist with the following traits:

» **Training and experience in pain management:** Ask prospective therapists whether they've worked with clients to help manage their pain, what training and certifications they have in this area, and how successful they've been. They can share stories without sharing confidential patient information.

» **Training and experience in the therapeutic model you think would be most effective for you:** If you have a specific therapy you want to try, be it CBT, psychodynamic therapy, mindfulness (which we discuss briefly in Chapter 4), or something else, choose a therapist who's trained in that model.

» **Knowledge and appreciation of the mind-body connection:** You want a therapist who understands and appreciates the different aspects of back pain management — medical treatments, psychological therapy, physical therapy, diet, lifestyle, sleep, and so on. Your therapist can help ensure that you're covering all the bases.

>> **Willingness to collaborate:** Your therapist should be willing to work with your other providers to deliver holistic and integrated treatment. Perhaps more importantly, your therapist should treat *you* as a key member of your pain management team and not merely a passive recipient of care.

TIP

Think of your treatment providers as partners, not healers. You're going to manage your pain, and they're going to help in various ways.

>> **Sensitivity to your treatment philosophy and preferences:** A good therapist listens to what you're saying and is willing to adapt their approach to your needs and preferences. You need to be able to trust your therapist, but they should trust and respect you as well.

REMEMBER

Your relationship with your therapist and your approach to treatment is likely to evolve over time. Be patient, but also be prepared to make changes if something isn't working. You don't want to shift gears too early or too often, but you also don't want to keep doing therapy that's not working or that doesn't resonate with your sensibilities. Finding the right balance isn't always easy; it takes confidence, mutual respect, and creativity.

Keep in mind that the mind-body connection we discuss in Chapter 4 works both ways. Improving your physical health with diet, exercise, and healthy lifestyle choices can have an enormous positive impact on your mental health and well-being.

4

The Part of Tens

Discover ten tips to empower yourself to stick with the program.

Challenge everything you think you know about back pain with ten hard-to-believe facts.

IN THIS CHAPTER

» **Accepting short-term sacrifice for long-term gains**

» **Balancing consistency with variety**

» **Making your routine fun**

» **Motivating yourself**

» **Energizing with music**

Chapter **20**

Ten Tips for Sticking with the Program

ace it — if healthy living were easy and fun, everybody would look like Jason Momoa or Gal Gadot. Building and maintaining a healthy body and a strong back requires hard work and discipline. Sticking with a health and fitness program is often the most challenging aspect of it.

The best path to success is to make healthy living a habit, and that requires changes in mindset and behavior — two of the most difficult changes imaginable. In this chapter, we share ten tips to set you on the right path and keep you in success mode.

Commit to 90 Days of Suck

A new habit takes 90 days to form, and that first 90 days is probably going to suck. As soon as your routine becomes a habit, though, sticking with it becomes easier. And, as we discuss in Chapter 4, when it leads to a change in identity ("I'm strong and healthy"), exercise is no longer a burdensome chore but a part of who you are.

REMEMBER

The old Joe Weider Triple Threat weight training program was based on 12-week cycles for a reason. After steady weight training for 12 weeks (about 90 days), you experience a noticeable difference in strength and physique. The fact that physical and behavioral changes both occur in that 90-day time frame is interesting. It sends a clear message that if you want to achieve transformative change in health and fitness, you must commit to 90 days of suck.

Be Consistent

Consistency reinforces thoughts and behaviors to the point of creating habits. Structure your days and each week to ensure that you're attending to everything that contributes to your health and fitness, including exercise, sleep, social engagement, intellectual stimulation, play, relaxation and reflection, and time to eat in a calm setting. You can add variety within this structure, but a structured routine enables you to maintain consistency and reveals aspects of your life that may require some attention.

Mix It Up

The old saying that "Variety is the spice of life" is true. Although we encourage you to be consistent, we also recommend varying your diet and activities to maintain interest and engagement. For example, consistency may involve eating a whole-food diet, but that doesn't mean eating the same thing every day. Likewise, exercising five days a week doesn't require doing the same exercise all five days. Even if you limit yourself to the exercises we present in Chapters 8 and 9, you can — and should — alternate those exercises so that you're developing different muscle groups.

REMEMBER

Changing routines challenges different parts of your body in different ways. It also subjects you to a steep improvement curve of mastering a new routine, which is beneficial for both mind and body.

Trick Yourself

Your mind is easily fooled and distracted. Unfortunately, it's usually distracted in the wrong direction and focused on unhealthy things, like cravings for sugary, salty, and starchy foods. The good news is that you have the power to fool your mind and redirect its attention to something else. Whenever you have a craving for something unhealthy, tell yourself you'll have it a little later. If the craving returns, tell yourself that you'll have it a little later. Keep telling yourself that, and if you do it long enough, you'll eventually realize that you don't need it, and the craving will pass.

TIP

Cut up some celery and carrots and snack on those instead of on sugary or starchy foods. Often, these healthy snacks are enough to keep intense cravings at bay. You can also trick your mind by dishing up on a smaller plate or bowl (and not going for seconds).

Another way to trick yourself is to break repetitions down into smaller groups, which can make doing lots of reps seem less daunting. For example, instead of counting off your reps from 1 to 20, 30, 50, or 100, count in sets of 10:

> 1, 2, 3, 4, 5, 6, 7, 8, 9, 10
>
> 1, 2, 3, 4, 5, 6, 7, 8, 9, 20
>
> 1, 2, 3, 4, 5, 6, 7, 8, 9, 30
>
> . . . and so on

If your goal is to row 800 strokes, count up to 100 eight times. We don't know the psychology behind why this works, but it does seem to help.

Partner Up

Peer pressure has a bad rap. It's usually associated with peers pressuring you to do something bad. But peer pressure can be beneficial, especially on those days you don't feel like exercising. Having someone to exercise with compels you to stick with the program. It also makes your journey to health and fitness more enjoyable.

If you don't have anyone in mind who is available to exercise with, consider enrolling in an exercise class or joining a gym, where you're likely to meet others who share your goal of becoming healthier and more fit. Adult basketball, volleyball, and pickleball leagues are other options to consider.

TIP

Have some fun by challenging one another and celebrating when you achieve your respective milestones.

Make It Fun

Some exercises are just plain boring. You can make them feel less boring by listening to your favorite music (see the later section, "Crank Up the Tunes") or by watching TV or listening to a podcast or audiobook. Other forms of exercise can be fun, such as playing basketball or volleyball, hiking in nature, or dancing. Look for ways to make your boring exercises less boring and incorporate fun physical activities into your day.

REMEMBER

Any physical activity with a purpose can make it more engaging, such as cleaning house, gardening, washing and vacuuming your vehicle, or walking or riding your bicycle to the grocery store instead of driving your car. When you have a sense of purpose, the physical exercise you're getting seems less like a workout. You may not even realize that you worked out until you wake up the next morning with sore muscles (that's a good thing!).

Track Progress and Celebrate Wins

Keep a notebook or create a separate file on your computer to track your progress. Set short- and long-term goals, as we explain in Chapter 4. Keep a log of your mood, weight, activities, and progress. These details alone are highly motivational. In addition, when you achieve a goal, celebrate. Treat yourself to something like a bath bomb, tickets to a concert, or something else you'll enjoy.

WARNING

Don't celebrate by doing something unhealthy, such as binging on your favorite junk food or TV series. Try to treat yourself with something healthy or at least health-neutral.

Make Healthy Choices Convenient

Make healthy choices as convenient as possible. You're more likely to exercise if everything you need is within easy reach, such as a home gym, a small set of kettlebells, or a pullup bar mounted in a doorway. If you need to drive a half-hour to a gym, that's an obstacle to exercise. Likewise, keep healthy food choices convenient. Keep a bag of chopped vegetables or chopped salad in your fridge, along with fresh fruits. Buy bags of nuts instead of bags of chips or packages of cookies. You're going to eat and drink what's convenient, so make sure that what's convenient is healthy.

TIP

Make unhealthy choices as inconvenient as possible. Don't bring junk food into your home or allow anyone else to do so. People who give you cakes, cookies, candy, donuts, and chips aren't doing you any favors.

Be Patient

Although the onset of your back pain may have seemed sudden, it probably developed over a long time, probably as a result of several factors. Rebuilding strength and mobility will take time. Rome wasn't built in a day. Imagine you're on an ocean liner heading across the vast expanse of the Pacific Ocean. A small change in course doesn't seem like much, but over several thousand miles, it can make a huge difference in where you end up. The small positive changes you make in your life can have a dramatic impact on your pain and on how healthy your back is, but these changes take time to produce noticeable changes.

REMEMBER

Setbacks are common. Don't let them discourage you. Rest for a day or two and make adjustments if necessary to get back on course, but don't give up.

Crank Up the Tunes

Music releases dopamine, a hormone that helps with motivation and habit formation. Use music to motivate yourself. Consider choosing music that resonates with your workout. Play calm, soothing music during yoga, heavy metal when you're pumping iron, and rap as you hit a heavy bag, for example. The right music gets your heart pumping, boosts your mood, energizes your training session, and makes the time pass more quickly.

IN THIS CHAPTER

» **Debunking back pain myths**

» **Fixing the problem even when you can't tell what's wrong**

» **Understanding why high-impact exercise can be good for your back**

» **Knowing the potential drawbacks of a back pain diagnosis**

» **Accepting the fact that your doctor may not have the answer**

Chapter **21**

Ten Hard-to-Believe Back Pain Facts

Start telling people that your back hurts, and you'll have no shortage of experts telling you what to do and sharing what they know. Unfortunately, much of what most people know about back pain is wrong. In this chapter, we bust several common myths and share some eye-opening facts about back pain so that you can get closer to being your own expert.

Your Back Pain Is Never in Your Back

If you think your back pain is in your back, you're mistaken. It's in your brain. If you receive a spinal block covering the painful area, you won't feel a thing. The pain is gone. If the pain were in your back, you'd still feel it.

The fact that you feel pain in your brain doesn't mean "it's all in your head," but it does mean that, to some degree, your mindset can impact the intensity of the pain and how it affects your ability to function and play a more active role in managing it. For more about the mind-body connection and how to use it to manage your back pain, see Chapter 4.

Sciatica Is Rarely Caused by Pressure on the Sciatic Nerve

The sciatic nerve is comprised of several nerve roots that exit separately from the spine and merge near where the upper thigh meets the hip. With sciatica, pain radiates down your leg, but it typically originates higher up, closer to the spine. The pressure isn't on the sciatic nerve but on the nerve roots that feed into it.

REMEMBER

Pressure on a nerve root is called *radiculopathy,* which is the accurate term for spinal-induced leg pain.

Your Back Should Be Straight Even When It's Bent

Whenever you bend over, you should maintain a neutral spine, as we explain in Chapter 7. Your upper back shouldn't be humped like a camel's. We know it sounds weird to say, "Don't bend when you bend over," but you can do so by hinging at the hip.

To hip-hinge, bend your knees slightly and thrust your butt back as though you're trying to sit on a chair that's too far behind you. Check out the photos in Chapter 7 to find out how to bend over while keeping your back straight (spine in a neutral position).

Six-Pack Abs Don't Mean You Have a Strong Core

Don't trust what you see when you look in a mirror. Those well-toned abs and obliques can be deceiving. Yet, that's the look most people are going for when they work out. Unfortunately, those workouts commonly neglect what we like to refer to as the *hidden core* — the back muscles, especially those that run along the spine and support it directly.

When you're building a strong core, don't neglect your back muscles. Strong back muscles support the spine, improve your posture, restore musculoskeletal balance, and make you look as good from the back as you do in the mirror! Check out Chapters 8 and 9 for exercises that strengthen your hidden core.

Conventional Wisdom About Acute and Chronic Back Pain Is Wrong

Two common beliefs in the modern medical community — that acute back pain needs no treatment and that chronic back pain has no treatment — are both wrong. Doctors often advise patients with acute back pain not to worry about it; it'll get better on its own. Unfortunately, acute back pain rarely gets completely better and tends to recur. Thus, it does warrant treatment. If your back pain is acute, follow the self-help guidance we provide in Part 2 to help prevent the pain from recurring or getting worse.

The other false belief is that nothing can be done to treat chronic back pain that has no clear cause or that persists after the cause has been treated and the patient has had sufficient time to heal. The truth is that even when doctors and patients can't identify a clear cause of the pain, they can manage it effectively with healthy living, proper exercise, and a positive mindset.

Medical Technology Is Improving, But Patients Aren't

Despite advances in medical and surgical technology and improvements in imaging techniques, modern medicine hasn't become much more successful in treating back pain over the past several decades. The healthcare community needs a better approach to treating back pain — a personalized, whole-health approach that actively engages the patient in the process.

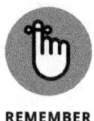

REMEMBER

No doctor can eliminate a patient's back pain. The best a doctor can do is diagnose and treat any identifiable pain generator. The patient needs to do the rest — eat a healthy diet, exercise, manage stress, and so on.

Doctor Doesn't Always Know Best

The old saying "Doctor knows best" isn't always true. In many cases, especially when it comes to back pain, the doctor doesn't know at all. To compound the problem, doctors have trouble admitting that they don't know. So, they try to help in any way they can — by prescribing medication or shots to treat the pain, by performing surgery on what they think *might* be causing the pain, or by recommending a half-dozen other treatments that relieve the pain partially or temporarily, if at all. Yes, NASA landed a man on the moon in the 1960s, and now, well into the 21st century, doctors still don't know why many of their patients' backs hurt.

REMEMBER

The good news is that you don't have to know the reason your back hurts to do something about it. Improving your overall health and building back strength and mobility by following our advice in this book will do wonders to alleviate your back pain.

Stress Can Be Good

Stress has a bad reputation, but stress isn't all bad. Emotional stress can build character. Physical stress can make you stronger. Stress can be negative or positive:

>> **Distress** comes from overwhelming demands, lack of control, and long-term exposure to emotional pressure. It can wear you down mentally and physically. It can even kill you.

>> **Eustress** challenges the mind and body in ways that build strength and resilience and improve performance.

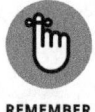

REMEMBER

A common misconception is that impact exercise, such as running, is not good for your back, but that's not true. Impact exercise makes bones stronger. I (Pat) have seen dozens of MRIs of runners and non-runners over the course of many years, and runners are less prone to degenerative spinal conditions than non-runners. Likewise, if you look at the MRIs of identical twins, one of whom weighs considerably more than the other, the spine of the one who weighs more typically has less degeneration. The spine adapts to the stress; it gets stronger as a result.

Surgery Is Merely Preparation for Physical Therapy

Surgeons hate this hard-to-believe fact, but it's true — the biggest benefit of spinal surgery is that it provides enough pain relief for enough time to enable the patient to return to physical activity and exercise. It's the physical activity and exercise, along with improving the patient's mindset and outlook, that lead to sustained back pain relief.

WARNING

Don't think of back surgery as a cure or an end in itself. It is a means to an end. If you don't follow up with self-help to improve your overall health and build back strength and mobility, the benefits of your surgery are likely to be fleeting.

Diagnosis Can Be Dangerous

A back pain diagnosis can be wonderful if it identifies an injury or anomaly that can be remedied, but it can be dangerous, as well. Here are a few potential downsides of a back pain diagnosis:

>> An obsession to find a cause can lead doctors and patients on a wild goose chase, resulting in false hope, questionable diagnoses, and unnecessary, ineffective, and possibly harmful treatments.

>> A diagnosis can present an incomplete or oversimplified understanding of the cause, leading to ineffective or incomplete treatment.

>> A diagnosis can trigger the chameleon effect, a phenomenon in which the patient develops symptoms of the condition they've been diagnosed with even when they don't have that condition.

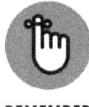
REMEMBER

If a comprehensive search for the pain generator fails, usually, the best approach is to abandon the search and treat the patient. Exploring ways to improve the patient's overall health and strengthen the back does no harm and has the potential to resolve much, if not all, of the pain.

Index

everyday changes
  about, 83–84
  adding movement, 101
  adjusting diet, 85–90, 100
  avoiding smoking and vaping, 90–91
  building mental health, 94–96
  building social well-being, 94–96
  exercising, 93–94
  getting more sleep, 91–92
  at home and work, 102–106
  improving overall health, 84–100
  lifestyle, 100
  managing stress, 96–99
Evil Bone Water, 211
exercise. *See also specific exercises*
  about, 28
  importance of, 93–94
  in movement, exercise, analgesics, and
    treatment (M.E.A.T.), 105
  using as a snack, 101
"expert" fallacy, 235
expertise
  developing, 265
  from physical therapists, 264
explosive power, as a component of muscular
    fitness, 16
exposure therapy, CBT and, 296
extension, 239

F

facet joints
  about, 38–39
  as pain generators, 22
  targeting, 260
facetogenic pain, 44
facets, disc pain compared with pain in, 43–44
fascia
  about, 41
  defined, 108
  massaging, 204–207
  targeting, 260
fascial adhesions, 41

fascial connection tightness, 54
fascial tightness, 41
fat deposition, 88
fats, healthier, 85, 86
fear of activities, back pain and, 75
fever, back pain and, 74
fiber, 90
fibromyalgia, 55
fight or flight response, 223–224
finding pain generator, 22–24, 246–247
fitness
  components of, 16–18
  gauging susceptibility to back pain using, 24
5-4-3-2-1 Grounding Exercise, 60
Flexeril (cyclobenzapine), 256
flexibility
  about, 17
  physical therapists and, 269
  prioritizing strength and mobility over, 118–120
flexion, 239
Flexion-distraction technique (Cox Technique), 277
floor lever, 171
fluoxetine (Prozac), 257
flying monkeys, 175
foam rollers, 204–206
food allergies, 88
food sensitivities, 88
foraminal stenosis, 285
foundations
  about, 117–118
  ankles, 126
  back-building using bodyweight, 130–152
  bent-over twists, 124–125
  bird dog, 132–133
  bridges, 139–143
  building endurance, 120–121
  building strength, 120–121
  cat and cow, 137–138
  child's pose, 137
  cobra stretch, 136
  crawls, 145–146
  cross-elbow-to-knee crunch, 131

H

hamstrings, foam roller for, 206

hand levers, 147–148

hands-on physical therapists, 269

hanging abs, 186–187

hardness, of foam rollers, 204

The Harvard longitudinal study, 94–95

health

  improving overall, 84–100

  restoring, 14–15

healthcare system, dysfunction of, 229–230

heat, as a conventional approach to back pain management, 12

heating pads, 209–210

heredity, gauging susceptibility to back pain using, 24

herniated discs, 37, 46–47, 52

hidden core, 108–110, 130

high-intensity interval training (HIIT), 16–18, 121

hip exercises, 126–127

hip flexors, foam roller for, 206

hip pain, as a non-spinal condition causing back pain, 53

hip-hinge, 113–115

Hippocrates (physician), 88, 89

hip-pop, 167

home, making changes at, 102–106

hot tubs, 210

household chores, 101

"How to Quit Using Tobacco," 91

hybrid callisthenics, 121

hydration, importance of, 102

hypertrophy, 38, 120

hypoxemia, 217

I

icons, explained, 3

Icy Hot, 211

identity, for habit formation, 100

illness, combatting, 14–15

implanting pain relief devices, 287–288

Important/Not Urgent (Schedule), in Eisenhower Matrix, 98–99

Important/Urgent (Do), in Eisenhower Matrix, 98–99

improving

  overall health, 84–100

  posture, 40

  weight management, 41

increasing blood flow, 41

infections

  abdominal, 52

  in discs, 38

  as a spinal condition, 48

inflammation

  in discs, 38

  of facet joints, 38

  as a non-spinal condition causing back pain, 53

informed decisions, making, 280

innervate, 37

insulin, 88

insurance providers, 234

integrative practitioner, 232

inter segmental movement, 109

internist, 231

intervertebral discs, 35

intrathecal pump, 288

intravertebral discs, 36–38

inversion tables, 213–214

J

job, gauging susceptibility to back pain using, 24

joints

  limbering up, 126–129

  role in chronic back pain, 27

judicial function, 30, 204, 251

K

kettlebell clean, 194–195

kettlebell push-ups, 172–173

kettlebells, back-building using, 154–171

kidney stones, 52

knees, 126
kyphoplasty, 286–287
kyphosis, 47–48, 285
kyphotic curve, 110

L

lacrosse balls, for massage, 206–207
lactose, 88
laminotomy, 284
Lao Tzu (philosopher), 271
lateral raises, 173–175
latissimus dorsi (lats)
  about, 112
  foam roller for, 205–206
leg pain, acute back pain with, 78
leg weakness, back pain and, 74–75
length, of foam rollers, 204
length of time, back pain and, 74
lifestyle factors
  as a cause of back pain, 10
  changes in, 100
lifting, neutral spine and, 112
ligaments, as pain generators, 22
limbering up joints, 126–129
listen, willingness to, of physical therapists, 268
lizard crawl, 146
longitudinal study, 94–95
long-term effects, from vaping, 91
lorazepam (Ativan), 299
lordotic curves, 110
lower back, 34
lumbar spine (lower back), 34, 205
lying down, neutral spine and, 112
Lyrica (pregabalin), 299

M

magnetic resonance imaging (MRI), 240–241, 247
maintaining neutral spine, 110–112
Maslov principle, 290

massage
  adding to physical therapy, 266–268
  back muscles and fascia, 204–207
massage gun, 207
massage therapist, 232
material, of yoga/physio balls, 212
mattresses, 102
measurable, in SMART goals, 68, 69
mechanical stress, in discs, 38
medial branch, 260
medical conditions, as a cause of back pain, 11
medical imaging
  about, 237–238
  computed tomography (CT) scan, 240
  diagnosis and, 238
  discography, 242–243
  magnetic resonance imaging (MRI), 240–241
  single photon emission computed tomography (SPECT) scan, 242
  X-rays, 238–239
medical massage, 267
medical technology, 313–314
medications
  about, 254
  anti-depressants, 256–257
  anti-inflammatory, 254–255
  anti-seizure, 257
  cannabinoids, 258
  as a conventional approach to back pain management, 12
  muscle relaxers, 256
  narcotics, 255–256
  non-steroidal anti-inflammatory drugs (NSADIs), 254
  psych, 298–300
  steroids, 255
  topical analgesics, 256
meditative breathing, 222–223
menopause, 88
mens sana in corpre ano, 63
mental health, building, 94–96

self-efficacy, 14, 65–66, 154, 268, 289

self-help, augmenting with professional care, 18–19

self-massage, 118

self-reliance, 14

Seroquel (quetiapine), 299

serotonin-norepinephrine reuptake inhibitors (SNRIs), 257, 298–299

sertraline (Zoloft), 257

setting goals, 66–70

The Seven Habits of Highly Effective People (Covey), 58, 99

shoulder pain, as a non-spinal condition causing back pain, 53

shoulders
  about, 127, 128
  core and, 112–113

side bends, 124

side crunch, 162–163

side twists, 122, 123

Sinequan (doxepin), 257

single kettlebell rows, 196–197

single leg bridge, 141–142

single photon emission computed tomography (SPECT), 51, 242

single-arm deadlift, 165–166

single-photon emission computed tomography (SPECT), 287

sitting
  neutral spine and, 112
  role in back pain, 28

six-point crawl, 145

60-second abs, 161–162

size, of yoga/physio balls, 212

skepticism, about doctors, 12–13

skipping rope, 121

sleep
  as a cause of back pain, 10
  CBT and enhancement of, 297
  importance of, 90, 91–92
  mindfulness for improving, 60
  on your back, 102–103

sleep apnea, 218

sleep test, 219

SMART goals, 66–70

SMARTER goals, 69–70

smoking, 90–91

snacks
  healthier, 90
  using exercise as, 101

snake, 138

social well-being, building, 94–96

a sound mind in a sound body, 63

spasms, of muscles, 40

specific, in SMART goals, 68, 69

specific adaptation to imposed demand (SAID), 97, 200

speed
  as a benefit of pain relief, 261
  of deep-breathing, 221

spinal canal, targeting, 260

spinal column, decompressing, 211–215

spinal conditions
  about, 45
  arthritis, 46
  bulging discs, 46–47
  degenerative disc disease, 46
  herniated discs, 46–47
  infection, 48
  osteoporosis, 47–48
  sacroiliac pain, 51
  spinal fracture, 48–49
  spinal stenosis, 50
  spondylolisthesis, 50–51

spinal cord stenosis, as pain generators, 23

spinal fracture, 48–49

spinal injections, as a conventional approach to back pain management, 12

spinal manipulation, 277

spinal nerves, 41–43

spinal stenosis, 50, 260, 284

vertebrae, as pain generators, 22
vertebral bodies (bones), 35, 36
vitamin D, 103
Voltaire (philosopher), 271
Voltaren, 211

W

walking, 101
warming up, 121–129
Warning icon, 3
water, 28, 85
wavelengths, for red light therapy, 209
websites
  American Cancer Society, 91
  Cheat Sheet, 4
  "How to Quit Using Tobacco," 91
weight
  gauging according to movement, 155
  gauging susceptibility to back pain using, 24
  of yoga/physio balls, 212
weight loss, back pain and, 74
weight management, improving, 41
weighted workouts, 199
wet cupping, 208
where to start
  about, 71
  conducting preliminary self-assessment, 72–78
  determining approach to back pain, 78–79
  rational frame of mind, 72

whiplash, 54–55
whirlpools, 209–210
whole foods, 28, 85, 89
wins, celebrating, 308
work, making changes at, 102–106
workouts, sample, 151–152, 199–202
workstation modifications, 103–104
worry, 78–79
wrist rolls, 128

X

Xanax (alprazolam), 299
X-rays, 238–239
X-roll, 134–135

Y

yard work, 101
yellow flags, 75, 291–292
yoga ball, stretching back with, 212–213

Z

Zanaflex (tizanidine), 256
Zoloft (sertraline), 257
zombie roll, 135
Zyprexa (olanzapine), 299

Dedications

From Pat: To Cathy, my inspirational wife, and to my greatest contribution to this world, our children, Chris and Jaqui

From Phil: To my parents, Patricia and Philip A. Ross, Jr., for instilling in me the drive and determination to always believe in myself and my abilities

About the Authors

Dr. Patrick Roth is a neurosurgeon with over 30 years of experience treating back pain. He believes that the strength of a surgeon lies in his humanity rather than in his hands. Early in his career, he obsessed over deciphering back pain generators and mastering technology to provide minimal access surgery to address those generators. Over time, he recognized that a more holistic approach was more effective.

Dr. Roth is the author of two previous books related to back pain: *The End of Back Pain* (HarperOne, 2014), which explores the power of the mind/body synergy in the treatment of back pain, and *The Me in Medicine: Reviving the Lost Art of Healing* (Changing Lives Press, 2018), which explores the power of narratives in medicine. He teaches a new and innovative course at the Hackensack Meridian School of Medicine called "Human Dimension," which is focused on each student's humanity and the social determinants of health. He has served as the chairman of neurosurgery at Hackensack University Medical Center for more than a decade and also serves as the founding chairman of neurosurgery at the School of Medicine. He has trained dozens of residents over his career.

Dr. Roth completed his residency in neurosurgery at Tufts Medical Center in 1994. In 2019, he added a master's degree in public health from Columbia University to better understand where he could add value to the care of patients with back pain. He is the founder of New Jersey Brain and Spine, the largest subspecialized neurosurgical group in the state. Despite being a surgeon, he has harbored a lifelong distrust of fee-for-service medicine and of how surgeons select their cases, and he is proud of being a "one and done" surgeon — one job, one wife, and one house.

Phil Ross, MS, also known as Master Phil, The Kettlebell King, is a college professor, presenter, author, publisher, actor, 9th Degree Black Belt with the East/West MAA, Brazilian Jiu Jitsu Black Belt, Master Kettlebell Instructor, Bodyweight Specialist, and Master Blade Wielder.

He obtained his undergraduate degree from the University of Maryland, College Park campus, and was selected as the speaker at the graduate commencement at American Military University, where he secured his master's degree in sports and health sciences. He is also a graduate of the ACUE program for education. He is a certified personal trainer, master RKC kettlebell instructor, certified USA boxing coach, and certified functional movement specialist; he holds numerous certifications in fitness, strength, and martial arts, and he's a board member of the Industry Advisory Council for Collaborative Institutional Training Initiatives for APUS.

A lifelong combat athlete and fitness pundit, he has competed on the National Level in Submission Fighting, Kickboxing, Full Contact Karate, Taekwondo, and Olympic Style Wrestling, and has garnered titles in bodybuilding and power-lifting. He is the owner of The BodyBell Method and Survival Strong certifications, which are divisions of Master Phil Industries.

He has authored *A Guide to Street Survival and Strength* (Master Phil Industries, LLC, 2024), *Ferocious Fitness* (Dragon Door Publication, Inc., 2016), *Exercise Snacks: Fitness 5 Minutes at a Time* (WP Lighthouse, 2024), and *The Kettlebell Workout Library Manual* (Amazon Kindle, 2023). Additionally, he has created and produced the *Kettlebell Secrets* video training series, *Survive a Violent Environment (S.A.V.E.)*, the #1 Rated Self-Defense and Fitness Video series (2007), and a library of instructional videos on his YouTube channel, `https://www.youtube.com/@TheMasterPhil`.

Authors Acknowledgements

Publishing is a team sport, and the publication of this book is no exception. Special thanks to Wiley senior acquisitions editor Tracy Boggier for choosing us to author this book and for laying the groundwork to make it happen. Her patient and steady hand helped guide the project during its initial stages over a very rocky road. Special thanks also to wordsmith Joe Kraynak (`joekraynak.com`), who spun our early drafts of chapters into pure gold and guided us through the writing process from start to finish.

Thanks, Rick Kughen, our development editor, for painstakingly shepherding our manuscript through the editorial and production process, juggling all the pages, photos, and illustrations; ensuring that they got placed properly; making sure that everything fit the way it should; and sharing his insights from the perspective of a back pain patient. Rick also served as our copy editor, picking through our manuscript word by word, eliminating errors, and ensuring that our ideas and instructions were expressed as clearly as possible.

A special thank you goes out to the models featured in our book: Jasmine Quinones, Jaylin Akridge, and Adrienne Ross. Your commitment and professionalism during our photoshoot were impeccable.

Last, but not least, we thank our technical editor, Arnold Criscitiello, M.D., for checking the accuracy of the information and guidance we present throughout the book, generously sharing his own insights, and giving our readers a second opinion. His input made what we believe is a great book even better!

Publisher's Acknowledgments

Executive Editor: Tracy Boggier
Development Editor: Rick Kughen
Copy Editor: Rick Kughen
Technical Editor: Arnold Criscitiello

Production Editor: Tamilmani Varadharaj
Cover Image: © PeopleImages/Getty Images